CASE REVIEW
Head and Neck Imaging

Series Editor

David M. Yousem, MD, MBA
Professor of Radiology
Director of Neuroradiology
Russell H. Morgan Department of Radiology and Radiological Science
The Johns Hopkins Medical Institutions
Baltimore, Maryland

Other Volumes in the CASE REVIEW Series

Brain Imaging
Breast Imaging
Cardiac Imaging
Emergency Radiology
Gastrointestinal Imaging
General and Vascular Ultrasound
Genitourinary Imaging
Musculoskeletal Imaging
Nuclear Medicine
OB/GYN Ultrasound
Pediatric Imaging
Spine Imaging
Thoracic Imaging
Vascular and Interventional Imaging

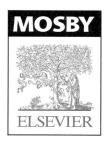

David M. Yousem, MD, MBA
Professor of Radiology
Director of Neuroradiology
Russell H. Morgan Department of Radiology and
    Radiological Science
The Johns Hopkins Medical Institutions
Baltimore, Maryland

Ana Carolina B. S. da Motta, MD
Russell H. Morgan Department of Radiology and
    Radiological Science
The Johns Hopkins Medical Institutions
Baltimore, Maryland

WITH 443 ILLUSTRATIONS

CASE REVIEW

Head and Neck Imaging

SECOND EDITION

CASE REVIEW SERIES

MOSBY
ELSEVIER

1600 John F. Kennedy Blvd.
Suite 1800
Philadelphia, PA 19103-2899

HEAD AND NECK IMAGING: CASE REVIEW   ISBN-13: 978-0-323-02989-6
                                                       ISBN-10: 0-323-02989-2

NOTICE

Knowledge and best practice in this field are constantly changing. As new research and experience broaden our knowledge, changes in practice, treatment and drug therapy may become necessary or appropriate. Readers are advised to check the most current information provided (i) on procedures featured or (ii) by the manufacturer of each product to be administered, to verify the recommended dose or formula, the method and duration of administration, and contraindications. It is the responsibility of the practitioner, relying on their own experience and knowledge of the patient, to make diagnoses, to determine dosages and the best treatment for each individual patient, and to take all appropriate safety precautions. To the fullest extent of the law, neither the Publisher nor the Editors assume any liability for any injury and/or damage to persons or property arising out or related to any use of the material contained in this book.

Library of Congress Cataloging-in-Publication Data

Yousem, David M.
    Head & neck imaging : case review / David M. Yousem.—2nd ed.
        p. cm.—(Case review series)
    Rev. ed. of: Head & neck imaging. 1998.
    ISBN 0-323-02989-2
    1. Head—Imaging—Case studies. 2. Neck—Imaging—Cases studies.
I. Title: Head and neck imaging. II. Yousem, David M. Head & neck imaging.
III. Title. IV. Series.
    RC936.Y68   2006
    617.5'10754—dc22   2005054406

Acquisitions Editor: Meghan McAteer
Editorial Assistant: Ryan Creed

Working together to grow
libraries in developing countries

www.elsevier.com | www.bookaid.org | www.sabre.org

ELSEVIER   BOOK AID International   Sabre Foundation

Printed in the United States of America.

Last digit is the print number: 9   8   7   6   5   4   3   2   1

In memory of my Fa-ja…

And to my mentors, my peers and my students

DMY

To
God, who guides me through my life
Mom and Dad, who helped me be who I am
The wonderful people that I have crossed paths
with during these years

ACM

I have been very gratified by the popularity of the Case Review Series and the positive feedback the authors have received on publication of their first edition volumes. Reviews in journals and word-of-mouth comments have been uniformly favorable. The authors have done an outstanding job in filling the niche of an affordable, easy-to-read, case-based learning tool that supplements the material in *THE REQUISITES* series. While some students learn best in a noninteractive study-book mode, others need the anxiety or excitement of being quizzed, being put on the hot seat. Recognizing this need, the publisher and I selected the format of the Case Review Series to simulate the Boards experience by showing a limited number of images needed to construct a differential diagnosis and asking a few clinical and imaging questions (the only difference being that the Case Review books give you the correct answer and immediate feedback!). Cases are scaled from relatively easy to very difficult to test the limit of the reader's knowledge. A brief authors' commentary, a cross-reference to the companion *REQUISITES* volume, and an up-to-date literature reference are also provided for each case.

Because of the success of the series, we have begun to roll out the second editions of the volumes. The expectation is that the second editions will bring the material to the state-of-the-art, introduce new modalities and new techniques, and provide new and even more graphic examples of pathology.

This volume of the Case Review Series, *Head and Neck Imaging*, is the first of the second editions. Dr. Motta and I have chosen to replace all 200 cases from the first edition with 200 new cases. In this way both editions remain valuable, and there is no overlapping of images between editions. The emphasis remains on cross-sectional imaging, with new cases introducing more three-dimensional techniques. The head and neck region remains one of the most challenging to a resident or fellow, and our goal was to provide a mix of cases that would make addressing lesions of this region less intimidating. We believe that the second edition of *Head and Neck Imaging: Case Review* will be a valuable resource to all of our readers.

David M. Yousem, MD, MBA

This is the second edition of the *Head and Neck Imaging: Case Review,* but it should not be considered just a freshening up of an older version. In this book we supply 200 **new** cases with no overlapping images from the previous edition even though, obviously, we had to cover many of the same entities. We tried to add in a bit more 3D imaging and dropped most of the plain film and ultrasonography and nuclear medicine studies, leaving those modalities to be covered by dedicated books devoted to those techniques. There is greater emphasis on differential diagnoses and more detail on treatment or workups of the pathologic entities. The material has been modernized as we have consulted clinical colleagues freely and frequently for guidance.

I think that the readers will, once again, enjoy the Case Review approach, as it really simulates the real-world scenario of going through the worklist, case by case, and trying to nail down the diagnoses. As it turns out, the head and neck area is often the most feared region of the body to evaluate (I see a lot of neck cases left over for me by my colleagues from the previous day... and nearly all of the TMJ MRI scans!), which is why a case review book on the topic is so valuable.

This book was written between two salient events in my life. On October 9, 2004, I completed (barely) my first (and last) Ironman competition in Cambridge, Maryland. It was the culmination of a lot of training and competitions, starting with 10K runs, half-marathons, marathons, sprint triathlons, Olympic triathlons, and half Ironman events. What an accomplishment... which landed me in the ED for 3 hours receiving 4 liters of fluid before my kidney function returned. Anyway, I digress.... Immediately after the Ironman I went through a furious 3 months of writing up the cases that I had been collecting over the past 4 years. I set a goal of getting the manuscript in by January 2005 and doing editing during that month. I achieved that goal (but only through the invaluable help of my co-author Carol Motta, who helped save my life), so I was flying pretty high in early 2005 with an Ironman and another book under my belt.

From the highs to the lows.... On February 10th I was diagnosed with prostate cancer. Now mind you, I am a wee 46 years old with a PSA of 0.3, but my internist (bless his heart, Dr. David Roberts) felt a nodule on the right side of my prostate and I insisted on a biopsy rather than serial (ughgggghhhh) rectal exams of my prostate. Boy was I shocked when it came back positive. In March 2005 I underwent a radical prostatectomy and all that entails... if you men out there know what I mean :-). All signs point to a complete resection with no spread.

In June 2005 my Dad died. Another crushing event. A huge influence in my life and a great role model of integrity.

Why do I disclose such personal stuff in the Preface of this book? Because my motto has always been to live life to its fullest, never be complacent, and keep contributing to the world in the best way you can. One of the ways I contribute to the community is through my teaching, and one of the best ways to get the teaching more widely disseminated is through writing books. That's why I love doing *THE REQUISITES* and these Case Review books. God willing, I will keep doing them for many more years to come. And hopefully you will keep reading (fine print... BUYING) them!

This is also the time to thank the special people in my life. I don't want this to sound like a last will and testament after the sobering news about my prostate gland, but I want to make sure that Marilyn and Ilyssa and Mitch know how much I love them. I do the best I can to decrease the impact of the Ironman training and the writing of my books on them; I hope that it's true that quality is sometimes more important than quantity. Mom, Sam and Penny, Bailey, Emilie, and Jack—quality as well.

Bob Grossman has been my mentor for many many things in my life and I will always use him as my svengali. For a best friend, go no further than Norm Beauchamp, true blue and a sincere heart. To my gang: Scott G, Scott M, Marty, Ronenn, Coos, Bart, Jeff, Steve, Todd, Barry—thanks for the support through these recent tough times. Loevner, you'll always be special to me. You go girl! Jon, thanks for being the kind of boss and friend that any academician would love to have.

To Meghan and Hilarie: thanks for having faith in me that I could bring another "best-seller" home… and more to come.

To the very special people in my work life that put a smile on my face each day:

Melinda—Thank you for transcribing the tapes that I made traveling back and forth to work day after day in October, November, and December 2004. *You made* this book—thank you for being such a caring friend too. You have a great heart.

Rena—You've been with me so long it's hard to imagine succeeding at work without you. You are a pillar of strength.

Carol—Thank you for your inspiration and breathing life into this book… not to mention the office. You make life fun.

To my clinical and radiology colleagues at JHMI, thank you for helping me professionally, intellectually, and spiritually.

To my "twin soul": You make me smile when I think about the future. We really are in orbit together. Our lives will always be intertwined. Thank you for making me believe that there is life after love and love after life.

To my readers: I hope you like this book. Feedback?

To all (as always):

Live, love, learn, and leave a legacy.

Dave Yousem
September 2005

Being invited to help Dave write *Head and Neck Imaging: Case Review*, second edition, was something that I never expected. I was deeply honored and touched, as Dave is one of the most brilliant neuroradiologists in the world and he belongs to a renowned institution, Johns Hopkins University. I dreamed for many years of visiting or working at Hopkins, and this all began when I came to attend the AFIP course (great, fantastic course, where I met many nice people—especially Mr. Carl Williams and Dr. Kelly Koeller… such cuddly guys!) in 2002. At that time my friend Gilberto Szarf was doing his Body Imaging fellow at Hopkins and introduced me to Dave.

And God made his ways and my life crossed Dave's life and we became very gooooooood (my Brazilian way of emphasizing very special things) friends. Dave is a wonderful guy with lots of energy, laughs, encouragement (he's very good at doing this), who owns a big, gigantic heart and is very, very demanding!!! (yep, coach! You know you're an "iron monster"). I'll always be there for you!

So, here I am now at Hopkins, and I feel very blessed that everything has gone just *perfectly*! (although the beginning was pretty tough—missing my family, friends, my country, *the food* !!!). And yes, I'm a very affectionate crying baby— I'm the youngest child!

As Dave has already covered all the modifications and updates related to the book, I'll cover the very gooooood part of this preface, which is thanking some important people that accompanied me during this walk.

My "crazy," funny, and wonderful family (Mom, Dad, Clau, Wagner, Theo, Cainha, Duda, Mimi)—my treasure! They always supported me in the good and bad moments (especially those! Thanks Mom and Dad!) that I passed through. And my lovely and amorous uncle Sérgio Dias.

To my great radiology Brazilian friends Pierpaolo Martelli, Frederico Benevides, Simone Caetano, Erica Endo, Rodrigo Vaz de Lima, and my buddies from SPR (Regina, Marcel, Marcelo, Paulo, Heitor, Pri, Vânia, Dri). Thanks for being there and encouraging me… always!

Thanks to my amazing Brazilian stepfamily (Ale, Pri, Quinha, tia Marly, tio José Carlos) that "adopted" me as part of their family.

Thanks to my fond and supportive friend Emanoela Cemin for being a big part of my life. I love you! You're awesome! And I know you'll never forget me even so far away!

Thanks to my Brazilian buddy Luciano Farage, who shares my office at Hopkins and supports my craziness!!! (my candango's big head).

Thanks to my beloved friend Walter Marcellus Anetzeder and his parents, Walter and Amélia, for all their blessed thoughts and prayers.

A big, huge thanks to my special friend, confidant, and stepsister Melinda (big monster) and all her family (Dan, Jacob, Mr. Mervin, Mrs. Georgette) for turning my blue days in the USA into the most shiny days that I'd ever expect! I love you so much! You're my American family!!!

A lovely thanks to my colleagues at Hopkins, especially Rena (so cheerful!), crazy Ovsev and the IT guys (love you!!! Chris, Adam and sweetie Shanelle) for all your help whenever I needed IT.

Thanks to my mentors Dr. Henrique Carrete Jr. and Dr. Nitamar Abdala (from Escola Paulista de Medicina), who made me fall in love with neuroradiology and taught me much more than that—taught the meaning of the words "believe" and "friendship." To Dr. Nelson Fortes and Dr. Lázaro do Amaral (from MedImagem), who patiently tried to clarify all my doubts. I know guys—I ask a lot! And to Dr. Douglas Racy and Dr. Sérgio Lima for giving me the opportunity of studying in such an amazing place—MedImagem.

Thanks to all the staff of Escola Paulista de Medicina, my special and sweet home, from which I graduated and completed my residency, especially Celinha, Rosa, Marilene, Valéria, Denilson, Sandra, Ana, Bubaloo, and Paty. You made my days in the residency happier!

Thanks to my Reiki master Nelson Hashimoto for always trying to keep my aura very bright! Yep—I really need this! *Forever!*

And a special thanks to a wonderful guy who appeared recently in my life, but he and his family took my heart... Mr. Bill Mowrey (and his world's most famous crabcake. *Yummy!*).

"Plagiarizing" Dave's advice but in my own way, I would say: believe in your dreams, try to reach them, listen to your heart, don't let empty people put you down, don't put others down in your quest to achieve your goals, and don't forget the most important things in your lives: happiness, health, love, friends, and family!

"Every man must decide whether he will walk in the light of creative altruism or the darkness of destructive selfishness. This is the judgment. Life's most persistent and urgent question is, 'What are you doing for others?'" (Martin Luther King, Jr.)

Ana Carolina B. S. da Motta
September 2005

Opening Round Cases

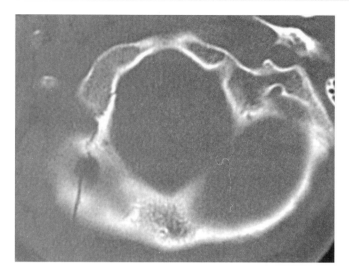

1. What is the shape of most skull base fractures?

2. What are the potential risks and complications of skull base fractures?

3. Identify the mechanism of injury in this case.

4. How often are skull base fractures missed on facial bone films?

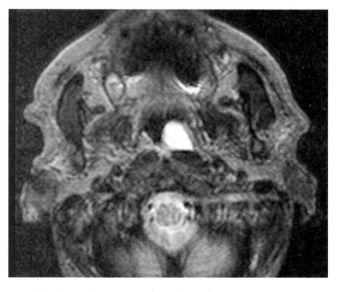 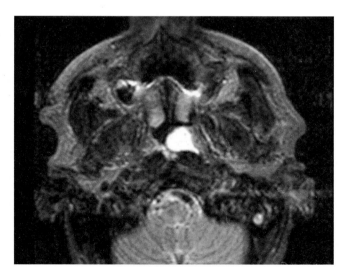

1. Which is this more likely to be: a mucus retention cyst or a Tornwaldt cyst? Why?

2. How do Tornwaldt cysts arise?

3. How do mucus retention cysts arise?

4. What is the typical history for a Tornwaldt cyst?

CASE 1

Skull Base Fracture

1. Most are shaped in arcs, with the top of the arc the most anterior aspect of the skull.

2. CSF leaks, dissections, pseudoaneurysms, meningitis, optic canal hematomas affecting the optic nerves.

3. Compression (axial loading) injury.

4. >50%.

Reference

Bloom AI, Neeman Z, Slasky BS, et al: Fracture of the occipital condyles and associated craniocervical ligament injury: incidence, CT imaging and implications, *Clin Radiol* 52:198–202, 1997.

Cross-Reference

Neuroradiology: THE REQUISITES, pp 842–843.

Comment

This patient shows evidence of bilateral occipital condyle fractures. This is a frequently missed diagnosis on plain films (owing to bony overlap) and on CT scans (because the emergency department radiologist is concentrating so much on the cervical spine that he or she disregards the skull base).

Fractures of the skull base may sweep in an arc from posterior to anterior to posterior when they involve the sphenoid bone. In so doing, the fractures may affect the carotid or optic canals.

Occipital condyle fractures usually occur after motor vehicle accidents or sports injuries. Most patients present with loss of consciousness, neck pain, headache, reduced range of motion, and cranial nerve deficits (hypoglossal nerve injury most common).

Fifty percent of occipital condyle fractures are missed on plain films. Associated C1 and C2 fractures are present in >10% of cases.

The classification of occipital condyle fractures by Anderson and Montesano is as follows:

I—impacted comminuted fracture without displacement of fragments into the foramen magnum due to axial loading force

II—linear skull base fracture extending into an occipital condyle due to a direct blow to the cranium

III—fracture with avulsion of condylar fragments with displacement into the foramen magnum due to lateral inclination and rotation injury

Only class III fractures are unstable, but they also are the most common type.

Notes

CASE 2

Mucus Retention Cyst of the Nasopharyngeal Mucosa

1. Mucus retention cyst, because it is off midline, is associated with the eustachian tube, and was not bright on T1W scans.

2. Retraction of nasopharyngeal mucosa during notochord regression into the clivus.

3. Obstruction of tiny minor salivary glands.

4. They are most often asymptomatic.

Reference

Robson CD: Cysts and tumors of the oral cavity, oropharynx, and nasopharynx in children, *Neuroimaging Clin N Am* 13:427–442, 2003.

Cross-Reference

Neuroradiology: THE REQUISITES, pp 642–644.

Comment

The images show a cystic lesion off midline closely apposed to and along the plane of the eustachian tube. The lesion was bright on T2W and FLAIR images, as one would expect for a mucus-filled structure. It should not enhance and is smooth in outline. In the sinus, this is a mucus retention cyst. Here it is the same.

Although Tornwaldt cysts are more common than mucus retention cysts in this location, they are almost always in the midline. They are more commonly bright than dark on T1W scans on the basis of higher protein concentration. Tornwaldt cysts, although usually discovered incidentally, rarely may cause chronic halitosis or be so large as to obstruct the eustachian tube, leading to serous otitis media.

Rarely one might see a cephalocele, craniopharyngioma, or teratoma in the nasopharynx that can manifest as a cystic mass in the nasopharynx.

Notes

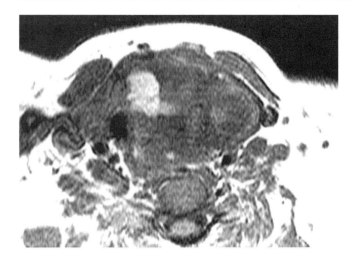

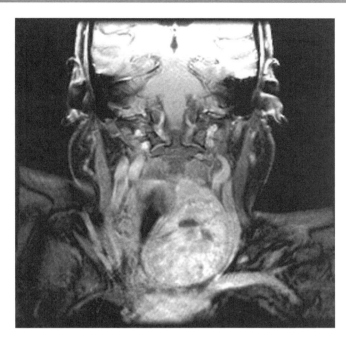

1. Name the two most common symptoms associated with this lesion.

2. How are most goiters discovered radiographically?

3. Is the goiter or the surgery for the goiter more likely to cause a recurrent laryngeal nerve palsy?

4. How often do multinodular goiters extend substernally?

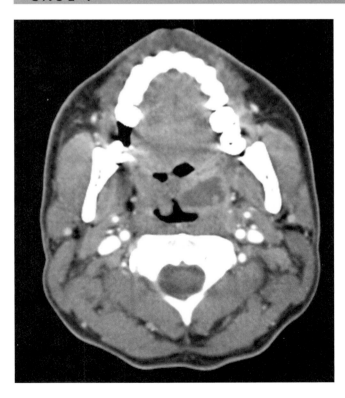

1. Where is this lesion located?

2. What is the differential diagnosis?

3. Name the usual pathogen involved.

4. What is Lemierre syndrome?

CASE 3

Multinodular Goiter

1. Neck mass and dyspnea.

2. From chest radiographs showing tracheal deviation.

3. Usually it is the surgery that results in a higher rate of vocal cord paralysis than the goiter itself, with total thyroidectomy (2.4%) having three times the rate of partial thyroidectomy (0.8%).

4. 37%.

Reference

Misiolek M, Waler J, Namyslowski G, et al: Recurrent laryngeal nerve palsy after thyroid cancer surgery: a laryngological and surgical problem, *Eur Arch Otorhinolaryngol* 258:460–462, 2001.

Cross-Reference

Neuroradiology: THE REQUISITES, p 739.

Comment

Multinodular goiter is a common finding on CT scans of the head and neck, particularly in women. Important findings to address with multinodular goiters are the extent of tracheal and esophageal deviation, and substernal and upper neck extension. If one sees bilateral abnormalities in the thyroid glands—whether the abnormalities are focal calcifications, cysts, or areas of mixed densities—more than likely the process is multinodular goiter. The debate about the significance of a dominant nodule in a goitrous gland has been resolved: It should be treated as a potential cancer just as if it occurred in a virgin gland free of any disease.

It is rare in the United States to see the various forms of acute thyroiditis, especially if they are asymptomatic. Hashimoto thyroiditis is an exception because it may antecede goiter formation. Hashimoto thyroiditis is usually more diffuse, symmetric, and without areas of cyst formation, hemorrhage, or calcification. This entity is due to the attack by antithyroid autoantibodies. Lymphomas, especially of the MALT type (mucosa-associated lymphoid tissue) occur more frequently in patients with Hashimoto thyroiditis.

There is currently a debate regarding the need for total versus partial thyroidectomy for treatment of goiters. The rationale for subtotal thyroidectomy in part revolves around the lower incidence of the most common surgical complication from thyroidectomy surgery—recurrent laryngeal nerve palsy. As noted earlier, the risk nearly triples if one attempts a total thyroidectomy. Some studies have reported complication rates of 6% to 7%. A higher probability of this complication occurs after secondary or repeat procedures of the thyroid and in malignant cases.

Notes

CASE 4

Peritonsillar Abscess

1. The space between the tonsil and the pharyngeal constrictor muscle.

2. Tonsillar abscess versus carcinoma; rarely fistula from branchial cleft cyst.

3. *Streptococcus.*

4. *Lemierre syndrome* refers to streptococcal pharyngitis leading to a peritonsillar abscess from *Fusobacterium necrophorum.* This leads to jugular thrombophlebitis and septic thromboemboli to the lungs with pneumonia.

Reference

Fujimoto M, Aramaki H, Takano S, Otani Y: Immediate tonsillectomy for peritonsillar abscess, *Acta Otolaryngol Suppl* 523:252–255, 1996.

Cross-Reference

Neuroradiology: THE REQUISITES, pp 651–653.

Comment

The distinction between tonsillar inflammation and peritonsillar abscesses is one that is not moot. Exudative tonsillitis is usually evident clinically because one sees pus formation arising from the tonsils. This clinical presentation may be seen most commonly in children and young adults, in whom pharyngitis and tonsillitis are the most common head and neck infections (along with middle ear disease). A patient with a peritonsillar abscess presents with symptoms of pain, otalgia, trismus, fever, neck stiffness, odynophagia and signs of fever, uvular deviation, palate swelling, and tonsil asymmetry. The most common source of peritonsillar abscess is still tonsillitis.

There is currently a debate as to whether a trial of antibiotics and percutaneous intraoral drainage versus immediate tonsillectomy surgery is warranted in children with peritonsillar abscesses. Early surgery may reduce the rates of parapharyngeal abscesses and mediastinitis, which are among the worst complications of tonsillitis. A parapharyngeal abscess warrants early surgery. Nonetheless, the surgeon, if required to do so, would drain a peritonsillar abscess intraorally, whereas a parapharyngeal abscess requires drainage via a cervical approach; this is an important distinction to make.

Quinsy is another term for a peritonsillar abscess. Quinsy occurs when infection spreads from the tonsillar bed to the surrounding tissues.

Notes

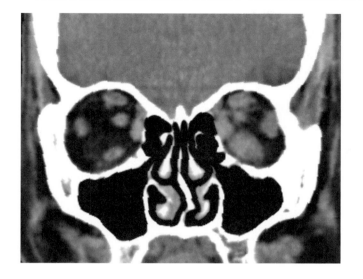 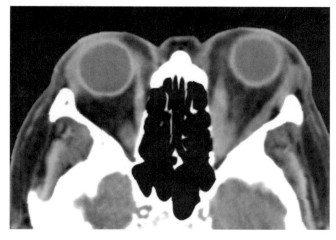

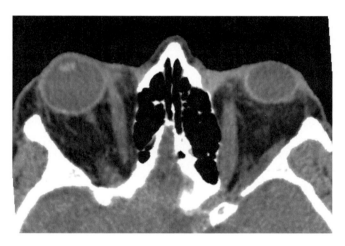 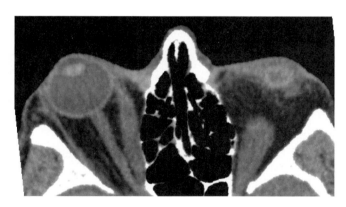

1. Identify the possible hormonal states in which thyroid ophthalmopathy may occur.

2. Which is most common?

3. What is the most common orbital manifestation of thyroid eye disease?

4. Name the most common cause of unilateral exophthalmos.

CASE 5

Thyroid Eye Disease

1. Hyperthyroid, euthyroid, hypothyroid.

2. Hyperthyroid.

3. Exophthalmos, increased orbital fat volume.

4. Thyroid eye disease.

References

Ben Simon GJ, Syed HM, Douglas R, et al: Extraocular muscle enlargement with tendon involvement in thyroid-associated orbitopathy, *Am J Ophthalmol* 137:1145–1147, 2004.

Nishida Y, Tian S, Isberg B, et al: Significance of orbital fatty tissue for exophthalmos in thyroid-associated ophthalmopathy, *Graefes Arch Clin Exp Ophthalmol* 240:515–520, 2002.

Cross-Reference

Neuroradiology: THE REQUISITES, pp 503–504.

Comment

Thyroid eye disease is the most common cause of bilateral (bottom figures) *and* unilateral (top figures) proptosis in adults.

The term *thyroid eye disease* is used because too often students of the entity believe that the disease is associated only with the hyperthyroidism of Graves disease. Although this is the most common scenario for thyroid ophthalmopathy, the manifestations may arise after Graves disease has been treated and the patient is euthyroid or hypothyroid. Other terms used include thyroid-associated orbitopathy, Graves orbitopathy, and Graves ophthalmopathy.

Classically the inferior and medial rectus muscles are affected early and often. Tendinous sparing is supposed to differentiate thyroid eye disease from orbital pseudotumor, but it is an overstated sign because tendons are involved in about 8% of thyroid eye disease cases. The most common orbital manifestation of thyroid eye disease is an increase in the volume of the orbital fat leading to exophthalmos. Nishida et al found that the total orbital fatty tissue volume and the anterior orbital fatty tissue volume correlated more closely with the degree of exophthalmos than the extraocular muscle volume.

Indications for decompressive surgery for thyroid eye disease include (1) compressive optic neuropathy, (2) orbital apex compression, (3) vascular compromise, (4) exposure keratopathy, and (5) cosmesis. Surgical decompression may be performed endoscopically with either an orbital floor or medial-lateral decompression, usually via lamina papyracea end fracture. Medial-lateral decompression is favored due to lower rates of postoperative diploplia.

Notes

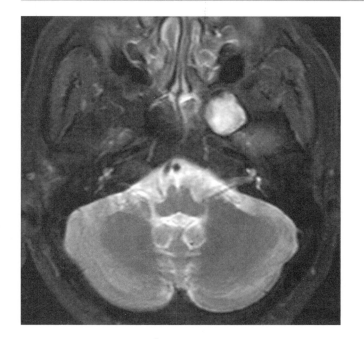

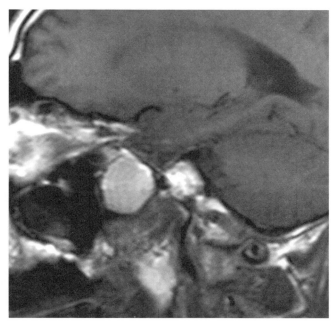

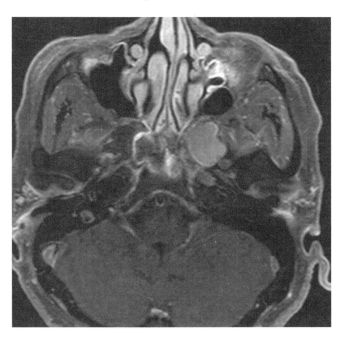

1. In this location, what is the differential diagnosis?

2. Why is this not a cephalocele?

3. What are the most common sites for mucoceles?

4. At what protein concentration does the signal intensity on a T1W scan convert from dark to bright on a 1.5 Tesla MRI scanner?

Mucocele

1. Mucocele, cholesterol granuloma, hemorrhagic cyst, melanoma metastasis.

2. Unlike this lesion, cephaloceles are not bright on pregadolinium T1W scans.

3. Frontal, ethmoidal (75%) > maxillary (20%) and sphenoid (5%).

4. 15%.

Reference

Serrano E, Klossek JM, Percodani J, et al: Surgical management of paranasal sinus mucoceles: a long-term study of 60 cases, *Otolaryngol Head Neck Surg* 131:133–140, 2004.

Cross-Reference

Neuroradiology: THE REQUISITES, pp 510, 562, 628.

Comment

Protein within the paranasal sinuses may have a variable appearance depending on its concentration. At low concentrations (<10%), the proteinaceous secretions are similar to water, and they appear dark on T1W scans and bright on T2W scans. As the concentration of protein increases, the signal intensity on the T1W scans increases to a point (15% to 25%) where the T1W and T2W scans show hyperintensity within the paranasal sinus. With increasing protein concentration, the next change is a diminution in the signal intensity of the secretions on the T2W scans, leading to a combination of bright on T1W and dark on T2W scans (30% to 35%). Finally, as more and more water protons are squeezed out of the hyperproteinaceous concretions, the signal intensity becomes dark on the T1W and the T2W sequences (>35%).

Mucoceles are most common in the frontal and ethmoid sinuses and are far less frequent in the sphenoid and maxillary sinus. Because the mucocele is due to obstruction of the egress of mucus from the sinus, one should look for a blockage at the frontal (ethmoidal) recess when dealing with mucoceles in these locations. In some cases, that obstruction is due to tenacious secretions or polyps, but in others it may be a postoperative phenomenon after endoscopic sinus surgery. Alternatively, one may have a neoplastic process (osteoma or carcinoma versus fibrous dysplasia) obstructing the ostium. The sinus expands over time with bony remodeling, leading to the typical appearance of the mucocele. In some cases, the bony walls may seem totally unapparent; however, there is usually a periosteal layer that is separating the mucocele from the brain, dura, and orbit.

Most mucoceles currently are treated via an endoscopic approach.

Notes

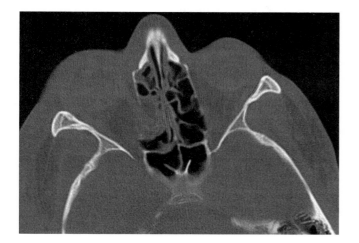

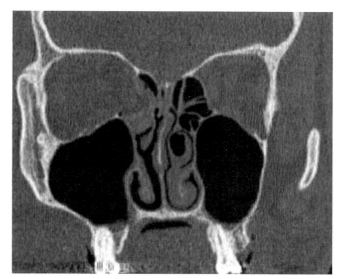

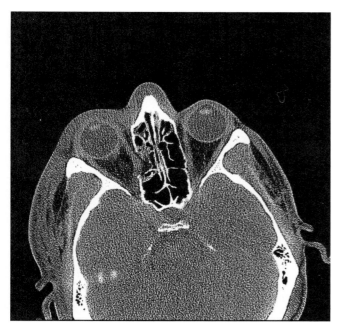

1. What is the most common site of an orbital fracture?

2. What is the least common orbital wall to be fractured?

3. Identify the two clinical features that lead to a more aggressive treatment of orbital fracture.

4. Name the most common causes of decreased visual acuity in patients with orbital trauma.

Orbital Wall Fracture

1. Orbital floor.

2. Orbital roof.

3. Double vision with limited mobility or decreased visual acuity.

4. In order of declining frequency, retrobulbar hemorrhage, optic nerve thickening presumably secondary to edema, intraorbital emphysema, optic nerve impingement, detached retina, and ruptured globe.

Reference

Lee HJ, Jilani M, Frohman L, Baker S: CT of orbital trauma, *Emerg Radiol* 10:168–172, 2004.

Cross-Reference

Neuroradiology: THE REQUISITES, pp 266–268.

Comment

Pertinent findings when describing orbital fractures include the presence of displacement of the fractured fragments, herniation of fat or muscular tissue defect, retrobulbar hematoma, and involvement of the region of the entry of the anterior or posterior ethmoidal arteries. Surgical reconstruction with small pins and screws is used to decrease the risk of diplopia associated with displacement of the globe or deformation of the extraocular muscles. Cosmetic deformities also may be addressed with these surgical corrections.

The terms *Bombay door* and *trapdoor* have been used to refer to the displacement of fracture fragments associated with orbital floor trauma. The Bombay door has two components of the fracture, which are oriented inferiorly, often transmitting the infraorbital nerve along with fat and other orbital content. The trapdoor has a single rotation of axis for the fracture fragment. It is important to recognize the normal infraorbital canal in the floor of the orbit to ensure that one does not misdiagnose a fracture when dealing with simply the infraorbital nerve canal. The presence of air-fluid levels in the sinuses is a strong indicator of acute fractures in a patient with facial trauma. Nonetheless, because of the potential tamponade of vessels by the orbital fat through the fracture fragments, one occasionally sees an acute orbital floor fracture without air-fluid levels and blood in the maxillary sinus.

Numerous fracture complexes involve the orbits. Le Fort type I fractures affect the maxilla bilaterally, sparing the orbital walls. Le Fort type II fractures cross the floors of the orbits but also involve the medial orbital walls. Le Fort type III fractures (craniofacial dissociation) extend across the lateral orbital walls into the medial orbital walls. Le Fort fractures may occur unilaterally or bilaterally. Most Le Fort fractures also are characterized by fractures of the pterygoid plate region.

Zygomaticomaxillary complex fractures involve the orbital rim (and frequently the orbital floor) and lateral orbital wall. These are usually due to dissociations of the zygomaticofrontal, zygomaticomaxillary, and zygomatic arch regions. The zygomaticofrontal suture region involves the lateral orbital wall, and the plane of the fracture involves the floor of the orbit. This fracture also is called a *tripod fracture* or *trimalar fracture.*

Notes

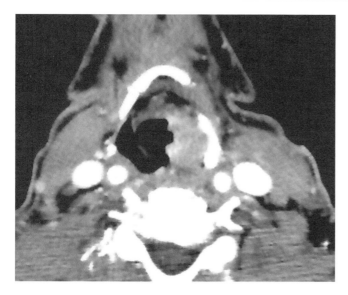

1. In what part of the larynx is this lesion?
2. What is the most common histology in this location?
3. What is the most common sarcoma in this location?
4. What percentage of laryngeal cancers are supraglottic?

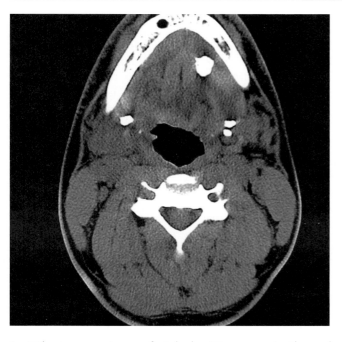 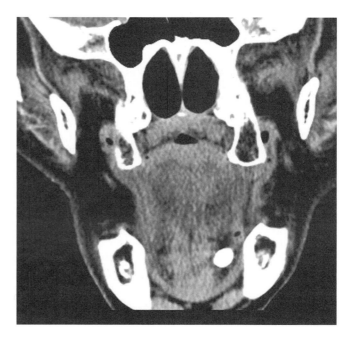

1. What percentage of sialadenitis occur in the submandibular gland?
2. What percentage of submandibular stones are radiopaque on plain films?
3. What percentage of submandibular sialadenitis are due to stone disease?
4. How accurate is magnetic resonance sialography for detecting salivary stones?

Aryepiglottic Fold Squamous Cell Carcinoma

1. Supraglottic larynx.
2. Squamous cell carcinoma.
3. Chondrosarcoma.
4. 30%.

Reference

Greene FL, Balch CM, Fleming ID, April F (eds): *AJCC Cancer Staging Manual,* 6th ed, New York, Springer-Verlag, 2002.

Cross-Reference

Neuroradiology: THE REQUISITES, pp 672–676.

Comment

The aryepiglottic fold is a portion of the supraglottic larynx. Tumors in this location may grow quite large and may fill the space between the aryepiglottic fold and the piriform sinus posterior wall. When this happens, it is difficult to determine whether the tumor is arising from the hypopharynx–piriform sinus versus the supraglottic larynx–aryepiglottic fold. Although this determination is a quandary for the radiologist when there is no air space identified between the pharyngeal wall and epiglottic fold, under endoscopy the anatomy is easy to discern because the surgeon usually is able to pass a small endoscope either lateral to the mass (identifying an aryepiglottic fold origin) or medial to the mass (identifying it as a piriform sinus lesion).

The staging of supraglottic carcinoma is derived in part from the extent of the lesion, the mobility of the larynx, and the degree or presence of cartilaginous invasion. Unresectability usually is defined by extension to the prevertebral musculature, encasement of the carotid artery, or extension to the mediastinum.

T staging is as follows:

T1—tumor limited to one subsite of supraglottis, normal vocal cord mobility

T2—tumor invades mucosa of more than one adjacent subsite of supraglottis or glottis or region outside the supraglottis (mucosa of base of tongue, vallecula, medial wall of piriform sinus) without fixation of the larynx

T3—tumor limited to larynx with vocal cord fixation or invades postcricoid area, preepiglottis, paraglottic space, or minor thyroid cartilage erosion (e.g., inner cortex)

T4a—tumor invades through the thyroid cartilage or invades adjacent tissues (trachea, soft tissues of neck, deep muscle of the tongue, strap muscles, thyroid, or esophagus) or both

T4b—tumor invades prevertebral space, encases carotid artery, or invades mediastinal structures

Notes

Submandibular Gland Calculus

1. 10%.
2. 70%.
3. 90%.
4. >90%.

Reference

Becker M, Marchal F, Becker CD, et al: Sialolithiasis and salivary ductal stenosis: diagnostic accuracy of MR sialography with a three-dimensional extended-phase conjugate-symmetry rapid spin-echo sequence, *Radiology* 217:347–358, 2000.

Cross-Reference

Neuroradiology: THE REQUISITES, pp 700–703.

Comment

Why are so many more calculi found in the submandibular gland versus the parotid gland? A variety of factors may influence this frequency, including the higher pH of the submandibular glands saliva, causing a more favorable environment for calcium phosphate and calcium oxalate crystal formation. In addition, the saliva is more mucoid, making it thicker and more likely to precipitate.

The duct of the submandibular gland is wider than that of the parotid gland, and it must course in an uphill fashion to get to the floor of the mouth, which leads to a higher rate of stasis within the duct. The duct may be traumatized in the floor of the mouth, which could lead to irritation and spasm, increasing the likelihood of stasis.

The treatment of submandibular gland calculus disease is manifold. At the outset, the clinician simply may provide the patient with a secretagogue to encourage increased saliva production and flow. The submandibular gland duct subsequently may be dilated by the clinician with various dilators and stents to assist in stone passage.

One also can marsupialize the duct and probe it or perform ductoplasty to try to enlarge the duct to encourage stone passage. Glandular removal in general is a last resort because stone disease often is bilateral and because having a dry mouth predisposes to irritation and other complications.

Notes

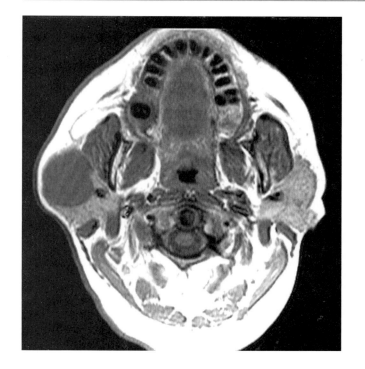

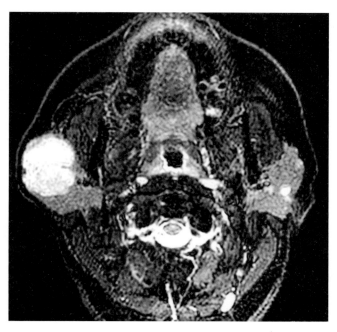

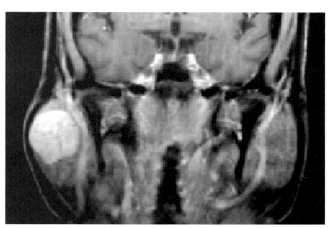

1. What percentage of this type of tumor are bright on T2W scans?

2. What percentage of pleomorphic adenomas are in the parotid gland?

3. In the head and neck, where are the most common sites for myoepitheliomas?

4. Why remove a benign pleomorphic adenoma of the parotid gland?

Pleomorphic Adenoma

1. >95%.

2. 84%.

3. Parotid and palate.

4. There is a reasonably high rate (15% to 20%) of malignant degeneration over time.

Reference

Kinoshita T, Ishii K, Naganuma H, Okitsu T: MR imaging findings of parotid tumors with pathologic diagnostic clues: a pictorial essay, *Clin Imaging* 28:93–101, 2004.

Cross-Reference

Neuroradiology: THE REQUISITES, pp 706–710.

Comment

Pleomorphic adenomas are the most common benign tumors in the sublingual glands, submandibular glands, parotid glands, and minor salivary glands. They represent 80% of the benign tumors of the parotid gland, which represent 80% of all tumors of the parotid gland. This means that 64% of all tumors of the parotid glands are pleomorphic adenomas.

Pleomorphic adenoma is the most common variety of benign adenomas of the salivary glands. Oxyphilic adenomas and monomorphic adenomas are other varieties, which are rarely identified. Pleomorphic adenoma is characterized by extreme brightness on a T2W scan and enhancing avidly with contrast material. The lesions show well-defined margins with an element of lobulation to them. Although they occur rarely, calcification and cyst formation may be present in pleomorphic adenomas. This begs the question: if one sees a cystic lesion or calcified lesion in the parotid gland, should one consider a pleomorphic adenoma? Absolutely.

One feature of pleomorphic adenoma that should be recognized is its tendency to accumulate contrast material over time if one performs a dynamic CT scan or MRI.

When describing pleomorphic adenomas, it is important to be precise with respect to whether or not the tumors are in the superficial or deep portion of the gland; this is defined by the plane of the stylomandibular tunnel. It is truly defined by the plane of the facial nerve, but because radiologists have a difficult time identifying the facial nerve within the gland, we use the stylomandibular tunnel.

In general, tumors that are superficial to the facial nerve are treated with an incision in front of the ear, whereas tumors that are entirely deep to the facial nerve and in the deep lobe of the gland are approached via a submandibular cervical incision. Tumors that span the superficial and deep portions of the gland generally are approached with a superficial incision with careful identification of the facial nerve. Facial nerve palsy is the dreaded complication of parotid gland surgery, and surgeons spend a lot of time dissecting the facial nerve from the stylomastoid foramen through the parotid gland to the superficial facial muscles and structures to prevent this complication.

Pleomorphic adenomas have the potential for malignant degeneration, which is why they are removed in their entirety by the head and neck surgeon. In addition, pleomorphic adenomas show a propensity for seeding along the surgical track. At one point, this propensity led to some element of consternation with regard to fine-needle aspiration of the lesion for histologic examination. Subsequent studies have shown, however, that with needles ≤18G in size the possibility of seeding by the needle track is infinitesimal.

In most cases, fine-needle aspiration is performed with either a 22G or 25G needle. The risk of injury to the facial nerve by fine-needle aspiration also is quite small and should not preclude the transparotid approach to a deep lobe mass.

Notes

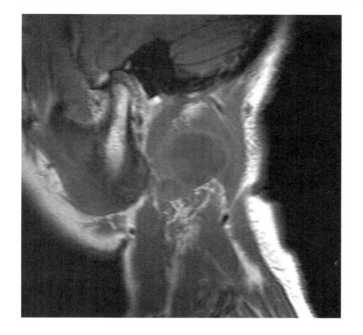

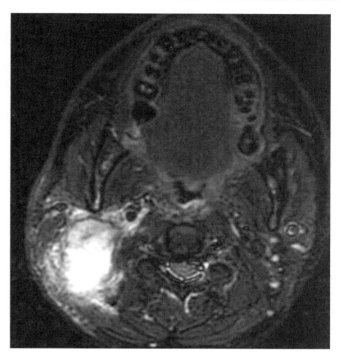

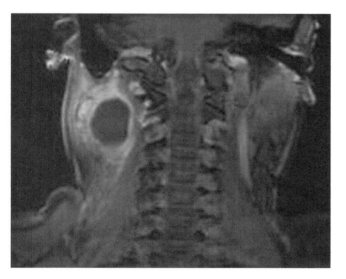

1. Name the two biggest risk factors for this lesion.

2. What is the most common organism?

3. What percentage of skeletal infections secondary to intravenous drug abuse are represented by cervical vertebral osteomyelitis?

4. Identify the microorganism that patients with sickle cell disease are susceptible to with respect to osteomyelitis.

Perivertebral Abscess

1. Intravenous drug abuse and postoperative status.

2. *Staphylococcus aureus.*

3. 2% to 4%.

4. *Salmonella.*

Reference

Alcantara AL, Tucker RB, McCarroll KA: Radiologic study of injection drug use complications, *Infect Dis Clin North Am* 16:713–743, 2002.

Cross-Reference

Neuroradiology: THE REQUISITES, p 733.

Comment

How does one distinguish between a retropharyngeal process versus a perivertebral collection? The best way to make this distinction is to determine how the longus colli muscles are displaced. If the longus colli muscles are displaced posteriorly, this indicates that the lesion is coming from the pharyngeal or the retropharyngeal space. If the abnormality is intrinsic to the longus colli–longus capitis muscle complex or if the longus colli–longus capitis muscle complex is displaced anteriorly, it identifies the mass as a perivertebral mass.

This distinction is not moot. Most pharyngeal processes are secondary to squamous cell carcinoma of the mucosa and the retropharyngeal lymphadenopathy associated with it. Occasionally, sarcomas may occur in this location as well. Infections include retropharyngeal abscess and necrotizing lymphadenitis of the retropharyngeal space. Peritonsillar collections also manifest in this fashion.

Perivertebral space lesions include lesions related to the spinal column. Anterior osteophytes and ligamentous calcification are common perivertebral space abnormalities. On the neoplastic front, one should consider metastases to the vertebral bodies and primary vertebral body bone tumors, which include myeloma, chordomas, lymphoma, and sarcomas of the bone. Infections include discitis, osteomyelitis, and perivertebral abscess collections. The differential diagnosis is markedly different between the two spaces, and the location of the longus colli–longus capitis muscle complex becomes more important.

Notes

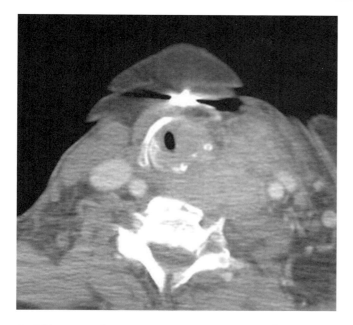

1. What are the most common sources for tumors eroding the laryngeal cartilages?

2. What inflammatory conditions can cause laryngeal cartilage erosion?

3. How often does thyroid carcinoma invade the larynx-trachea-esophagus axis?

4. Name the most common site for arthritis of the larynx.

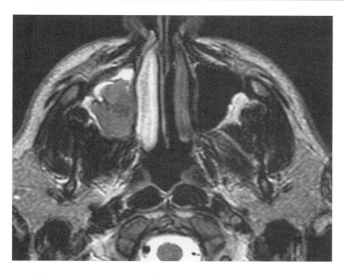 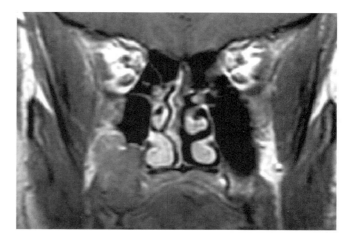

1. What percentage of sinonasal cancers are adenocarcinomas?

2. Identify industry workers at risk for adenocarcinomas of the sinuses.

3. Where do most adenocarcinomas arise in the sinonasal cavity?

4. What are the most common intracranial manifestations of sinonasal undifferentiated carcinoma metastases?

CASE 12

Thyroid Carcinoma Invasion into the Larynx

1. Laryngeal squamous cell carcinomas, thyroid carcinomas, laryngeal chondrosarcomas, and nodal metastases.

2. Granulomatous infections (tuberculosis, leprosy, sarcoidosis, Wegener granulomatosis, syphilis), radiation chondronecrosis, rheumatoid arthritis, trauma, foreign body reaction, ingested toxins, and relapsing polychondritis.

3. 5–10%.

4. The cricoarytenoid joint.

Reference

Machens A, Hinze R, Lautenschlager C, et al: Thyroid carcinoma invading the cervicovisceral axis: routes of invasion and clinical implications, *Surgery* 129:23–28, 2001.

Cross-Reference

Neuroradiology: THE REQUISITES, pp 740–745.

Comment

Medullary carcinoma of the thyroid gland is more likely to invade the larynx than papillary carcinoma, but the increased prevalence of the latter leads to the overall increased incidence in papillary carcinoma. Although increased T stage increases the risk of laryngeal invasion by thyroid cancer, increased N stage increases the risk of esophageal infiltration.

Circumferential involvement of adjacent laryngeal cartilage >90 degrees by thyroid carcinoma is accurate to 94% in predicting tumor invasion. Invasion is more common when the thyroid cancer is a recurrence rather than primary disease in most series. Aggressive resection and iodine therapy may still be curative.

Notes

CASE 13

Sinonasal Undifferentiated Carcinoma

1. 10% to 20%.

2. Shoemakers, woodworkers.

3. The ethmoid sinuses.

4. Direct invasion and dural metastases.

Reference

Phillips CD, Futterer SF, Lipper MH, Levine PA: Sinonasal undifferentiated carcinoma: CT and MR imaging of an uncommon neoplasm of the nasal cavity, *Radiology* 202:477–480, 1997.

Cross-Reference

Neuroradiology: THE REQUISITES, pp 634–635.

Comment

Sinonasal undifferentiated carcinomas are aggressive malignancies associated with a poor prognosis. These carcinomas most commonly occur in the ethmoid sinus and show early bone destruction. Involvement of the adjacent structures of the nose, skin, orbit, and calvaria is common even at presentation. The imaging appearance is similar to that of a squamous cell carcinoma gone wild (no videos please), often with necrosis. They enhance heterogeneously. Males are affected in a ratio of 3:1 over females. When patients present, most tumors are >4 cm with subsequent extension into the anterior cranial fossa in 70% and orbital invasion in 40%. Median survival is 10 months.

Notes

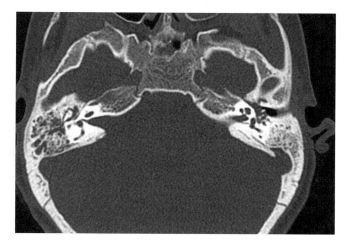

1. What is the most common indication for surgery for otomastoiditis?
2. What is the most common CT finding for this complication?
3. Identify the three routes of spread of infection from the middle ear to the intracranial space.
4. What is the most likely source of mastoiditis and facial nerve palsy?

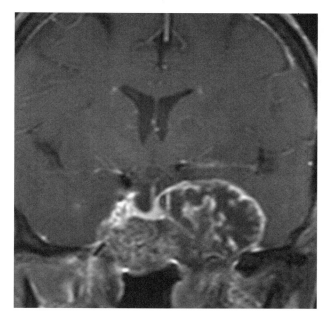 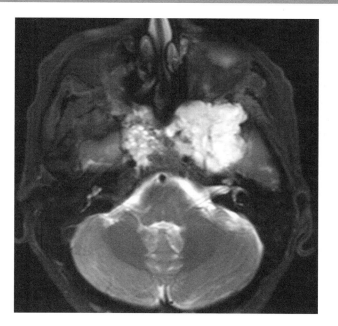

1. What is the classic site of origin of this lesion?
2. What percentage of lesions arise in the head and neck?
3. What is a chondroid chordoma?
4. Name the classic histologic finding of the chordoma.

CASE 14

Otomastoiditis

1. Mastoidectomy for subperiosteal abscess.

2. Cortex erosion.

3. (1) Direct extension, (2) hematogenous spread, (3) thrombophlebitis.

4. Cholesteatoma.

Reference

Migirov L: Computed tomographic versus surgical findings in complicated acute otomastoiditis, *Ann Otol Rhinol Laryngol* 112:675–677, 2003.

Cross-Reference

Neuroradiology: THE REQUISITES, pp 575–583.

Comment

Opacification of the middle ear and mastoid air cells is a common finding in children with ear pain and fever and in patients being instrumented in the ICU. Presumably the nasogastric tubes and orotracheal tubes that are placed can cause either lymphoid proliferation or intrinsic obstruction of the eustachian tube, which may lead to fluid backing up into the mastoid or middle ear air cells. Nonetheless, the adage is that one should always consider the possibility of an obstructing nasopharyngeal carcinoma if one finds recurrent otomastoiditis in an adult.

Another scenario in which fluid in the middle ear and the mastoid air cells is seen frequently is when a patient has undergone radiation therapy. There is seepage of fluid from the irritated mucosa.

It has been observed that patients who have carbon monoxide poisoning also seem to have a higher rate of mastoid air cell opacification. The exact etiology of this is unknown.

In many instances of obstructive cases, one is dealing with noninfected fluid rather than a bacterial purulent infection. Obstructive causes result in a serous otitis media and mastoiditis, as opposed to the infectious etiology usually caused by streptococcal organisms.

Notes

CASE 15

Chondrosarcoma of Skull Base

1. Petrooccipital fissure.

2. 6.5%.

3. A low-grade chondrosarcoma.

4. Physaliphorous cell.

Reference

Rosenberg AE, Nielsen GP, Keel SB, et al: Chondrosarcoma of the base of the skull: a clinicopathologic study of 200 cases with emphasis on its distinction from chordoma, *Am J Surg Pathol* 23:1370–1378, 1999.

Cross-Reference

Neuroradiology: THE REQUISITES, pp 557–559.

Comment

Chondrosarcomas of the skull base have more favorable long-term prognoses than chordomas because they are usually low-grade neoplasms. Five- and 10-year survivals after surgery and proton-beam radiation therapy are >95%, as opposed to 51% 5-year and 35% 10-year survival with chordomas. Prognostic factors that portend local radiation failure for skull base chondrosarcomas include older age (>52), larger diameter (>45 mm), and greater volume (>28 mL). Carbon ion radiotherapy is popular now.

Classic teaching is that chondrosarcomas have a more eccentric positioning than chordomas and have more popcorn-style calcification in their matrix. Most stain positively for S-100, and none show keratin staining.

Mean age of patients with skull base chondrosarcomas is 39. There is a slight female predominance.

Notes

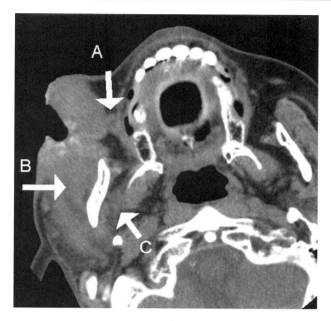

1. Identify the most common site of head and neck cancer.

2. What is the most common histology of skin cancer?

3. What is the rate of growth of aggressive basal cell carcinoma?

4. What muscles delineated by the letters A, B, and C are infiltrated with cancer?

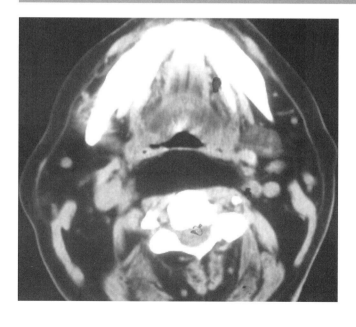
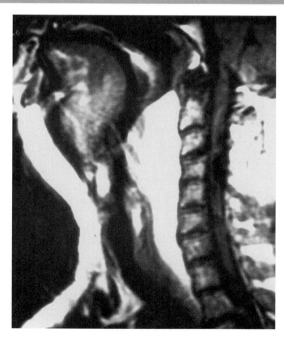

1. What are the echogenicity characteristics of this lesion?

2. What is typical of a myxoid liposarcoma?

3. Name four fat-containing tumors in the neck.

4. What is a lipoblastoma?

CASE 16

Skin Cancer

1. The skin.

2. Basal cell carcinoma.

3. 10%.

4. *A* = orbicularis oris; *B* = masseter; *C* = lateral pterygoid.

Reference

Walling HW, Fosko SW, Geraminejad PA, et al: Aggressive basal cell carcinoma: presentation, pathogenesis, and management, *Cancer Metastasis Rev* 23:389–402, 2004.

Cross-Reference

Neuroradiology: THE REQUISITES, p 662.

Comment

Facts about basal cell carcinoma include the following:

It is the most common skin cancer in whites.
The major risk factor is ultraviolet sunlight exposure.
The most common head and neck site is the nose (67%), followed by the orbit (19%, with medial orbit, 10 times more common than lateral orbit), and the ear (13%).
Ten percent of basal cell carcinomas show aggressive growth, and of these, 3% show perineural invasion.
With perineural invasion, the 5-year prognosis, which normally is >90% with basal cell carcinoma, decreases to 50%.
The 5-year local control rates without salvage therapy are 87% with microscopic perineural invasion and 55% with clinical perineural invasion.
Of local failures, 88% occur in patients with positive margins.
Recurrences occur in regional lymph nodes in 50% of cases with perineural invasion.

Notes

CASE 17

Lipoma

1. Hyperechoic to muscle, well defined, compressible.

2. More of a fluid density to it.

3. Lipoma, liposarcoma, teratoma, lipoblastoma, hibernoma.

4. A tumor of immature embryonic white fat occurring in young children with a mixture of fat and nonadipose tissue.

Reference

Murphey MD, Carroll JF, Flemming DJ, et al: From the archives of the AFIP: benign musculoskeletal lipomatous lesions, *Radiographics* 24:1433–1466, 2004.

Cross-Reference

Neuroradiology: THE REQUISITES, pp 117–118, 431–432.

Comment

Lipomas are the most common benign mesenchymal tumors of the head and neck. They have density and signal intensity characteristics typical of those of fat. Lipomas are said to increase in size as individuals gain weight; however, the change should be relatively minor. If one does see a lipoma that is increasing rapidly in size, one should consider the possibility of liposarcoma. The standard teaching is that liposarcomas may look nearly identical to lipomas, but the liposarcomas I have seen almost always have a strandiness to the fat or a focal nodule, which would suggest the possibility of sarcomatous etiology.

The most common locations for head and neck lipomas are in the soft tissue of the neck, particularly in posterolateral subcutaneous tissue, the nape of the neck, and the supraclavicular regions.

Lipomas are soft, painless, and mobile clinically. Multiple lipomas occur in 5% of individuals, and 13% of all lipomas arise in the head and neck. Most lipomas are isoechoic to hyperechoic relative to muscle.

Madelung disease (multiple symmetric lipomatosis) represents diffuse fatty deposition throughout the neck and is more frequent in alcoholics. Enlargement of the chin and neck occurs in a symmetric diffuse pattern. The fat is not encapsulated.

Notes

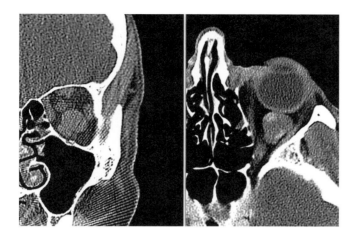

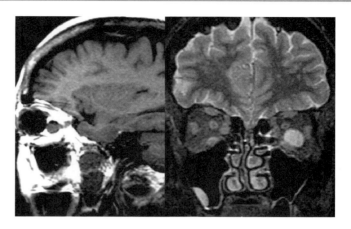

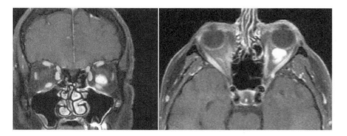

1. What is in the differential diagnosis?

2. What percentage of orbital hemangiomas are intraconal?

3. What is meant by an orbital hemangioma?

4. What is the grade for this vascular lesion of the orbit?

C A S E 1 8

Orbital Hemangioma

1. Varix, schwannoma/neurogenic tumor, meningioma, leiomyoma, metastasis, optic nerve glioma, lymphoma, hemangioma.

2. 80%.

3. It is a low-flow congenital vascular malformation.

4. Type 3.

Reference

Tanaka A, Mihara F, Yoshiura T, et al: Differentiation of cavernous hemangioma from schwannoma of the orbit, *AJR Am J Roentgenol* 183:1799–1804, 2004.

Cross-Reference

Neuroradiology: THE REQUISITES, pp 496–498.

Comment

Orbital cavernous hemangiomas are the most common masses in the orbit. They predominate in women (4:1 ratio) in their 40s and usually present with unilateral proptosis or visual disturbance or both. This is typically an intraconal process, which is well defined and may enlarge with a Valsalva maneuver or during pregnancy.

One grading system for vascular lesions of the orbit puts type 1 as no flow malformations, such as lymphangiomas; type 2, venous flow lesions, such as varices; type 3, low-flow lesions, such as cavernous hemangiomas (which are also known as venous malformations, making this classification a bit suspect); and type 4, high-flow lesions such as true arteriovenous malformations.

The differential diagnosis often includes a cranial nerve schwannoma because cranial nerves III, IV, V, and VI have branches within the orbit. Both conditions are hyperintense, both are well defined, and both enhance. It was shown that on dynamic scanning, hemangiomas begin with a central spot or point of enhancement, which spreads peripherally, whereas orbital schwannomas usually enhance initially on the periphery. Both may remodel bone.

Other masses that can occur in the orbit include leiomyomas, meningiomas, dermoids, pseudotumors, and lacrimal fossa masses.

Orbital hemangiomas show avid contrast enhancement. Occasionally, one may see calcifications within the lesion because it truly represents a venous vascular malformation, and there may be phleboliths.

Notes

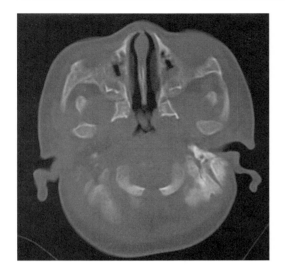
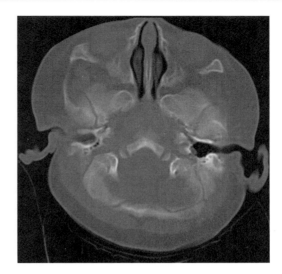
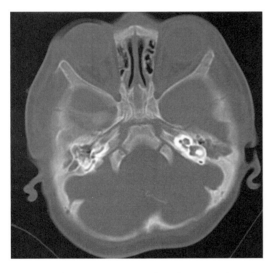
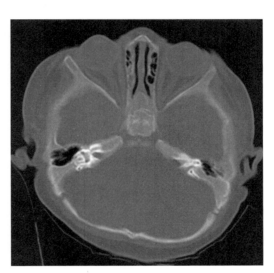

1. Which sinuses are the first to develop?

2. Which sinus is the last to develop fully?

3. At what age do the sinuses stop growing?

4. What is the hiatus semilunaris?

CASE 19

Sinus Development

1. Ethmoid and maxillary.

2. Frontal.

3. After puberty.

4. The air space above the uncinate process, connecting the infundibulum to the middle meatus.

Reference

Pohunek P: Development, structure and function of the upper airways, *Paediatr Respir Rev* 5:2–8, 2004.

Cross-Reference

Neuroradiology: THE REQUISITES, pp 611–614.

Comment

The paranasal sinuses develop from deepening of the nasal pits, separated from the oral cavity by the oronasal membrane. The nasal airways and sinuses show an exponential growth in the first 3 years of life, followed by a slower, more linear pattern reflecting the growth of the rest of the body. The maxillary sinuses grow first and influence the whole shape of the face. The frontal and sphenoid sinuses begin to develop around 2 years of age. At birth, most infants have aerated ethmoid and maxillary sinus air cells. There is a second growth spurt at 7 to 12 years of age.

The least bit of crying may result in congestion of the mucosa, which may appear to show opacification of the paranasal sinus; however, this may be a reactive change only. In patients with cystic fibrosis, the frontal sinus development may be arrested, and one should look for the presence of polyps specifically in this age and in this patient group. Chronic sinusitis may ensue.

Functional endoscopic sinus surgery in pediatric patients is common. In individuals who have anatomic variations that predispose them to sinusitis, endoscopic sinus surgery may be of considerable benefit in alleviating the chronic sinusitis.

Notes

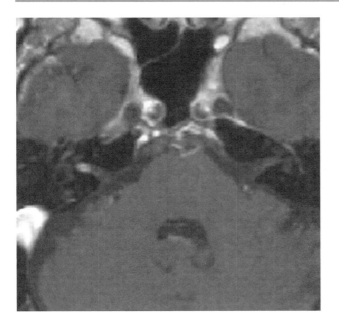 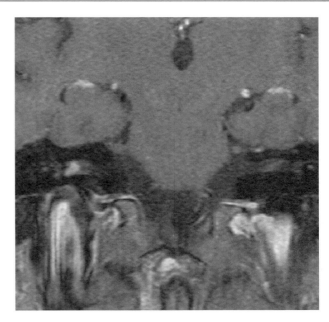

1. What is MISME?

2. What is the differential diagnosis for enhancing intracanalicular masses?

3. Identify the organism for Ramsay Hunt syndrome.

4. Is a schwannoma of the cerebellopontine angle or a meningioma more likely to show cyst formation?

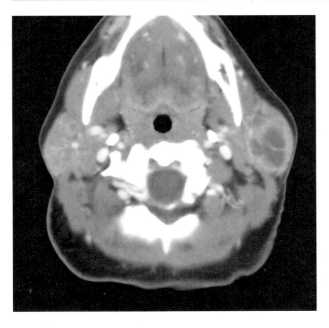 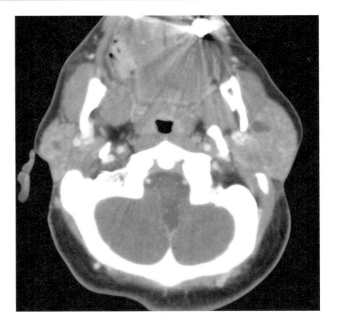

1. What is an ARPC?

2. What separates the superficial and deep portions of the parotid gland?

3. What percentage of HIV-positive individuals develop parotid lesions?

4. Name the three most common neoplasms in the tail of the parotid gland (in decreasing order of frequency).

CASE 20

Intracanalicular Vestibular Schwannoma

1. Multiple inherited schwannomas, meningiomas, and ependymomas; often a term used to describe neurofibromatosis 2.

2. Cranial nerve VIII schwannoma, cranial nerve VII schwannoma, subarachnoid seeding, vascular loop, meningioma, sarcoidosis, Bell palsy, Ramsay Hunt syndrome, polyneuritis.

3. Varicella zoster.

4. Schwannoma.

Reference

Asaoka K, Barrs DM, Sampson JH, et al: Intracanalicular meningioma mimicking vestibular schwannoma, *AJNR Am J Neuroradiol* 23:1493–1496, 2002.

Cross-Reference

Neuroradiology: THE REQUISITES, pp 106–107.

Comment

Approximately 20% of vestibular schwannomas are entirely intracanalicular. Debate continues as to the most common nerve that is affected by the vestibular schwannomas, with some saying it is the inferior vestibular nerve and others saying it is the superior vestibular nerve. Because the tumor is one of vestibular nerves, it should not be characterized as an acoustic schwannoma, as the cochlear nerve is uncommonly affected despite the hearing loss symptoms. High-resolution sagittal T2W scans through the plane of the internal auditory canal may define the origin of the neoplasm. Nonetheless, gadolinium-enhanced MRI remains the gold standard for imaging of these lesions.

Hearing preservation, when one is treating an intracanalicular vestibular schwannoma, is not guaranteed; in a meta-analysis, only 57% of cases showed functional hearing preservation. Facial nerve function is preserved in more than 95% of intracanalicular schwannomas.

Facial nerve symptoms are more common with intracanalicular meningiomas than schwannomas. Calcification, involvement of the adjacent bone, and a dural tail are telltale signs of meningiomas. Although most schwannomas displace the facial nerve superiorly and medially, most meningiomas of the internal auditory canal infiltrate and encase the facial nerve, leading to a worse postoperative facial nerve function rate.

Notes

CASE 21

HIV-Related Cyst

1. AIDS-related parotid cyst.

2. The facial nerve.

3. 5%.

4. Pleomorphic adenoma, Warthin tumor, lymphoma.

Reference

Hamilton BE, Salzman KL, Wiggins RH 3rd, Harnsberger HR: Earring lesions of the parotid tail, *AJNR Am J Neuroradiol* 24:1757–1764, 2003.

Cross-Reference

Neuroradiology: THE REQUISITES, pp 704–705.

Comment

Intraparotid cysts associated with HIV infection may be multiple and may be associated with solid nodules. These are usually lymphoepithelial. The question remains how these lymphoepithelial cysts develop. In most cases, they are believed to represent cystic change within lymph nodes or lymphoid aggregates rather than simple cysts. When the cysts are aspirated, they show HIV particles within them. The cysts may cause discomfort. Doxycycline sclerotherapy is often recommended. Patients who are HIV-positive also have a predilection for lymphoma development in the parotid glands. They also may have granulomatous infections that may involve the parotid gland, such as tuberculosis or fungal infections, including candidiasis. Rarely one may see Kaposi sarcoma of the skin grow into the adjacent parotid gland from the ear region.

Associated with HIV-related cyst and nodules in the parotid glands one may find posterior triangle lymphadenopathy and adenoidal hypertrophy, which also are indicative of HIV infection.

Notes

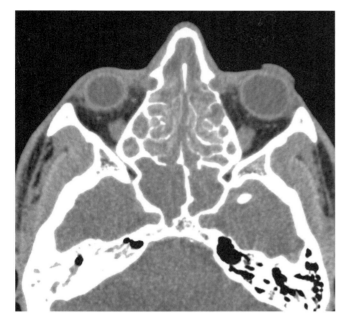 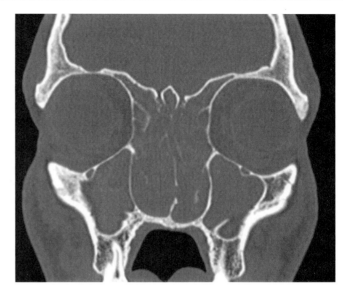

1. Name the most common causes of complete sinus opacification.

2. What is Kartagener syndrome?

3. What are some associations with sinonasal polyposis?

4. What is the sine qua non of polyposis on CT?

CASE 22

Sinonasal Polyposis

1. Bacterial sinusitis, fungal sinusitis, polyposis, and mucoceles.

2. Situs inversus, chronic sinusitis (often with polyps), and bronchiectasis.

3. Cystic fibrosis, allergic rhinitis, aspirin intolerance, asthma, and nickel exposure.

4. Enlargement of ostia and sinonasal passages.

Reference

Kaplan BA, Kountakis SE: Diagnosis and pathology of unilateral maxillary sinus opacification with or without evidence of contralateral disease, *Laryngoscope* 114:981–985, 2004.

Cross-Reference

Neuroradiology: THE REQUISITES, pp 629–631.

Comment

Sinonasal polyposis can occur in a variety of settings. In some cases, the polyps arise in a healthy individual with no predisposition to polyps. There may be a history of atopy, however, which might include dust, mites, and seasonal allergies.

Polyps occur in 36% of patients with aspirin intolerance and 7% of patients with asthma. The polyps are often multiple and bilateral. Of patients with widespread sinonasal polyposis, 4% to 20% have aspirin intolerance. Recurrences of polyps that have been removed are increased in individuals with aspirin intolerance.

Children with cystic fibrosis also have a predilection for chronic sinusitis and sinonasal polyposis. These individuals have abnormal sweat gland tests and present in their youth with recurrent sinusitis. Their frontal sinus development is decreased, but the remainder of their sinonasal cavity often is expanded because of the extensive polyposis. This is a genetic disorder, which is involved with the ciliary motility that leads to inadequate mucociliary clearance. Cystic fibrosis is the most common lethal hereditary condition in white Americans; the gene is characterized as the *cystic fibrosis transmembrane conductance regulator (CFTR)*. The gene's prevalence is approximately 1:3500 Americans. Death usually results from the pulmonary complications caused by the inability to clear mucus (just as in the sinuses), with a median age of death at 30 years. Genetic therapy shows promise.

Notes

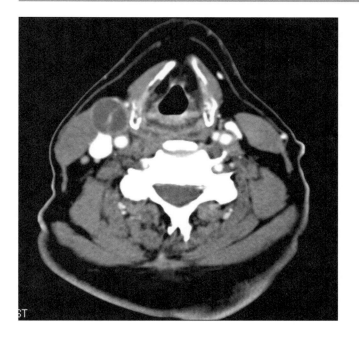
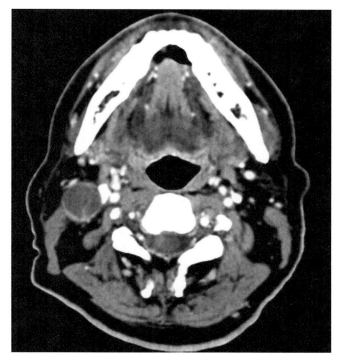

1. What are common primary sources for cystic nodal metastases?

2. What is the differential diagnosis?

3. How often is the nodal disease the source of the patient's presentation to the clinician's office as opposed to the aerodigestive mucosa primary tumor?

4. What is the staging of nodal disease in squamous cell carcinoma of the tonsil?

Cystic Nodes

1. Tonsil and thyroid gland.

2. Branchial cleft cysts, lymphangioma, abscess, and cystic nodal metastases.

3. 40%.

4. Staging is as follows:

NX—regional nodes cannot be assessed

N0—no regional node metastases

N1—metastasis in a single ipsilateral lymph node, ≤3 cm in greatest dimension

N2—metastasis in a single ipsilateral lymph node, >3 cm but ≤6 cm in greatest dimension; or in multiple ipsilateral lymph nodes, all ≤6 cm in greatest dimension; or in bilateral or contralateral lymph nodes, all ≤6 cm in greatest dimension

    N2a—metastasis in single ipsilateral lymph node >3 cm but ≤6 cm in greatest dimension

    N2b—metastasis in multiple ipsilateral lymph nodes >6 cm in greatest dimension

    N2c—metastasis in bilateral or contralateral lymph nodes, all ≤6 cm in greatest dimension

N3—metastasis in a lymph node >6 cm in greatest dimension

Reference

Greene FL, Page DL, Fleming ID (eds): *AJCC Cancer Staging Manual,* 6th ed. New York, Springer-Verlag, 2002.

Cross-Reference

Neuroradiology: THE REQUISITES, pp 681–690.

Comment

The lymph nodes from tonsil carcinoma are unique in that they may be cystic in appearance without showing early extracapsular spread. They may be quite large, bilateral, and multiple. The first echelon of nodal spread of tonsil carcinoma is to level II high jugular chain, then level III midjugular chain. As part of the oropharynx, tonsil carcinoma has a high rate of nodal spread (see below).

Primary Site	Nodes at Presentation
Nasopharynx	72–85%
Oropharynx	68–76%
Hypopharynx	59–65%
Supraglottis	55–80%
Oral Cavity	3–36%
Sinonasal	10–17%
Glottis	3–7%

Understanding nodes requires understanding the nomenclature of the location of nodes:

I—Contains the submental (Ia) and submandibular (Ib) triangles bounded by the anterior and posterior bellies of the digastric muscle, the hyoid bone inferiorly, and the body of the mandible superiorly.

II—Contains the upper jugular lymph nodes and extends from the level of the skull base superiorly to the hyoid bone inferiorly. IIa and IIb are split anteroposteriorly by their relationship to the spinal accessory nerve (sternocleidomastoid margin on imaging).

III—Contains the middle jugular lymph nodes from the hyoid bone superiorly to the level of the lower border of the cricoid cartilage inferiorly. IIIa and IIIb are split anteroposteriorly by their relationship to the spinal accessory nerve (sternocleidomastoid margin on imaging).

IV—Contains the lower jugular lymph nodes from the level of the cricoid cartilage superiorly to the clavicle inferiorly. IVa and IVb are split anteroposteriorly by their relationship to the sternoclavicular head of the sternocleidomastoid muscle.

V—Contains the lymph nodes in the posterior triangle bounded by the anterior border of the trapezius muscle posteriorly and the posterior border of the sternocleidomastoid anteriorly. Va are the nodes along the spinal accessory chain in upper V. Vb refers to more inferior nodes that run along the transverse cervical artery. Anatomically the differentiation is the omohyoid muscle inferior belly.

VI—Contains the nodes of central compartment from the hyoid bone to the suprasternal notch. The lateral boundary is the carotid sheath.

VII—Contains the lymph nodes inferior to the suprasternal notch in the superior mediastinum.

Notes

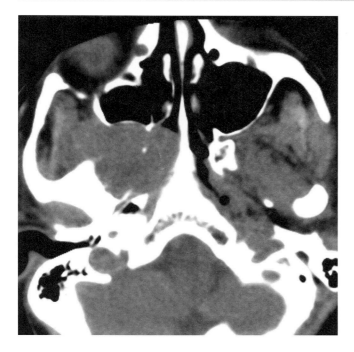 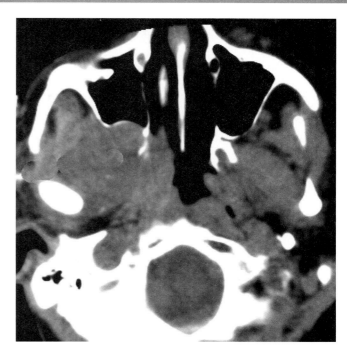

1. What is the sinus of Morgagni?

2. Name the three histologic varieties of nasopharyngeal carcinoma.

3. What percentage of American cases of nasopharyngeal carcinoma are keratinizing?

4. What is in the differential diagnosis of nasopharyngeal masses?

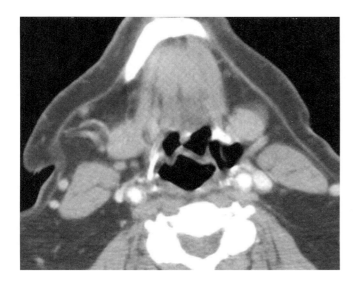 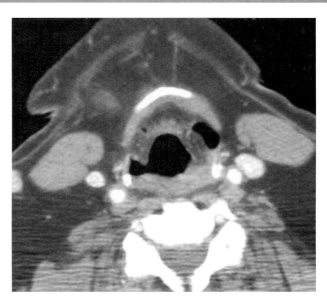

1. How often is this abnormality associated with laryngeal carcinoma?

2. How often is it bilateral?

3. What is pus in the saccule of the laryngeal ventricle called?

4. What percentage of laryngoceles are "mixed"?

C A S E 2 4

Nasopharyngeal Lymphoma

1. A natural dehiscence in the pharyngobasilar fascia that transmits the eustachian tube on the one hand and, unfortunately, nasopharyngeal carcinoma on the other hand.

2. Keratinizing squamous cell carcinoma, nonkeratinizing carcinoma, and undifferentiated carcinoma.

3. 75% in Americans, especially in whites. The other types are more common in Asians.

4. Lymphoma, rhabdomyosarcoma, juvenile angiofibroma, and minor salivary gland tumors.

Reference

Greene FL, Page DL, Fleming ID (eds): *AJCC Cancer Staging Manual,* 6th ed. New York, Springer-Verlag, 2002.

Cross-Reference

Neuroradiology: THE REQUISITES, pp 645–651.

Comment

Nasopharyngeal carcinoma is separated into three histologic subtypes: keratinizing squamous cell carcinoma, nonkeratinizing carcinoma (also known as transitional cell carcinoma/lymphoepithelioma/Rigaud), and undifferentiated carcinoma (also known as anaplastic carcinoma). Undifferentiated nasopharyngeal carcinoma is strongly associated with Epstein-Barr virus exposure and Chinese nationality.

The T staging and nodal staging of nasopharyngeal carcinoma is unique:

T staging:

T1—tumor confined to the nasopharynx
T2—tumor extends to soft tissue
   T2a—tumor extends to the oropharynx or nasal cavity or both without parapharyngeal extension
   T2b—with parapharyngeal extension
T3—tumor involves bony structures or paranasal sinuses or both
T4—tumors with intracranial extension or involvement of cranial nerves, infratemporal fossa, hypopharynx, orbit, or masticator space or both

N staging:

N0—no regional lymph node metastasis
N1—unilateral metastasis in lymph nodes, ≤6 cm in greatest dimension, above the supraclavicular fossa
N2—bilateral nodes ≤6 cm above supraclavicular fossa
N3—metastasis in lymph nodes >6 cm or to supraclavicular fossa or both
N3a—>6 cm in dimension
N3b—extension to the supraclavicular fossa

Notes

C A S E 2 5

Laryngocele

1. Approximately 5% to 10%.

2. Approximately 20%.

3. Pyolaryngocele or laryngopyocele.

4. Approximately 45%.

Reference

Alvi A, Weissman J, Myssiorek D, et al: Computed tomographic and magnetic resonance imaging characteristics of laryngocele and its variants, *Am J Otolaryngol* 19:251–256, 1998.

Cross-Reference

Neuroradiology: THE REQUISITES, pp 670–671.

Comment

Laryngoceles represent dilations of the saccule of the laryngeal ventricle. The dilated area may be filled with air, fluid, or purulent material. When filled with fluid, it is often termed a *saccular cyst,* whereas when filled with purulent material, it is often called a *pyolaryngocele.*

Although laryngoceles may occur on a physiologic basis in individuals with increased intralaryngeal pressure (e.g., trumpet players, glass blowers, wind instrument players), they also may occur due to an obstructing lesion at the origin of the saccule. This may result from inflammatory disease with a stricture, or it could be secondary to neoplasm. The reported incidence of carcinoma causing laryngoceles varies; in some series, it is 15%.

Classically, laryngoceles are separated into those that remain medial to the thyrohyoid membrane (internal laryngoceles), those that are external to the thyrohyoid membrane (external laryngoceles), and those that expand the internal and the external compartment (mixed laryngoceles).

Notes

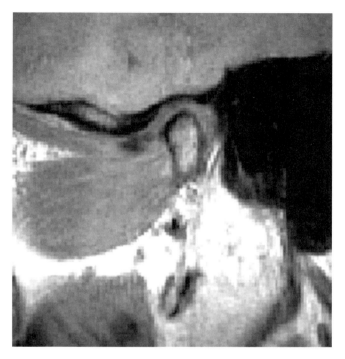
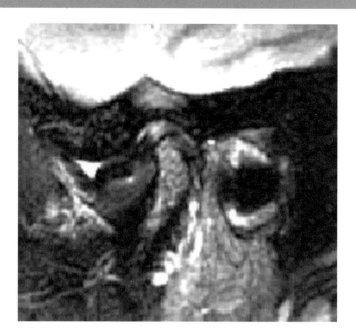

1. How many compartments are there to the temporomandibular joint (TMJ) bursa?
2. Explain the significance of TMJ effusions.
3. What are the demographics of TMJ pain syndrome?
4. Explain the significance of bilaminar zone high signal on T2W scans.

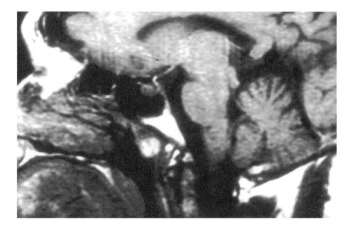

1. List all the names for this entity.
2. What is its significance?
3. What are the treatment options?
4. Why is this entity bright on T1W scans?

Temporomandibular Joint Effusion and Bilaminar Zone Inflammation

1. Two, but they are divided into four separate spaces.

2. They are highly correlated with pain.

3. >10:1 female-to-male ratio, and most are 20 to 45 years old.

4. Also highly associated with pain.

Reference

Yano K, Sano T, Okano T: A longitudinal study of magnetic resonance (MR) evidence of temporomandibular joint (TMJ) fluid in patients with TMJ disorders, *Cranio* 22:64–71, 2004.

Cross-Reference

Neuroradiology: THE REQUISITES, pp 714–718.

Comment

Several MRI findings may be associated with TMJ pain. Effusions, bilaminar zone high signal intensity, synovial proliferation, and mandibular condyle bone marrow edema have a better correlation with pain than mere anterior displacement of the meniscus of the TMJ. Some inflammatory arthropathies also should be considered when one has large joint effusions, including collagen vascular diseases and septic arthritis.

The likelihood of having a meniscus recapture is decreased when one has a large joint effusion. The likelihood of anterior meniscus displacement approaches 100% when one has synovial proliferation. Synovial inflammation is best seen on a gadolinium-enhanced study of the TMJ.

Notes

Tornwaldt Cyst

1. Tornwaldt cyst, Thornwaldt cyst, pharyngeal bursa cyst, nasopharyngeal bursa.

2. In most cases none.

3. Excision or marsupialization.

4. Presumably because of high protein content in the cyst.

Reference

Ikushima I, Korogi Y, Makita O, et al: MR imaging of Tornwaldt's cysts, *AJR Am J Roentgenol* 172: 1663–1665, 1999.

Cross-Reference

Neuroradiology: THE REQUISITES, pp 642–644.

Comment

Next to the mucus retention cyst, Tornwaldt cyst is the most common cyst identified in the head and neck. It is a cyst that resides in the midline of the nasopharynx and is thought to occur as a result of the retraction of the mucosa of the nasopharynx as the notochord ascends into the vertebral column. The mucosa leaves appose each other, and encysted fluid may be present. The curious finding in these cysts is that they often are bright on T1W scan; this is believed to be due to high protein concentration, which accounts for the occasional finding of dark signal intensity on T2W scan. Nonetheless most cysts are bright on T2W scans and T1W scans.

The nasopharyngeal Tornwaldt cyst has little clinical importance. Rarely it may be a source for persistent halitosis.

The differential diagnosis includes a nasopharyngeal cystic craniopharyngioma; however, these lesions should have more solid components and focal contrast enhancement. Mucus retention cysts occur in the nasopharynx and may simulate Tornwaldt cysts, but they are usually off midline along the course of the eustachian tube and are less likely to be bright on T1W scans.

Notes

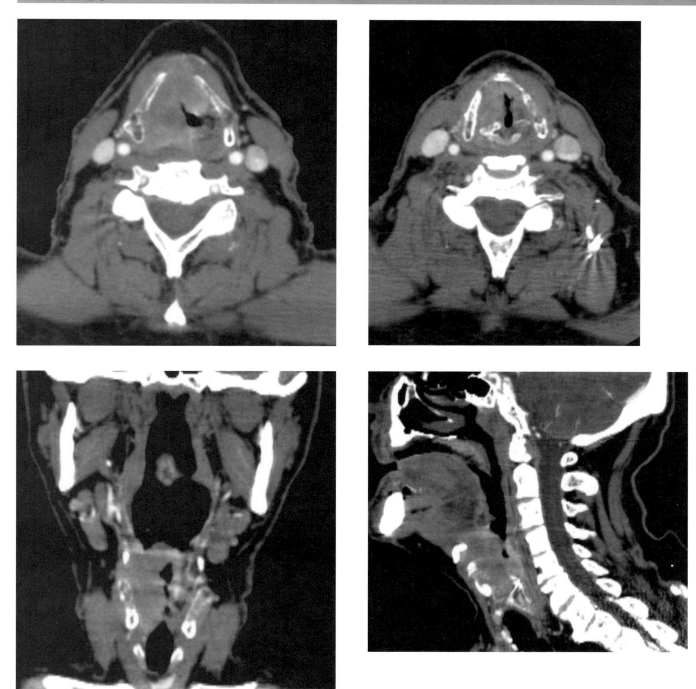

1. What is the main structure of the suprahyoid supraglottis?

2. Name at least three contraindications to supraglottic laryngectomy.

3. Are lymph nodes more common with glottic or supraglottic carcinomas?

4. What is this patient's chance of having a second primary tumor?

Supraglottic Carcinoma

1. The epiglottis.

2. Invasion of the thyroid or cricoid cartilage, fixation of the arytenoids, interarytenoid involvement, impaired vocal cord mobility, piriform sinus involvement, and base of tongue involvement.

3. Supraglottic by far.

4. 15%.

Reference

Yousem DM, Tufano RP: Laryngeal imaging, *Magn Reson Imaging Clin N Am* 10:451–465, 2002.

Cross-Reference

Neuroradiology: THE REQUISITES, pp 672–676.

Comment

The prognosis of supraglottic laryngeal carcinoma correlates well with tumor volume. If a supraglottic carcinoma is <6 mL in volume, radiation therapy locally controls disease in 89% of cases. If the tumor is >6 mL, the local control rate decreases to 52%. Factors that determine local control rate for glottic carcinoma are based less on volume and relate more to submucosal preepiglottic and paraglottic involvement and cartilaginous invasion. Nonetheless it seems that glottic lesions >3 mL in size do worse with radiation therapy.

In patients in whom surgical treatment of laryngeal carcinoma is contemplated, some critical issues include (1) the extent of the tumor across midline (precludes vertical hemilaryngectomy), (2) the presence of and degree of bulky preepiglottic fat or hyoid invasion (precludes supracricoid laryngectomy and supraglottic laryngectomy), (3) transglottic or paraglottic spread (precludes horizontal supraglottic laryngectomy), (4) interarytenoid or bilateral arytenoid invasion (precludes any supracricoid laryngectomy), (5) subglottic carcinomatous extension (precludes all laryngeal conservation surgeries), and (6) cricoid cartilage invasion (precludes all laryngeal conservation surgeries).

Notes

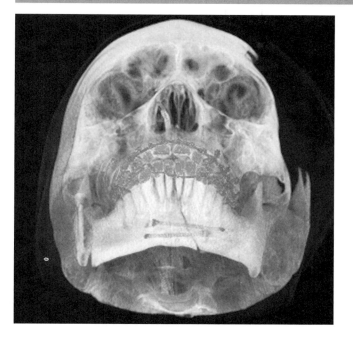 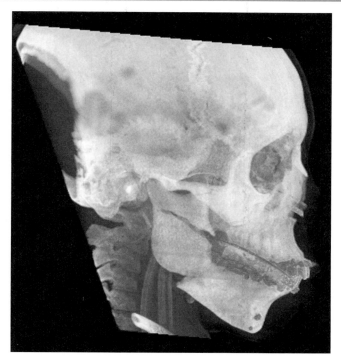

1. Name the two most common sites for mandibular fractures?

2. Which bones are most commonly grafted for mandibular reconstructions?

3. Name the two main neural canals in the mandible.

4. Why are three-dimensional reconstructions useful in facial trauma?

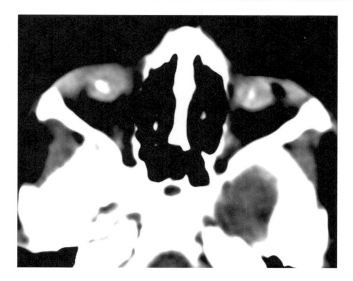

1. What is the most common entity associated with a small, calcified globe?

2. What is the most common pediatric entity associated with a normal-sized calcified globe?

3. What is the most common calcification in an adult with a normal-sized globe?

4. What is the most common cause of a large calcified globe?

Three-Dimensional Reconstruction of Mandibular Fracture

1. Body (symphyseal) and condyle (subcondylar).

2. Fibula and iliac crest.

3. Inferior alveolar canal and mental foramen.

4. To show extent of disease, degree of displacement, to provide a model for prostheses, to plan grafts, to compare with postoperative appearance, and to assess involvement of neural canals.

Reference

Tello R, Suojanen J, Costello P, McGinnes A: Comparison of spiral CT and conventional CT in 3D visualization of facial trauma: work in progress, *Comput Med Imaging Graph* 18:423–427, 1994.

Cross-Reference

Neuroradiology: THE REQUISITES, pp 268–269.

Comment

What is the value of creating three-dimensional images for clinicians? In addition to more graphically displaying the extent of injuries and the displacement of bone fragments, three-dimensional images and three-dimensional data sets are used to fashion reconstructive devices for various parts of the anatomy. Temporomandibular joint prostheses may be fashioned in a manner that takes into account the normal variation of anatomy of an individual. A three-dimensional representation of the skull before surgery for craniosynostosis may provide before and after pictures that one can assess for improvement in cosmesis, the need for further reconstruction, and the effectiveness in a developing technique. When one is performing orbital reconstructive surgery, the extent of deformation of the walls and the need to elevate orbital floor fractures are well visualized in this fashion. In patients who require mandibular advancement, the extent of the maldevelopment is best seen when one has three-dimensional images, particularly if there is any evidence of asymmetry from right to left.

Notes

Phthisis Bulbi

1. Phthisis bulbi.

2. Retinoblastoma.

3. Optic nerve head drusen.

4. Axial myopia with a drusen or chronic retinal-uveal detachment.

Reference

Osborne DR, Foulks GN: Computed tomographic analysis of deformity and dimensional changes in the eyeball, *Radiology* 153:669–674, 1984.

Cross-Reference

Neuroradiology: THE REQUISITES, p 490.

Comment

Phthisis bulbi is the end stage of any long-standing injury to the globe that results in what one sees on CT as a calcified, small, irregularly shaped globe. In most instances in young patients, the etiology is orbital trauma. The patient may have had globe rupture with extensive hemorrhage that could not be reinflated or simply severe perforation with nonfunctioning retinal tissue. Bilateral phthisis bulbi may be the result of retinopathy of prematurity with small, calcified globes or retinopathy of diabetes mellitus with extensive recurrent retinal detachment or choroidal detachment and ischemic retinopathy. Radiation damage to the globes also may create bilateral phthisis bulbi. Bilateral involvement with a TORCH (Toxoplasmosis, Other [congenital syphilis and viruses], Rubella, Cytomegalovirus, and Herpes simplex virus) infection while in the uterus can result in bilateral phthisis bulbi.

Effectively the globe is nonfunctioning, and the individual is blind in that eye.

Notes

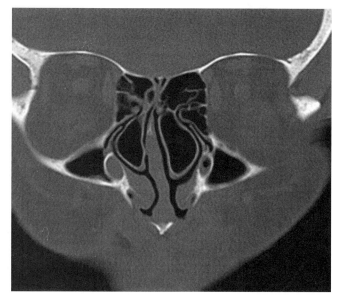

1. Identify the anatomic variation shown on the scan.
2. What is the drainage of this variation?
3. What is the incidence of an agger nasi cell?
4. What is the incidence of a Haller cell?

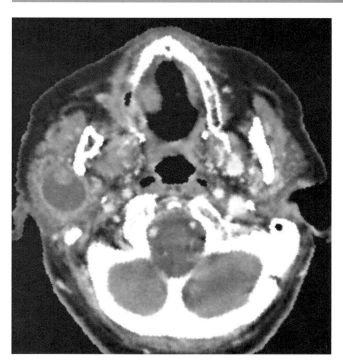

1. Name four potential etiologies of parotid cysts.
2. What parotid cyst is associated with AIDS?
3. What other disease entity is associated with the same type of cyst?
4. Name the two most common cystic neoplasms of the parotid gland.

Concha Bullosa

1. Concha bullosa.

2. Usually to anterior ethmoid air cells.

3. 50%.

4. 15% to 20%.

Reference

Kantarci M, Karasen RM, Alper F, et al: Remarkable anatomic variations in paranasal sinus region and their clinical importance, *Eur J Radiol* 50:296–302, 2004.

Cross-Reference

Neuroradiology: THE REQUISITES, pp 611–614.

Comment

A concha bullosa is a normal variation that occurs in the paranasal sinuses in which the middle turbinate is aerated. The middle turbinate may have two attachments to it—one that is attached to the cribriform plate superiorly and one that is attached to the basal or ground lamella, which is the medial orbital wall–lamina papyracea. If just the vertical attachment of the turbinate is aerated, it is frequently termed a *lamellar cell.* When the turbinate and the vertical attachment are aerated, it is truly called a *concha bullosa.* The significance of the concha bullosa is that, when large, it may obstruct the infundibulum or middle meatus of the ostiomeatal complex, leading to a predisposition to sinusitis. When two mucosal surfaces to the paranasal sinuses are apposed, this leads to stasis of the flow of secretions resulting from the ineffectiveness of the mucociliary clearance. The theory behind functional endoscopic sinus surgery is to maintain the patency of all these narrow airways of drainage so that the large paranasal sinuses may have free clearance of the mucus secretions.

Sinusitis may affect the concha bullosa, and one might see opacification of the middle turbinate air cell. Usually these drain via the anterior ethmoid air cell complex into the middle meatus. Rarely one also may see a mucocele of the concha bullosa.

Agger nasi cells represent anterior ethmoid air cells that are located anterior, lateral, and inferior to frontal recess. Haller cells are infraorbital ethmoidal cells that develop into the floor of the orbit (i.e., the roof of maxillary sinus) adjacent to and above the maxillary sinus ostium. Uncinate aeration occurs in 2% to 5% of cases. Inferior turbinate aeration is present in <1% of cases.

Notes

Parotid Cyst

1. Mucus retention cysts, first branchial cleft cysts, sialocele, and lymphoepithelial cyst.

2. Lymphoepithelial cyst.

3. Sjögren syndrome.

4. Pleomorphic adenoma and Warthin tumors.

Reference

Som PM, Brandwein MS, Silvers A: Nodal inclusion cysts of the parotid gland and parapharyngeal space: a discussion of lymphoepithelial, AIDS-related parotid, and branchial cysts, cystic Warthin's tumors, and cysts in Sjogren's syndrome, *Laryngoscope* 105:1122–1128, 1995.

Cross-Reference

Neuroradiology: THE REQUISITES, pp 700–705, 746.

Comment

Cysts in the parotid gland may arise from a variety of causes. Although benign lymphoepithelial lesions (BLELs) are the most common cysts attributed to HIV positivity, a few caveats are in order: (1) A patient need not have full-blown AIDS but may be HIV positive only and have BLELs. (2) Lymphoepithelial nodules and aggregates may be present in addition to cysts with HIV positivity. (3) BLELs also are seen with Mikulicz and Sjögren syndrome. Clinically the patient's glands are enlarged, swollen, and mildly painful. BLELs should never cause cranial nerve VII palsies. When BLELs are solid, one should consider in the differential diagnosis Sjögren syndrome, sarcoidosis, mononucleosis, mastocytosis, lymphoma, and Rosai-Dorfman disease. Five percent of HIV-positive individuals have parotid BLELs.

Treatment of HIV-related BLELs includes antiviral agents, doxycycline sclerotherapy, and rarely surgery.

First branchial cleft cysts arise just outside or within the parotid gland.

Notes

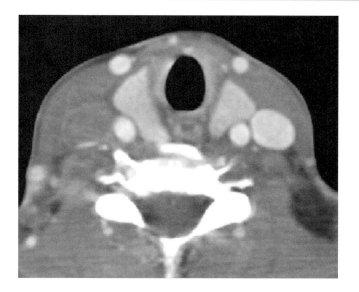

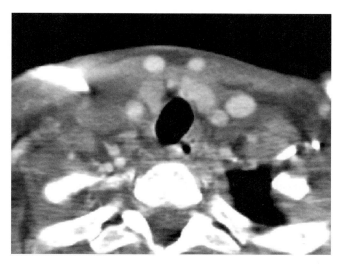

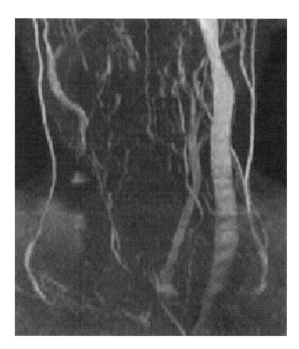

1. What is the cause of this patient's palpable mass in the supraclavicular fossa?

2. Name the most common cause of internal jugular vein thrombosis.

3. What stage of hemorrhage is rarely seen in thrombosed vessels but is common in intraparenchymal hematomas?

4. What is Trousseau's syndrome?

Jugular Venous Thrombosis

1. Jugular vein thrombosis on the right side.

2. Indwelling catheter.

3. Hemosiderin.

4. Large vein thrombosis associated with visceral cancers, usually pancreatic, and histologically usually adenocarcinoma.

Reference

Nguyen-Dinh KV, Marsot-Dupuch K, Portier F, et al: Lemierre syndrome: usefulness of CT in detection of extensive occult thrombophlebitis, *J Neuroradiol* 29: 132–135, 2002.

Cross-Reference

Neuroradiology: THE REQUISITES, p 725.

Comment

Jugular venous thrombosis most often occurs in the setting of an indwelling catheter or hypercoagulable state. There may be an inflammatory component that is associated with the thrombosis, in which case one should use the term *thrombophlebitis.* This condition may cause an adjacent cellulitis or myositis. As opposed to intracranial, intraparenchymal hematomas, the evolution of hemorrhagic blood products within the lumen of a blood vessel has different characteristics. It is rare to see a hemosiderin deposition within a blood vessel. The time of the evolution of clot from deoxyhemoglobin to methemoglobin also is more variable than the traditional 3 to 5 days described for intraparenchymal hematomas. The subacute hematoma also persists for a longer time. The evolution of deoxyhemoglobin to methemoglobin is said to occur from the periphery and move centrally when one is dealing with an intraparenchymal hematoma; however, it seems to move centrally to peripherally when one is dealing with an intraluminal clot.

One medication that seems to have a predilection for causing venous thrombosis is asparaginase, which is sometimes used in acute leukemia patients. Asparaginase destabilizes the antithrombin, plasminogen, and fibrinogen cascades and causes a significant thrombosis somewhere in the body in 1% to 2% of patients undergoing induction therapy. The mechanism may be through vitamin K effects.

Trousseau syndrome, also known as migratory thrombophlebitis, occurs in about 10% of patients with pancreatic adenocarcinoma. This syndrome is treatable with heparin therapy because it seems to be due to an acceleration of platelet-aggregating factors and procoagulants. Lemierre syndrome represents an anaerobic oropharyngeal infection leading to septic thrombophlebitis of the internal jugular vein.

Notes

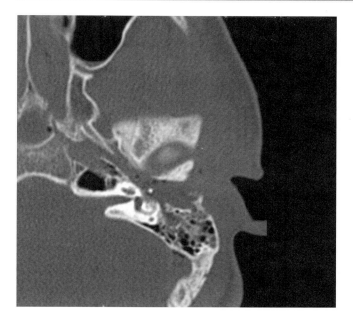 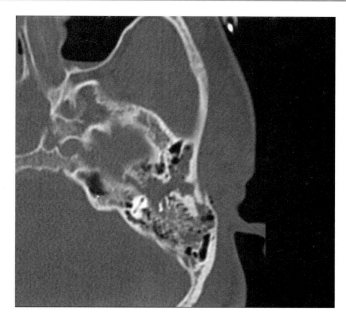

1. Which type of fracture, longitudinal or transverse, is more common?

2. Which fracture type has a higher rate of facial nerve injury?

3. Which fracture type has a higher rate of labyrinthine injury?

4. Which fracture type has a higher rate of ossicular injury?

Temporal Bone Fracture

1. Longitudinal.

2. Transverse.

3. Transverse.

4. Longitudinal.

Reference

Ozturan O, Bauer CA, Miller CC 3rd, Jenkins HA: Dimensions of the sinus tympani and its surgical access via a retrofacial approach, *Ann Otol Rhinol Laryngol* 105:776–783, 1996.

Cross-Reference

Neuroradiology: THE REQUISITES, pp 565–607.

Comment

Numerous complications may occur as a result of temporal bone fracture. Each of these complications should be considered by the radiologist interpreting the temporal bone CT scan to define the presence of these abnormalities. Temporal bone fractures may cause ossicular disruption or dislocation or both, which may affect the joint between the malleus and the incus and the incus and the stapes. The incus is the most vulnerable ossicle as a result of its tenuous ligamentous attachments. Incudostapedial dislocation is the most common type of posttraumatic ossicular disruption, followed by *combined* incudomalleolar and incudo-stapedial disruptions. Dislocation of the ossicles can lead to conductive sensory hearing loss. This hearing loss may be difficult to differentiate from the conduction loss associated with the hemotympanum and mastoid/middle ear fluid, which occurs in association with these fractures as well.

Facial nerve paralysis may occur secondary to temporal bone fracture resulting from either transection of the nerve or, more commonly, contusion injuries to the nerve. The labyrinthine and tympanic course of the facial nerve should be observed carefully for the presence of fracture lines extending across this plane.

CSF leak can occur after temporal bone fractures. This leak results in persistent meningitis and possibly even seizure. One should look for fluid in the tegmen tympani mastoid air cells or fracture extension to the roof of the temporal bone. Occasionally MRI may be useful in determining whether or not an encephalocele, which contains brain tissue, is herniating through the fracture site.

Perilymphatic fistula also can be a complication of a temporal bone fracture. In this case, there is communication between the middle ear cavity and the labyrinthine structures most commonly associated with a fracture extending to the vestibule or lateral semicircular canal. This situation can result in chronic labyrinthitis and dizziness and even labyrinthitis ossificans. Secondary meningitis also may occur with temporal bone fractures in which hemorrhage and CSF accumulate in the labyrinth structures; this is another possible etiology for labyrinthine ossification.

Rarely pseudoaneurysms of the carotid arteries can occur with temporal bone fractures.

The hypotympanum consists of the sinus tympani, the facial nerve recess, and the intervening pyramidal eminence. The hypotympanum is a blind area for the otoscopist and an area where residual disease after cholesteatoma surgery often resides. The subiculum connects the sinus tympani to the round window and the ponticulus connects the sinus tympani to the oval window. The sinus tympani lies between the ponticulus and the subiculum, which block it from view.

Notes

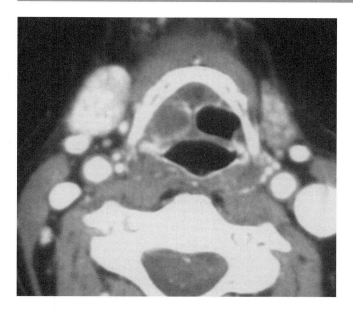

1. Where is this lesion located?

2. What is the most common cyst in this location?

3. Where is the highest proliferation of minor salivary glands in the head and neck?

4. What are typical symptoms for this lesion?

Vallecular Cyst

1. The right vallecula.

2. Mucus retention cyst.

3. The palate.

4. Asymptomatic usually; may have obstruction, dysphagia or voice changes.

Reference

Cuillier F, Samperiz S, Testud R, Fossati P: Antenatal diagnosis and management of a vallecular cyst, *Ultrasound Obstet Gynecol* 20:623–626, 2002.

Cross-Reference

Neuroradiology: THE REQUISITES, pp 669–670.

Comment

Most vallecular cysts present clinically in infants, with upper airway obstructive symptoms (including apnea and failure to thrive) predominating. The differential diagnosis includes cystic pleomorphic adenomas (because this is a lesion of minor salivary glands), thyroglossal duct cysts, dermoids, teratomas, and lymphatic vascular malformations. Laryngomalacia may coexist, and death resulting from asphyxia from this combination has been reported.

The cysts look like any mucus retention cyst: low density on CT, bright on T2W MRI, and enhancing only peripherally.

Treatment is via marsupialization or CO_2 laser.

Notes

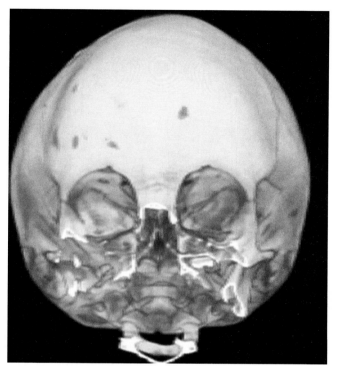 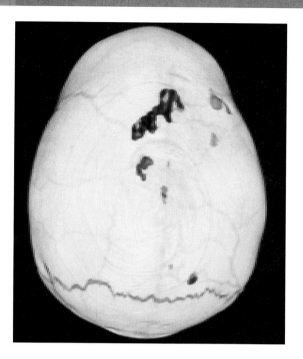

1. What is the most common suture to fuse inappropriately?
2. What is the most frequent cause of infantile head shape deformity?
3. What sutural closure can cause the "harlequin eye"?
4. Are males or females more frequently affected by craniosynostosis?

Sagittal Suture Craniostenosis

1. Sagittal suture.

2. Sleeping on one side all the time.

3. Unilateral coronal suture closure.

4. Males.

Reference

Robin NH: Molecular genetic advances in understanding craniosynostosis, *Plast Reconstr Surg* 103:1060–1070, 1999.

Cross-Reference

Neuroradiology: THE REQUISITES, pp 438–440.

Comment

The sagittal suture is the most common suture to close prematurely in children. This premature closure results in scaphocephaly or dolichocephaly. It occurs in about 1:4200 births.

Trigonocephaly is the term used for metopic suture premature closure. The appearance is that of a ridge down the middle of the forehead like a type of dinosaur.

The harlequin or winking eye is seen with unilateral coronal suture closure. When bilateral, this suture closure results in a foreshortened head in an antero-posterior dimension called *brachycephaly.* Lambdoid sutural closure causes plagiocephaly.

Syndromes associated with craniosynostosis usually lead to multiple sutural closures, not only one. Common syndromes include the following:

Apert syndrome: craniosynostosis, midfacial hypo-plasia, syndactyly; autosomal dominant mode of transmission

Crouzon syndrome: maxillary hypoplasia, shallow orbits and ocular proptosis, deformed forehead; autosomal dominant mode of transmission, but 50% represent sporadic mutations, whereas 40% are familial

Pfeiffer disease: acrocephaly, broad thumbs and great toes, syndactyly of the hands; autosomal dominant mode of transmission

Saethre-Chotzen syndrome: acrocephaly, hyper-telorism, nasal septal deviation, lid ptosis, mild syn-dactyly of the hands and feet; variable expression

The diagnosis of craniosynostosis syndromes is based on clinical findings; however, DNA-based testing of the *FGFR1* (fibroblast growth factor receptor), *FGFR2,* and *FGFR3* genes may be diagnostic (see table).

Disease Name	Gene	Mutation Detection Rate
Pfeiffer syndrome (all types)	FGFR1	67%
Apert syndrome		>98%
Beare-Stevenson syndrome		
Crouzon syndrome	FGFR2	>50%
Jackson-Weiss syndrome		
Pfeiffer syndrome (all types)		67%
Crouzon syndrome with acanthosis nigricans	FGFR3	100%
Muenke syndrome		100%

Source: http://www.geneclinics.org/profiles/craniosynostosis/details.html

Notes

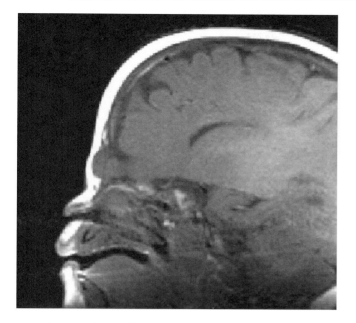

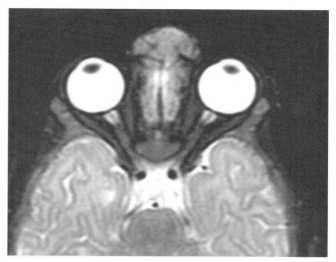

1. What is the difference between an encephalocele and a meningocele?

2. Name the most common associated intracerebral lesion associated with a frontal encephalocele.

3. Identify the most common orbital finding with a frontal encephalocele.

4. What is in the differential diagnosis?

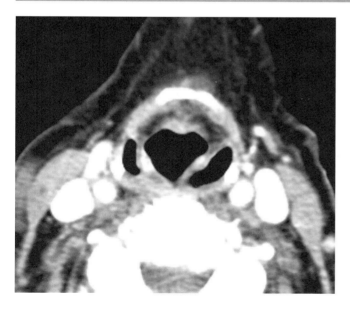

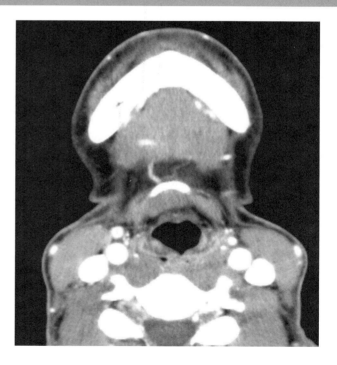

1. What is the differential diagnosis of this lesion?

2. What is the pathognomonic sign of a thyroglossal duct cyst (TGDC)?

3. How often is there functioning tissue in a TGDC?

4. How is the entity different from a lingual thyroid gland?

Frontal Encephalocele

1. The encephalocele has brain tissue in the protruding contents.

2. Agenesis of the corpus callosum.

3. Hypertelorism.

4. Dermoid, nasal glioma, venous vascular malformation, teratoma, rhabdomyosarcoma, and cephalohematoma.

Reference

Willatt JM, Quaghebeur G: Calvarial masses of infants and children: a radiological approach, *Clin Radiol* 59:474–486, 2004.

Cross-Reference

Neuroradiology: THE REQUISITES, pp 418–419, 616–617.

Comment

The nomenclature of cephaloceles separates them into basal and sincipital forms. The sincipital forms are cephaloceles that are visible to the external appearance. These are cephaloceles that protrude from behind the head (as in the Chiari III malformation) at the occipital–cervical spine junction or ones that protrude over the forehead or between the eyes. Occipital and frontonasal encephaloceles are the most common of the sincipital encephaloceles to involve the head and neck.

The basal encephaloceles are not visible to the external appearance. These encephaloceles usually herniate through defects along the sphenoid-ethmoid region and project into the sinonasal cavity or pharynx. Basal cephaloceles occur more commonly in the Southeast Asian population and are diagnosed later in life than sincipital cephaloceles.

Meckel-Gruber syndrome comprises the triad of occipital encephalocele, polycystic kidneys, and polydactyly. This syndrome has been mapped to a gene on chromosome 17. There may be associated cleft lip, cleft palate, pulmonary hypoplasia, Dandy-Walker syndrome, and genital ambiguity.

Dermoid cysts represent 20% of scalp masses in infants.

Notes

Thyroglossal Duct Cyst

1. Dermoid, abscess, necrotic node, sebaceous cyst, ranula.

2. The TGDC is often embedded in the strap muscles when in an infrahyoid location.

3. <5%.

4. The lingual thyroid gland is functioning tissue and is the only thyroid tissue in the body in 80% of cases. It is not cystic and appears in a suprahyoid location in the tongue base as a hyperdense mass on unenhanced CT.

Reference

Marianowski R, Ait Amer JL, Morisseau-Durand MP, et al: Risk factors for thyroglossal duct remnants after Sistrunk procedure in a pediatric population, *Int J Pediatr Otorhinolaryngol* 67:19–23, 2003.

Cross-Reference

Neuroradiology: THE REQUISITES, pp 738–747.

Comment

The TGDC is infrahyoid in 65% of cases, at the hyoid bone in 15%, and suprahyoid in 20%. As the TGDC migrates more inferiorly, there is a greater chance that it will be located off midline, which occurs in about 25% of cases. Although lingual thyroid glands, by virtue of the presence of the functioning tissue, have a reasonably high rate of nascent thyroid carcinoma, TGDCs are associated only rarely with thyroid cancer.

The thyroglossal duct begins at the foramen cecum of the base of the tongue in the midline. It is the means of migration of the thyroid tissue from the endoderm of the tongue, through the base of tongue looping around the hyoid bone and then leading to the low neck where the thyroid gland resides.

Typical age of presentation is in early childhood, and surgery may consist of simple excision or the definitive Sistrunk procedure with removal of the whole tracts and hyoid bone. TGDCs recur in 15% of patients; recurrences are best correlated with the presence of infection before surgery, age <2 years, and a multicystic appearance. In more than half of TGDCs, one sees high signal intensity on T1W scans, presumably owing to the high protein colloid amount.

Notes

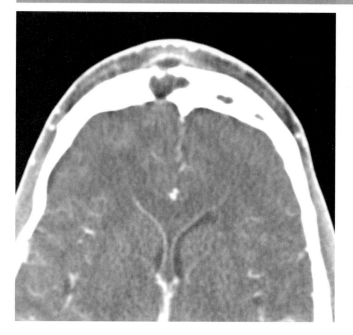 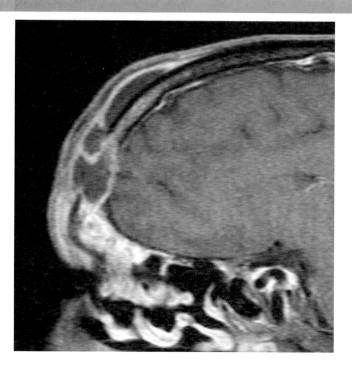

1. What is in the differential diagnosis of this lesion?

2. What are the potential complications of this entity?

3. Is this the most common site for a subperiosteal abscess as a complication of sinusitis?

4. Which would have a higher apparent diffusion coefficient: a mucous retention cyst or a squamous cell carcinoma of the frontal sinus?

Pott's Puffy Tumor

1. Mucocele, abscess, lytic metastasis

2. Meningitis, thrombophlebitis, subdural empyema, epidural abscess, sinus thrombosis, orbital cellulitis

3. No. Along the lamina papyracea is much more common.

4. A mucous retention cyst

Reference

Maeda M, Kato H, Sakuma H, et al: Usefulness of the apparent diffusion coefficient in line scan diffusion-weighted imaging for distinguishing between squamous cell carcinomas and lymphomas of the head and neck. *AJNR Am J Neuroradiol* 26: 1186–1192, 2005.

Cross Reference

Neuroradiology: THE REQUISITES, pp 626–627.

Comment

Patients with Pott's Puffy tumor present with a soft tissue swelling over the forehead, fever, erythema, headache, and congestion. Usually only the outer wall of the sinus has been violated, producing a subperiosteal abscess in the soft tissue, but occasionally, as in this case, the inner table may be violated as well. In this case one can see abnormal meningeal enhancement. It is in such cases that the potential for a host of intracranial complications of sinusitis must be addressed, and quickly.

The recent fascination with ADC values has extended to the head and neck. One would expect that hypercellular masses in the head and neck would show lower ADC values than inflammatory lesions or hypocellular masses. The only obfuscating factor would be the presence of purulent or hyperproteinaceous secretions, which may also show restricted diffusion (as demonstrated with intracranial abscesses). Maeda et al have published that the ADC values of squamous cell carcinomas can be distinguished from those of lymphoma by setting a threshold of 0.76×10^{-3} mm²/second, with an accuracy of 98%. The lymphoma ADCs are lower than those of the squamous cell carcinomas. There may also be a need to address the impact of keratin on ADC values.

Notes

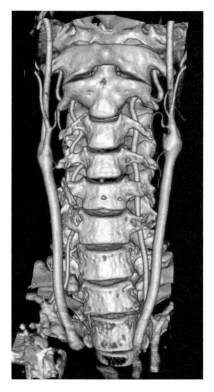 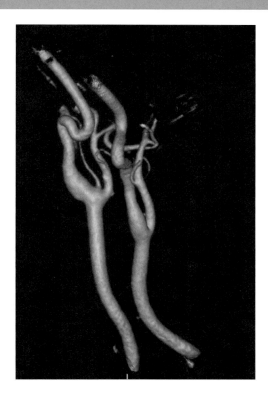

1. Using a 70% cutoff value for stenosis, what is the sensitivity of CT angiography in the carotid arteries for significant disease?

2. For calcified atherosclerotic plaque, which technique is better for evaluating the lumen—two-dimensional or three-dimensional CT angiography projections?

3. Which is more accurate for evaluating the carotid arteries in most head-to-head studies—CT angiography or magnetic resonance angiography?

4. Approximately what are the sensitivity and specificity of CT angiography for detecting aneurysms in patients with subarachnoid hemorrhage?

C A S E 4 0

CT Angiography

1. Approximately 95%.

2. Two-dimensional multiplanar analysis.

3. Magnetic resonance angiography (enhanced).

4. 90% and 90%.

Reference

Tomandl BF, Kostner NC, Schempershofe M, et al: CT angiography of intracranial aneurysms: a focus on postprocessing, *Radiographics* 24:637–655, 2004.

Cross-Reference

Neuroradiology: THE REQUISITES, pp 3–7.

Comment

CT angiography is in the process of revolutionizing vascular imaging in neuroradiology. Although one might have said the same for MR angiography in the 1990s, it seems that CT angiography has gained wider acceptance for use in the head, neck, and brain, in part because of the short scan time; wider availability of CT in the emergency department, the hospital and outpatient settings; and the potential for four-dimensional imaging, including the temporal component. Many institutions have replaced cervical carotid imaging by MR angiography with CT angiography. Reasons include the elimination of the multiple artifacts intrinsic to inflow phenomena on MR angiography and the disturbing difficulties with artifacts associated with turbulent flow on MR angiography. Nonetheless, CT angiography is not without issues. Extensive calcification of the wall of cervical carotid plaques makes postprocessing much more difficult than in patients with noncalcified atherosclerotic plaque. The initial fascination with three-dimensional volume imaging was soon diminished when one had to deal with the issue of stenosis with regard to wall plaque calcification. Two-dimensional multiplanar reconstructions and maximal intensity projection imaging with thin sections have become standard means of evaluating these types of plaques. In the emergency department, many institutions have adopted the policy of evaluating patients with subarachnoid hemorrhage using CT angiography first before conventional arteriography. Some neurosurgeons in North America and more broadly in Europe are now operating on aneurysms on the basis of good-quality CT angiography results.

Notes

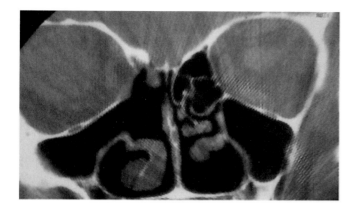

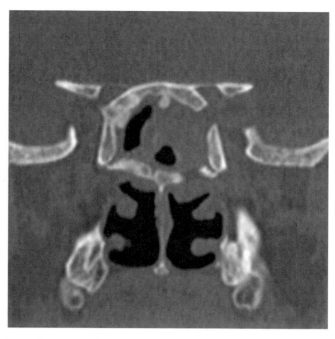

1. Which side of the nose shows more complications from functional endoscopic surgery, and why?

2. Name the two attachments of the middle turbinate.

3. What three structures are most commonly removed during functional endoscopic surgery?

4. What is the eponym for the most posterosuperior ethmoid air cell?

Complications of Endoscopic Sinus Surgery: Dehiscence of Cribriform Plate and Optic Canal Wall

1. The right side because right-handed individuals have a harder time working against their handedness (to the left side) as they face the patient (which would be the patient's right side).

2. The cribriform plate and the lamina papyracea.

3. The uncinate process, the ethmoidal bulla, and the middle turbinate.

4. Onodi cell.

Reference

Hudgins PA, Browning DG, Gallups J, et al: Endoscopic paranasal sinus surgery: radiographic evaluation of severe complications, *AJNR Am J Neuroradiol* 13: 1161–1167, 1992.

Cross-Reference

Neuroradiology: THE REQUISITES, pp 623–629.

Comment

Numerous things can go awry when performing functional endoscopic surgery. Perhaps the most common occurrence is injury to one of the anterior or posterior ethmoidal arteries. This injury may lead to excessive bleeding into the sinuses or, worse, hemorrhage that occurs into the orbits. Surgical clips along the superolateral walls of the ethmoid sinuses may suggest that this complication has occurred because this bleeding may be treated endoscopically.

Dehiscence of the walls of the lamina papyracea or cribriform plate may occur during the removal of the middle turbinate because it has attachments to both. This dehiscence may leave exposed periorbita medially, which puts the orbit at jeopardy for potential perforation or hematoma. With dehiscence at the cribriform plate, the main complication of concern is a CSF leak. Alternatively, over the long term, an encephalocele may develop.

Endoscopic surgery on the posterior ethmoidal and sphenoid sinuses may lead to injury to the optic nerves or the carotid arteries. For this reason, it is important to describe any congenital areas of dehiscent bone or thin bone within the sinuses so that the surgeon is aware of the potential risk.

Notes

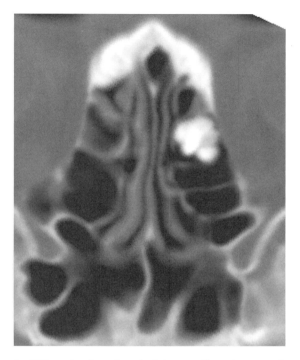
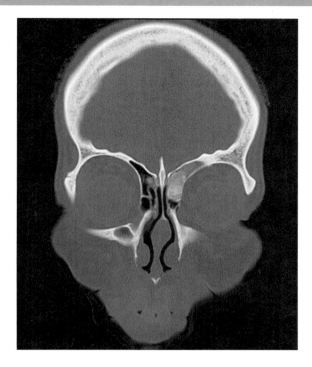

1. What is the classic history for sinonasal osteomas?

2. Name the other fibroosseous lesions of the sinuses.

3. Does fibrous dysplasia affect the maxilla more than the mandible?

4. What is Gardner syndrome?

Osteoma (Left) and Fibrous Dysplasia (Right)

1. Pain in the forehead with postobstructed secretions while the patient is on an airplane.

2. Osteoma, osteochondroma, osteoid osteoma, osteoblastoma, fibrous dysplasia, and ossifying fibroma.

3. Yes.

4. The association of adenomatous polyps throughout the gastrointestinal system, papillary carcinoma of the thyroid, hepatoblastoma, and osteomas of the mandible and paranasal sinuses.

Reference

Som PM, Lidov M: The benign fibroosseous lesion: its association with paranasal sinus mucoceles and its MR appearance, *J Comput Assist Tomogr* 16:871–876, 1992.

Cross-Reference

Neuroradiology: THE REQUISITES, pp 631–632.

Comment

Osteomas of the paranasal sinuses are potential pitfalls for the evaluation of a patient with sinonasal disease using MRI. The osteomas are dark in signal intensity on T1W, T2W, and post–gadolinium-enhanced scans and simulate an aerated paranasal sinus. Although one might identify the obstructed secretions around or blocked by the osteoma, the primary cause of the sinusitis would be inapparent on MRI. Osteomas occur in the frontoethmoidal region with less common involvement in the maxillary and sphenoid sinuses.

The classic description of presentation of a frontal osteoma is a patient who has severe sinus pain while flying in an airplane, presumably because of the atmospheric pressure changes associated with the osteoma and the blocked up paranasal sinus. Perforation to the intracranial compartment with a pneumatocele is rare. Mucoceles also may arise from obstruction by the osteoma.

There is an association of osteomas with colonic polyps with Gardner (autosomal dominant) syndrome. These osteomas are to be distinguished from hereditary exostoses, which project more commonly from long bones than from the paranasal sinuses. The osteomas in Gardner syndrome may occur elsewhere in the facial bones.

Osteochondromas are common benign tumors of bone that appear as bony outgrowths from the cortex and which arise from a cartilage cap. Their presentation is usually as a painless bony protuberance. Rarely there may be an association with Ollier syndrome, also known as hereditary multiple osteocartilaginous exostoses. This is an autosomal dominant condition in which the patient is at risk for one of the osteochondromas becoming malignant in adulthood. Red flags of conversion to chondrosarcoma would be progressive pain or sudden growth in tumor size. Resection of the low-grade chondrosarcoma is necessary because radiation and chemotherapy are less useful.

Nonossifying fibromas are common benign bone tumors in children in the extremities but rarely occur in facial bones.

Notes

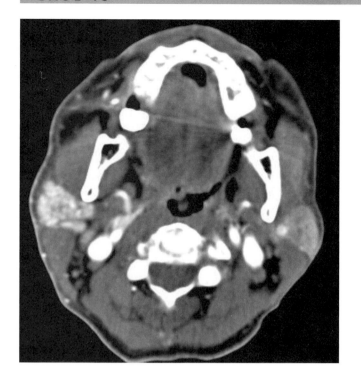

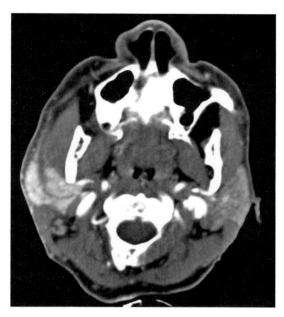

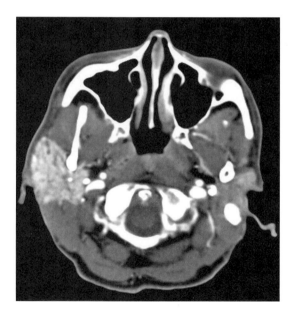

1. What is the chemical composition of a salivary gland calculus?

2. Do salivary calculi hurt more on eating or abstaining?

3. What gland harbors the most calculi?

4. What percentage of stones are opaque on plain radiography?

Parotid Duct Stone with Parotitis

1. Calcium phosphate or calcium oxalate.

2. While eating.

3. Submandibular gland.

4. 70% to 80%.

Reference

Gritzmann N, Rettenbacher T, Hollerweger A, et al: Sonography of the salivary glands, *Eur Radiol* 13: 964–975, 2003.

Cross-Reference

Neuroradiology: THE REQUISITES, pp 700–703.

Comment

A stone in the salivary gland is called *sialolithiasis,* and inflammation of the duct is called *sialodochitis.* Glandular parenchymal inflammation is termed *sialadenitis.* A dilated duct is called *sialoectasia.*

Submandibular gland and duct stones are more common than parotid stones. Sublingual and minor salivary gland calculi are rare. One should exclude calcifications in lymph nodes, tonsils, and vessels before suggesting calculi in these glands. The need for sialography to diagnose calculi is rare these days—unenhanced CT can detect most calculi reliably even if their density is minimally different from that of surrounding tissue. The accuracy of sonography in detecting sialolithiasis is approximately 90%. Nonopaque stones on plain radiography can be visualized if >2 mm. Enhancing vessels may simulate calculi, so unenhanced CT scans are best. Most submandibular calculi appear within the duct rather than in the glandular parenchyma.

Focal masslike firmness of the submandibular glands caused by chronic sialadenitis from calculus disease (Kuttner tumor) may simulate neoplasms. The pain and swelling of the gland with a calculus increase with eating. The closer the calculus is to the duct orifice, the easier the treatment, which may be managed with manual manipulation or surgical excision. Stones within the glandular parenchyma may necessitate glandular removal if the symptoms are such that the patient cannot tolerate the condition. Bilateral intraglandular sialolithiasis is problematic in that bilateral glandular removal may lead to a permanently dry mouth, which is uncomfortable for the patient and may lead to dental caries.

Notes

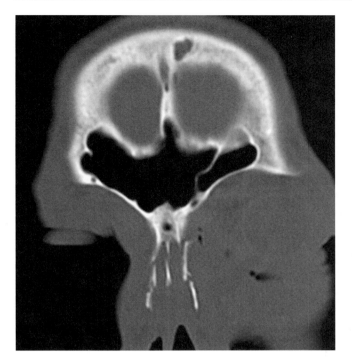

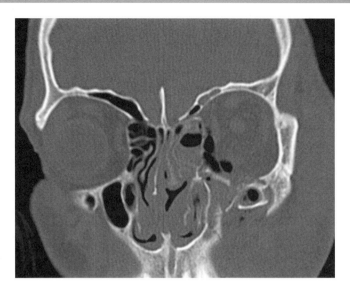

1. Name the most commonly fractured facial bone.

2. Name the second most commonly fractured facial bone.

3. Name the third most commonly fractured facial bone.

4. How often are vessels traumatized with penetrating wounds to the neck?

Facial Fractures

1. Nasal bone.

2. Orbital wall.

3. Mandible.

4. 20%.

Reference

Ofer A, Nitecki SS, Braun J, et al: CT angiography of the carotid arteries in trauma to the neck, *Eur J Vasc Endovasc Surg* 21:401–407, 2001.

Cross-Reference

Neuroradiology: THE REQUISITES, pp 263–264.

Comment

Three zones are usually identified with respect to vascular injuries to the head and neck. Zone 1 injuries are injuries from the clavicle to the cricoid cartilage and include the thoracic outlet vessels and supraaortic branches. Zone 2 lies from the cricoid to the angle of the mandible, and the vessels of concern are the carotids and to a lesser extent the vertebral arteries. Zone 3 goes from the angle of the mandible to the base of the skull, and the same vessels as for zone 2 are of concern.

Heretofore conventional arteriograms were performed to investigate injuries to these vessels. There is a fantastic potential for CT angiography to replace all of these diagnostic arteriograms for vessel surveillance (because >80% are negative for correctable lesions) and to limit the scope of arteriography to equivocal cases or to cases where endovascular therapy is required.

All of these injuries may be very serious and may include injuries to the airway and esophagus and pharynx. Some cases require immediate exploration, especially cases with a rapidly expanding hematoma, airway compromise or leak, or both.

See cases 1, 7, 29, 34, 48, and 56 for descriptions of other facial fractures.

Notes

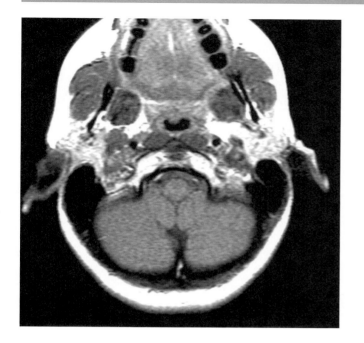
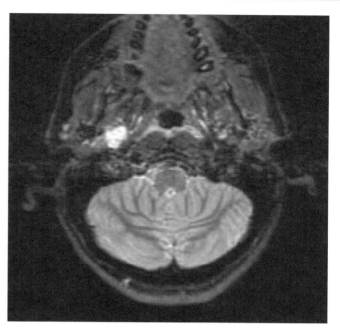
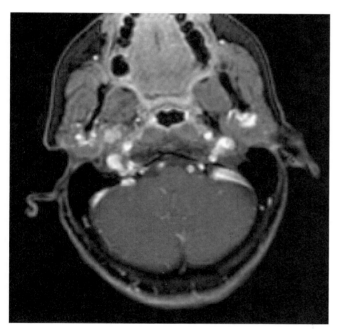

1. What is the most common parapharyngeal space primary tumor?

2. What is in the differential diagnosis for a lesion in this location?

3. Which branchial cleft cyst may arise in the parapharyngeal space?

4. What lower neck primary tumor has a predilection for parapharyngeal space adenopathy?

Parapharyngeal Space: Pleomorphic Adenoma

1. Pleomorphic adenoma.

2. Schwannoma, minor salivary gland malignancy, lymph node, venous vascular malformation, paraganglioma, sarcoma, nasopharyngeal carcinoma, branchial cleft cyst.

3. Bailey type 4 second branchial cleft cyst.

4. Thyroid malignancies.

Reference

Sherman PM, Yousem DM, Loevner LA: CT-guided aspirations in the head and neck: assessment of the first 216 cases, *AJNR Am J Neuroradiol* 25:1603–1607, 2004.

Cross-Reference

Neuroradiology: THE REQUISITES, pp 721–723.

Comment

Fine-needle aspiration (FNA) is an effective means for diagnosing most parapharyngeal masses. Advantages of FNA includes its low invasiveness, use of small needles in an area where several vascular structures are present, and the lack of a telltale scar from the procedure. The pain associated with the procedure is usually minimal when adequate local anesthetic is used. Neither sedation nor general anesthesia is required.

Non–image-guided FNA of *palpable* lesions has been well established as an accurate diagnostic tool in the head and neck, particularly in the salivary glands. FNA via a transoral approach for visible parapharyngeal space lesions has been described with an accuracy of 78% to 86% but a false-negative rate of 19% secondary to inadequate stabilization of the lesion at the time of aspiration, limits of the intraoral angles available to puncture the mass, and inability to make deep blind passes secondary to the underlying vessels.

Percutaneous image-guided FNA is not constrained by these limitations. Image-guided FNA can evaluate nonpalpable parapharyngeal lesions accurately, particularly lesions in a poorly accessible or deep location in the head and neck. Ultrasound-guided FNA is an established technique for lesion localization, particularly in evaluation of the thyroid gland and superficial cervical lymph nodes. Lesions deep to the bony structures of the face and air-containing spaces are not well localized by ultrasound but can be localized accurately and aspirated under CT guidance.

MRI-guided FNA has been performed with good results and minimal morbidity and provides excellent soft tissue resolution but does not provide bony detail. Although MRI has the advantage of absence of exposure to ionizing radiation, it has the disadvantages of limited availability, particularly open high-field MRI systems; longer image acquisition times; and the need for instruments compatible with a magnetic field. Although MRI guidance is likely to have an expanded role in the future, CT is currently the imaging modality of choice for biopsy of deep-seated or poorly localized head and neck lesions.

Notes

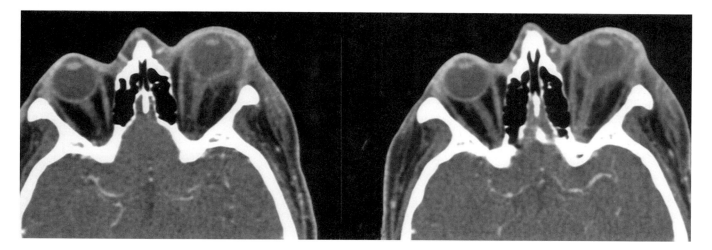

1. Name the demarcation between preseptal and postseptal orbital cellulitis.

2. What is the importance of making this distinction?

3. What are the most common sources of orbital cellulitis?

4. How does sinusitis spread to the orbit?

Postseptal Orbital Cellulitis

1. The orbital septum.

2. Orbital cellulitis represents a major threat to the survival of the eye, with issues of optic nerve ischemia, optic neuritis, vascular thrombosis, and spread to the cavernous sinus.

3. Sinusitis, trauma/iatrogenic (foreign bodies), and facial cellulitis.

4. Usually through the lamina papyracea; less commonly via veins.

Reference

Howe L, Jones NS: Guidelines for the management of periorbital cellulitis/abscess, *Clin Otolaryngol* 29: 725–728, 2004.

Cross-Reference

Neuroradiology: THE REQUISITES, pp 508–509.

Comment

The differentiation between preseptal (periorbital) cellulitis and postseptal (orbital) cellulitis is huge with respect to the danger to the eye from the disease. Although one could make an argument for outpatient treatment of patients with preseptal cellulitis, cases in which there are signs of retrobulbar involvement (diploplia, decreased acuity, abnormal pupil response, proptosis, ophthalmoplegia) require hospitalization with intravenous antibiotics and close observation.

Typical bacteria include *Staphylococcus, Streptococcus,* pneumococcus, and *Pseudomonas.* Because most cases are derived from sinus infections, antibiotic therapy is supplemented by nasal ephedrine drops, analgesics, and, as needed, surgical treatment for any complications.

This patient has tenting of the back of the globe indicating a globe under pressure and staphyloma formation. The scleral-uveal membranes are thinned and stretched. Breaks in Bruch membrane from the stretching of axial myopia may lead to choroidal atrophy and choroidal neovascularization culminating in choroidal detachments.

Notes

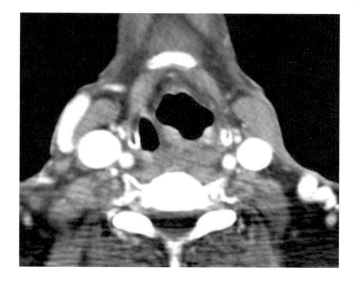

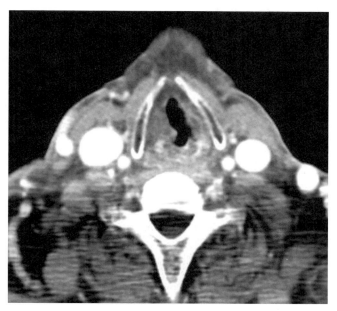

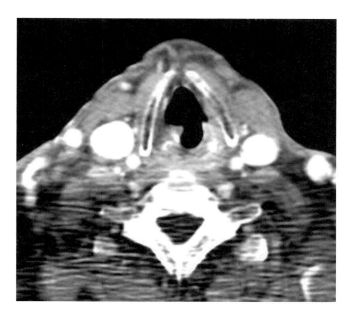

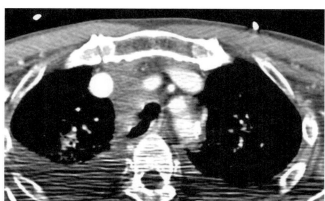

1. What is the matter with this larynx?

2. How would uvular deviation or soft palate paralysis help in evaluating this patient?

3. What is the most common feature of superior laryngeal nerve paralysis?

4. In what percentage of cases are the clinicians unable to determine a cause of vocal cord paralysis?

Vocal Cord Paralysis

1. There is vocal cord paralysis from a mediastinal mass.

2. It would suggest an upper vagus nerve etiology rather than a recurrent laryngeal nerve source of the vocal cord paralysis.

3. A normal larynx most commonly. Rarely there is arytenoid deviation or cricothyroid muscle atrophy (the only muscle it innervates).

4. 50%.

Reference

Richardson BE, Bastian RW: Clinical evaluation of vocal fold paralysis, *Otolaryngol Clin North Am* 37:45–58, 2004.

Cross-Reference

Neuroradiology: THE REQUISITES, pp 678–680.

Comment

Numerous findings might suggest vocal cord paralysis on a CT scan of the larynx. Look for medialization of the aryepiglottic fold, dilation of the ipsilateral piriform sinus, dilation of the ipsilateral vallecula, rotation and medialization of the arytenoid cartilage, medialization of the true vocal cord, dilation of the ipsilateral laryngeal ventricle, and atrophy of the cricoarytenoid muscle.

When a vocal cord paralysis occurs in association with a Horner syndrome or brachial plexopathy, one should consider mediastinal or lung apex lesions, which may affect the vagus nerve as it enters the mediastinum or the recurrent laryngeal nerve as it ascends in the tracheoesophageal groove. If one has pharyngeal paralysis or an absent gag reflex, one should consider upper vagus nerve lesions because those pharyngeal branches arise above the level of the hyoid bone. One would not expect recurrent laryngeal nerve isolated disease to cause pharyngeal abnormalities.

The most common cause of vocal cord paralysis is iatrogenic associated with thyroid or parathyroid surgery.

Notes

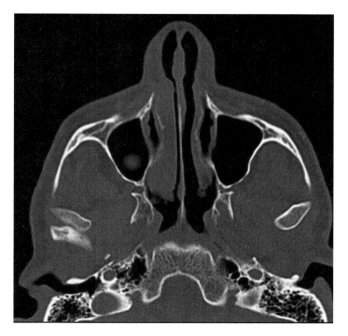
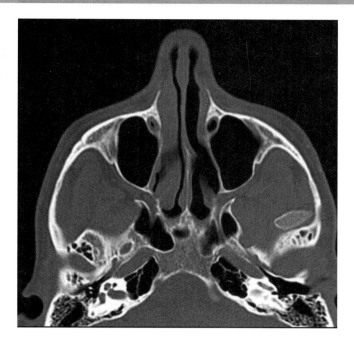

1. What is the cause of this patient's trismus?
2. Where is the mandible fractured most frequently?
3. Identify the most common setting in which the mandible is fractured.
4. What are the demographics of mandibular fractures?

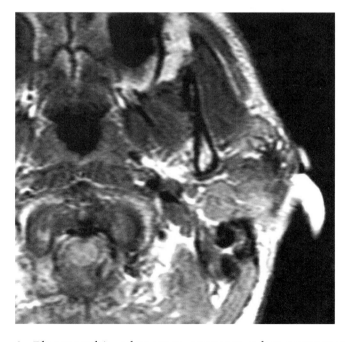
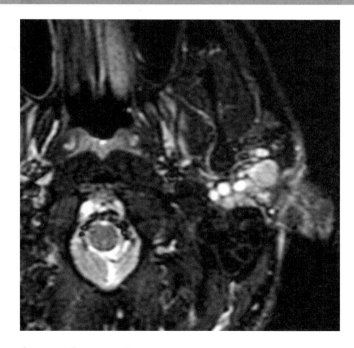

1. Pleomorphic adenomas compose what percentage of parotid masses?
2. Name the most common malignancy of the parotid gland.
3. Identify features that suggest a Warthin tumor.
4. Cystadenoma lymphomatosum is another term for what tumor?

CASE 48

Dislocated Mandible

1. Bilateral dislocated mandibles.

2. The parasymphyseal location.

3. Assaults and gunshot wounds.

4. 4:1 in favor of males.

Reference

King RE, Scianna JM, Petruzzelli GJ: Mandible fracture patterns: a suburban trauma center experience, *Am J Otolaryngol* 25:301–307, 2004.

Cross-Reference

Neuroradiology: THE REQUISITES, pp 268–269.

Comment

Be conscious of the appearance of the mandible during head CT evaluation of patients who have had craniofacial trauma. One should see the mandibular condyles centered in the glenoid fossa bilaterally. If one mandible is centered in the glenoid fossa but the other is not, one should be concerned about a fracture-dislocation of the mandible. If both mandibles are not in the cup of the glenoid fossa, one may have bilateral dislocation of the mandibles, which almost exclusively occurs anteriorly, or the patient may have had an open mouth during the CT scan. On opening the mouth, the mandibular condyles leave the glenoid fossa and project anteriorly under the articular eminence of the base of the temporal bones; this can be a potential pitfall. Most patients are not scanned with the mouth open, however, so one should suggest the possibility of mandibular trauma.

Fractures of the mandible are multiple in 68% of cases, especially parasymphyseal ones. Subcondylar fractures are the second most common sites. The angle of the mandible and the body of the mandible are more commonly fractured in assaults.

Isolated reports of intracranial dislocation of the mandible condyle have been published.

Notes

CASE 49

Pleomorphic Adenoma Seeding

1. 64%.

2. Mucoepidermoid carcinoma.

3. Older man with a heterogeneous mass in the tail of the parotid gland.

4. Warthin tumor.

Reference

O'Brien CJ: Current management of benign parotid tumors—the role of limited superficial parotidectomy, *Head Neck* 25:946–952, 2003.

Cross-Reference

Neuroradiology: THE REQUISITES, pp 706–712.

Comment

This is an example of a dreaded complication of surgery to remove a pleomorphic adenoma—seeding of the resection bed. Although seeding also used to occur when large-gauge aspiration biopsy needles (>14g) were used to sample parotid neoplasms percutaneously, that is no longer an issue in the 21st century.

Care is taken at surgical resection not to violate the capsule of the pleomorphic adenoma. The risk of seeding is greater with large (>25 mm) tumors because they generally have thinner capsules. Irrigation of the field may help prevent seeding, but this is partly the reason why some surgeons recommend parotidectomy over local excision of the lesion. Intraoperative tumor spill and inadequate resection (to a far greater extent) also are associated with an increase in the recurrence rate of pleomorphic adenoma. Radiation therapy reduces the risk of recurrence.

Facial nerve permanent paralysis and Frey (auriculotemporal/Baillarger) syndrome are other potential complications of surgery for parotid tumors. The former is estimated to occur in <5% of cases. Frey syndrome is a feeling of warmth and sweating on the ipsilateral face when there is a salivary stimulus. Salivation induces perspiration secondary to injured-disrupted autonomic nerve fibers.

Notes

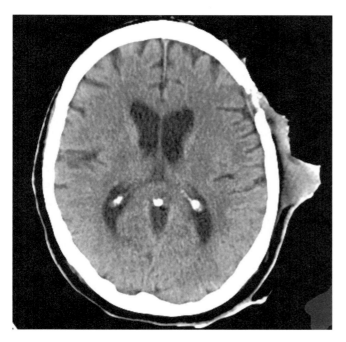
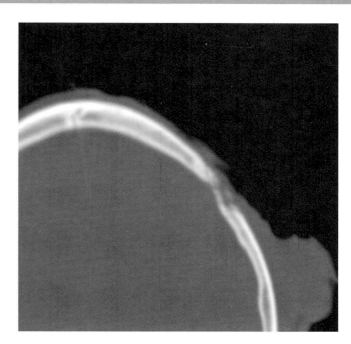

1. Identify the most common type of skin cancer in whites.
2. What physical features seem to indicate higher risk for skin cancers?
3. What is the most common skin cancer in African Americans?
4. What is mycosis fungoides?

Poorly Differentiated Squamous Cell Carcinoma of the Scalp

1. Basal cell carcinoma.

2. Fair skin, light hair, blue or green eyes.

3. Squamous cell carcinoma.

4. A cutaneous T cell lymphoma. It is a low-grade lymphoma that primarily affects the skin.

Reference

Williams LS, Mancuso AA, Mendenhall WM: Perineural spread of cutaneous squamous and basal cell carcinoma: CT and MR detection and its impact on patient management and prognosis, *Int J Radiat Oncol Biol Phys* 49:1061–1069, 2001.

Cross-Reference

Neuroradiology: THE REQUISITES, pp 569–570.

Comment

Cancers of the scalp usually are found in the sun-exposed portions of the hairline. The bottom lip, ears, and other sites of the face also may be highly represented among cases of skin cancers affecting the head and neck.

Basal cell carcinoma is the most common skin cancer affecting the head and neck, followed by squamous cell carcinoma and melanoma. Basal cell carcinoma is aggressive in less than 10% of cases and shows perineural involvement in 3% of the aggressive form. When perineural involvement is present, it may lead to involvement of cranial nerves V and VII. The prognosis of basal cell carcinoma decreases from >85% 5-year survival to 50% 5-year survival when perineural invasion is present.

Squamous cell carcinoma is more aggressive than basal cell carcinoma. Occasionally, one may see invasion through the skull (as in this case) from these aggressive lesions. The lymph node spread is usually to the collar nodes around the head and neck, but intraparotid lymphadenopathy also may be present in some cases.

Melanoma is the most common skin cancer to develop diffuse hematogenous spread. The depth and extent of the lesion determine the degree to which one might expect lymphadenopathy or distant metastasis. When there is bone involvement from a scalp cancer, the prognosis is much worse.

Notes

Fair Game Cases

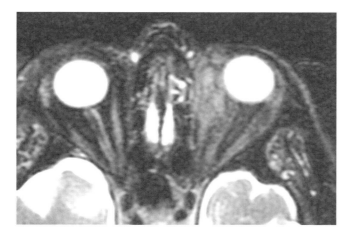

1. What is the differential diagnosis if this orbit is painless?

2. What is the differential diagnosis if the orbit is painful?

3. If the nasal septum is perforated as well, what are the top three diagnoses?

4. What is the typical signal intensity on T2W scans for Wegener granulomatosis?

Wegener Granulomatosis of the Orbit

1. Lymphoma, sarcoidosis, meningioma.

2. Orbital pseudotumor, postseptal cellulitis, Wegener granulomatosis.

3. Sarcoid, Wegener granulomatosis, lymphoma.

4. Low.

References

Fechner FP, Faquin WC, Pilch BZ: Wegener's granulomatosis of the orbit: a clinicopathological study of 15 patients, *Laryngoscope* 112:1945–1950, 2002.

Courcoutsakis NA, Langford CA, Sneller MC, et al: Orbital involvement in Wegener granulomatosis: MR findings in 12 patients, *J Comput Assist Tomogr* 21:452–458, 1997.

Cross-Reference

Neuroradiology: THE REQUISITES, pp 624–626.

Comment

Wegener granulomatosis is limited to the orbit in 80% of patients; 15% also may have sinonasal involvement. If the disease is limited initially to the orbit and treated appropriately, systemic disease is rare, but orbital involvement in systemic disease occurs in 50% of patients. Usual presenting symptoms are nonspecific and include lid swelling, eye pain, and blurred vision. Involvement, when not caused by direct spread from the sinonasal cavity, may be limited to the conjunctiva, scleral membranes, cornea, uveal tract, optic nerve or sheath or both, and extraocular muscles.

Treatment may be either surgical or medical (cyclophosphamide and prednisone).

Notes

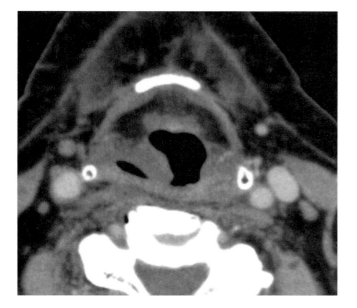

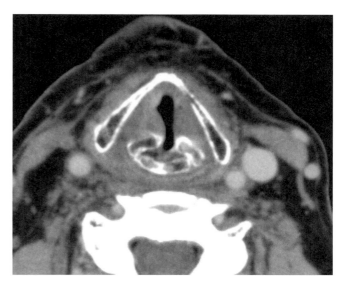

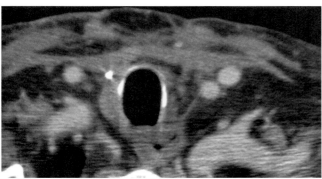

1. Describe the main findings in this case.

2. What are the most common etiologies for this phenomenon?

3. How is the entity treated?

4. Is the clinical symptom complex best approached with CT, MRI, or ultrasound?

Iatrogenic Vocal Cord Paralysis

1. Enlargement of the ipsilateral piriform sinus, adduction of the vocal cord, medialization of the arytenoid, atrophy of the cricothyroid muscle, postoperative appearance of the thyroid gland.

2. Iatrogenic (postoperative or intubation), idiopathic, thyroid/parathyroid neoplasms, and lymphadenopathy.

3. Thyroplasty.

4. CT because one has to go inferiorly into the chest under the aortic arch, and this is not well imaged with a neck coil or ultrasound.

Reference

Liu AY, Yousem DM, Chalian AA, Langlotz CP: Economic consequences of diagnostic imaging for vocal cord paralysis, *Acad Radiol* 8:137–148, 2001.

Cross-Reference

Neuroradiology: THE REQUISITES, pp 678–680.

Comment

The most common cause for vocal cord paralysis is thyroid surgery. Invariably the recurrent laryngeal nerve, which runs in the tracheoesophageal groove, is injured. Alternatively, with neck dissections, the vagus nerve is injured, but this is much less common than with thyroid/parathyroid operations.

Medialization thyroplasty and arytenoid adduction are effective treatments for medializing the paralyzed vocal cord, but the evidence does not support performing both procedures to improve voice quality. Thyroplasty alone improves the voice in >80% of cases. Even in long-standing vocal cord paralysis, medialization thyroplasty shows marked voice improvement. Thyroplasty may include placement of cartilage, Silastic, hyaluronic acid, Gore-Tex, or titanium material. Alternatively, one could inject the vocal cord with polytetrafluoroethylene (Teflon), collagen, fat, calcium hydroxyapatite gel, or hyaluronic acid. The most common cause for revison thyroplasty is undercorrection of the medialization procedure.

The average cost of finding space-occupying lesions in patients with vocal cord paralysis without suspicious antecedent clinical findings ($10,800) is >4.5 times higher than in patients with such a history ($2300). The benefits of obtaining negative findings and of detecting a few space-occupying lesions should be weighed against the costs of such a workup.

Notes

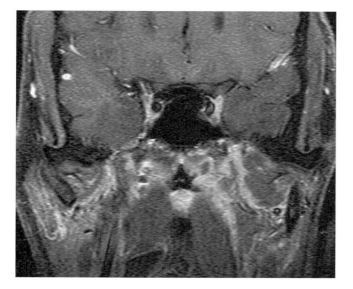
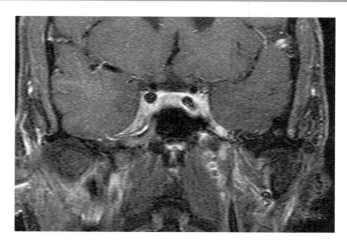
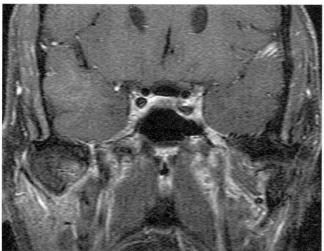

1. Of the big three (squamous cell, basal cell, and melanoma), which histology of skin cancer is the least likely to show perineural spread?

2. Which histology of salivary gland neoplasms is most likely to cause perineural spread?

3. What is the rate at which adenoid cystic carcinoma spreads via the nerves?

4. Which two cranial nerves show the highest rate of perineural spread from the parotid gland?

Perineural Spread of Neoplasm

1. Basal cell carcinoma.

2. Adenoid cystic carcinoma.

3. 50% to 60%.

4. Cranial nerves VII and V.

Reference

Chang PC, Fischbein NJ, McCalmont TH, et al: Perineural spread of malignant melanoma of the head and neck: clinical and imaging features, *AJNR Am J Neuroradiol* 25:5–11, 2004.

Cross-Reference

Neuroradiology: THE REQUISITES, pp 635–636, 710–711.

Comment

Perineural spread of cancer can occur with salivary gland, skin, or mucosal primary tumors in the head and neck. Although adenoid cystic carcinoma has the highest rate of perineural spread, nearly all histologies have shown a capacity for this phenomenon. In melanomas, the desmoplastic form predominates, and it usually follows cranial nerve V more often than cranial nerve VII. Only 5% of melanomas are of the desmoplastic variety.

Perineural spread is best shown by MRI; salient features include enhancement of the nerve, effacement of the skull base fat, thickening of the nerve, and demonstration of atrophy of the muscles innervated by the nerve. Enhancement of denervated muscles and high intensity signal on T2W images also may be seen. Although imaging is positive in only 50% of path proven cases, it does predict a worse prognosis, decreasing the 5-year survival by nearly 50%.

Basal cell carcinoma rarely is aggressive and shows perineural spread <1% of the time. Melanoma represents only 5% of all skin cancers but accounts for 65% of deaths from skin cancer; 20% of all melanomas arise in the head and neck.

Notes

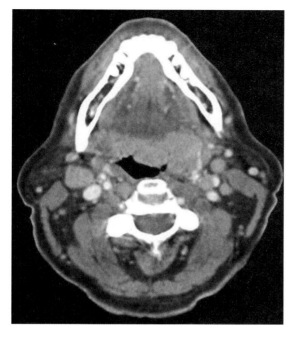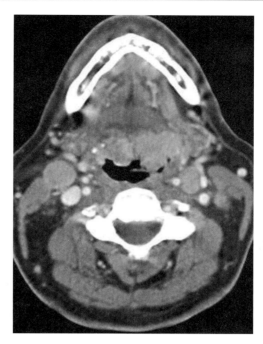

1. Identify the most common site of oropharyngeal carcinoma.
2. List the risk factors.
3. What are treatment decisions based on?
4. What is the 5-year prognosis?

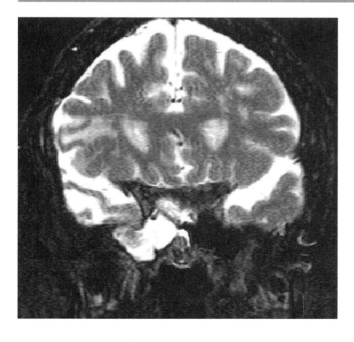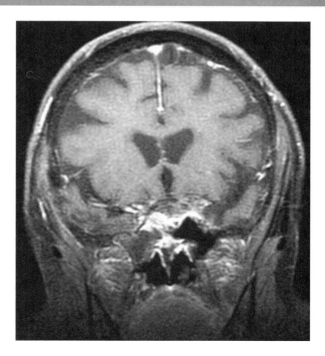

1. What is the differential diagnosis?
2. Identify typical symptoms.
3. List risk factors.
4. What is the best MRI technique for showing the pathology?

Tonsil Carcinoma

1. Palatine tonsil.

2. Smoking, alcohol consumption, chewing tobacco, and human papillomavirus exposure.

3. Extent to the tongue base, mandibular involvement, and extramucosal disease.

4. It depends on nodal staging, but 31% to 44% are typical values.

Reference

Johansen LV, Grau C, Overgaard J: Squamous cell carcinoma of the oropharynx—an analysis of treatment results in 289 consecutive patients, *Acta Oncol* 39:985–994, 2000.

Cross-Reference

Neuroradiology: THE REQUISITES, pp 657–658.

Comment

The term *reflex otalgia* applies to a referred pain in the ear in individuals with nasopharyngeal and oropharyngeal carcinomas. It is seen most often in individuals who have tumor involvement of structures innervated by the glossopharyngeal nerve.

According to the article by Johansen et al, clinical T stage and N stage, tumor size, gender, age, and pretreatment hemoglobin are significant prognostic parameters for squamous cell carcinoma of the oropharynx in a univariate analysis. Cox multivariate analysis showed that T stage, N stage, and gender were independent prognostic factors.

Treatment options are surgery and chemoradiotherapy.

Notes

Temporal Lobe Encephalocele

1. Meningocele, meningoencephalocele, arachnoid cyst of Meckel cave, mucocele, and lytic skull mass.

2. Seizures and rhinorrhea.

3. Trauma, prior surgery, Southeast Asian origin, and tegmen tympani erosion.

4. High-resolution T2W scan.

Reference

Yang E, Yeo SB, Tan TY: Temporal lobe encephalocoele presenting with seizures and hearing loss, *Singapore Med J* 45:40–42, 2004.

Cross-Reference

Neuroradiology: THE REQUISITES, pp 418–419.

Comment

Encephaloceles occur in 1:35,000 births. Temporal lobe encephaloceles often cause partial complex seizures early in life. They usually herniate into the petrous or mastoid portions of the temporal bone or into the paranasal sinuses. The distortion of the normal gray matter architecture is often visible in more subtle cases of mere tenting of the temporal lobe.

Morning glory syndrome is a congenital optic disc dysplasia (colobomas, detached retina, microophthalmia, and pigmentary retinopathy) often associated with craniofacial anomalies (cleft palate, hypertelorism, cleft lip) and basal encephaloceles.

Notes

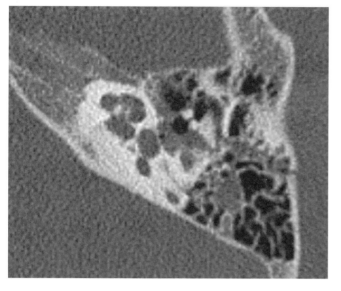

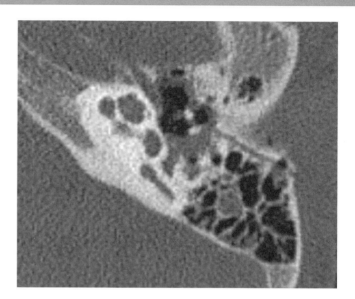

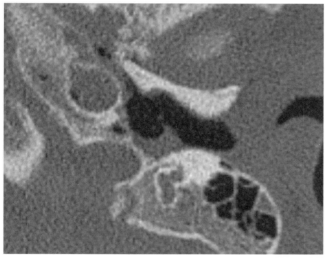

1. What are the salient findings in this case?

2. Name the four portions of the temporal bone.

3. Which temporal bone fracture has the highest rate of perilymphatic fistula?

4. Which temporal bone fracture has the highest rate of CSF leakage?

Temporal Bone Fracture

1. Fracture dislocation of the incudo-malleolar joint, hemotympanum, air in the carotid canal; no facial nerve or inner ear disruption.

2. Tympanic, mastoid, petrous, squamosal.

3. Vertical.

4. Vertical.

Reference

Schubiger O, Valavanis A, Stuckmann G, Antonucci F: Temporal bone fractures and their complications: examination with high resolution CT, *Neuroradiology* 28:93–99, 1986.

Cross-Reference

Neuroradiology: THE REQUISITES, pp 606–607.

Comment

Much has been said about the different forms of temporal bone fractures—fractures that traverse the long axis of the temporal bone (vertical fractures) and fractures that are in plane with the long axis (horizontal fractures). Most fractures actually are oblique in their orientation and so have features of both types.

Complications of temporal bone fractures include CSF leaks, hemotympanum, ossicular dislocation, facial nerve injury, perilymphatic fistula, injury to the cochlea and vestibule, and tympanic membrane disruption. One or more of these complications arise in 12% of all patients with temporal bone fractures. When facial nerve injury occurs, it usually does so at the geniculate ganglion level. In children, CSF leakage occurs in nearly 25% of cases. Nearly one third has an ossicular disruption.

The rate of bilateral temporal bone fractures is approximately 14%.

Notes

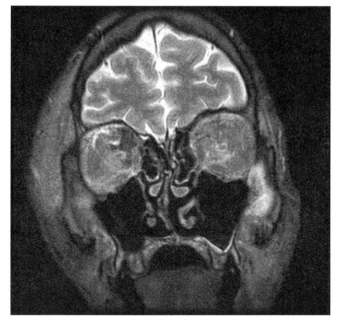
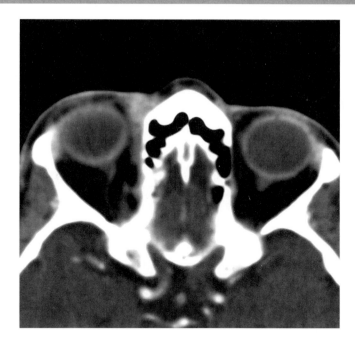
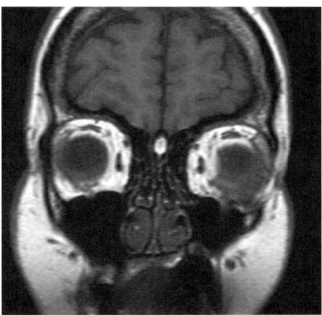

1. What is the differential diagnosis?
2. Name the most common site of orbital lymphoma.
3. Identify the most common clinical manifestation of orbital lymphoma.
4. What histologic type of lymphoma is most common in the orbit?

Multifocal Orbital Lymphoma

1. Lymphoma, pseudotumor, schwannoma, metastasis, and sarcoidosis.

2. Conjunctiva.

3. Soft tissue mass.

4. Non–Hodgkin B cell lymphoma.

Reference

Moon WJ, Na DG, Ryoo JW, et al: Orbital lymphoma and subacute or chronic inflammatory pseudotumor: differentiation with two-phase helical computed tomography, *J Comput Assist Tomogr* 27:510–516, 2003.

Cross-Reference

Neuroradiology: THE REQUISITES, pp 506–507.

Comment

Often the differential diagnosis in many infiltrative, mildly enhancing lesions in the orbit comes down to a question of orbital pseudotumor versus lymphoma. Moon et al published their findings in which increased CT attenuation between early-phase and late-phase enhanced axial scans was seen in 42% (n = 8) of lymphoma cases, and decreased CT attenuation was seen in 58% (n = 11). In 17 lymphomas (90%), the density decreased between late-phase axial and delayed coronal scans. Conversely, in seven cases of orbital pseudotumor (78%), the CT attenuation increased gradually over time from early-phase axial to delayed coronal scans. These authors advocate performing dynamic scans through the orbit with delayed imaging to distinguish between the entities.

In adults, 55% of nonocular orbital malignancies are from lymphomas with ever-increasing rates with each year. Lymphoma may be a manifestation of systemic disease or of localized primary orbital lymphoma. Treatment of orbital lymphoma is usually with low-dose radiation therapy, which leads to a rapid early response. Recurrence rates also are high (20%) and may include systemic disease.

Orbital lymphoma is usually of the non–Hodgkin B cell variety and reflects systemic disease at the time of diagnosis or subsequently in 75% of cases. The most common sites of involvement in the orbit are the conjunctivae and the lacrimal gland. Mucosa-associated lymphoid tissue (MALT) lymphoma may occur in the conjunctiva of the eye.

When one finds nasal septal perforation and an infiltrated process involving the orbit, one should consider a limited differential diagnosis, which includes Wegener granulomatosis, lymphoma, sarcoidosis, and fungal infection. Lymphoma, sarcoidosis, and Wegener granulomatosis may be associated with lymph node enlargement in the neck. This enlargement generally is not seen with fungal infection, unless the patient's underlying disease process is one that causes immunosuppression (e.g., HIV infection). The fungal infection that is most commonly associated with nasal septal perforation is a *Klebsiella* infection termed *rhinoscleroma*. Any aggressive infection, including aspergillosis and mucormycosis, may cause erosion of the nasal septum. Cocaine is the most common cause of nasal septum perforation.

Notes

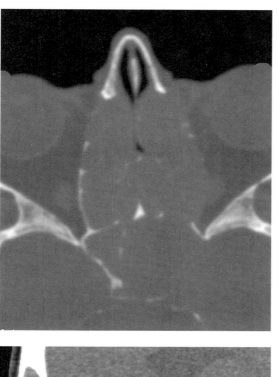
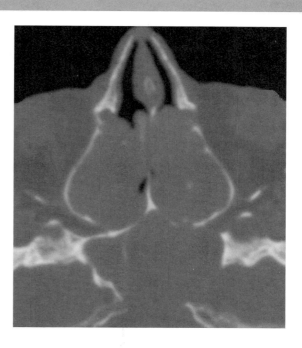
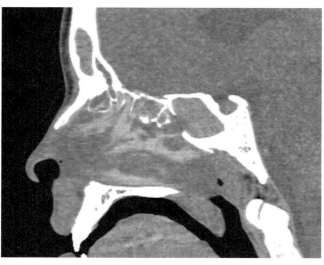
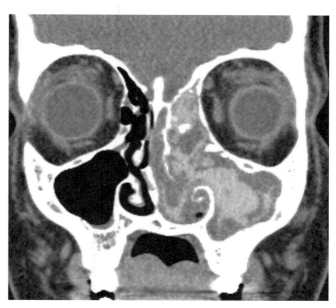

1. What is the differential diagnosis?

2. What features suggest a mucocele?

3. What features suggest allergic fungal sinusitis (AFS)?

4. How is AFS different from invasive fungal sinusitis?

Allergic Fungal Sinusitis

1. Polyps, mucoceles, AFS, and cystic fibrosis.

2. Expansion of the sinus, thinning of the bones, and obstruction of the ostia.

3. Abnormal density to the sinus secretions, remodeling and thinning of the bony sinus walls, erosion of the sinus walls, and abnormal signal intensity on MRI.

4. Invasive sinusitis usually means extension to the orbits to the cavernous sinus or the intracranial space. The bones are destroyed rather than expanded and thinned.

Reference

Mukherji SK, Figueroa RE, Ginsberg LE, et al: Allergic fungal sinusitis: CT findings, *Radiology* 207:417–422, 1998.

Cross-Reference

Neuroradiology: THE REQUISITES, p 627.

Comment

In AFS, no histologic evidence of fungal hyphae invasion into blood vessels, submucosa, or bone, which may be seen with the invasive form, is present. AFS usually involves multiple sinuses and often is bilateral.

AFS occurs in individuals who have a history of atopy/asthma but normal immunologic status. The patient develops sinonasal obstruction with the presence of polyps and expanded paranasal sinuses.

On CT, the sinuses are hyperdense, indicating hyperproteinemia and the fungi themselves. On MRI, one might find high signal intensity on T1W scan. The high signal intensity has been attributed to the hyphae of the sinus and the accumulation of manganese associated with the fungal sinusitis. Other possibilities include calcification or iron within the secretions, accounting for the low signal. The walls of the sinuses may be expanded in a fashion similar to that of mucoceles or polyposis. The pattern of signal intensity and the pattern of contrast enhancement are different from those of mucoceles, however, which in general are more homogeneous in their signal intensity and show only peripheral rim enhancement. Fungal sinusitis may have an irregular filiform pattern of contrast enhancement. The signal intensity is more heterogeneous.

Although the pathogens associated with AFS include *Mucor, Curvularia, Bipolaris,* and *Aspergillus,* this is not a disease entity in which there is the marked invasiveness typically seen in aggressive infiltrative fungal sinusitis. Typical invasive fungal sinusitis tends to involve the cavernous sinus and may extend to the walls of the cavernous carotid artery. Vascular complications of invasive fungal sinusitis include cavernous sinus thrombosis and vasculitis with development of infarctions.

Notes

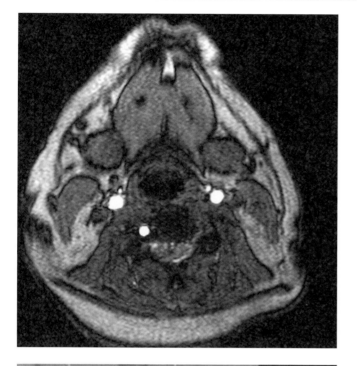

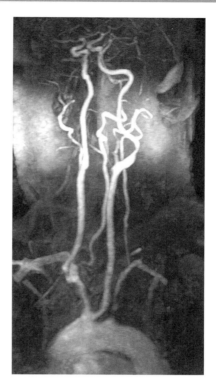

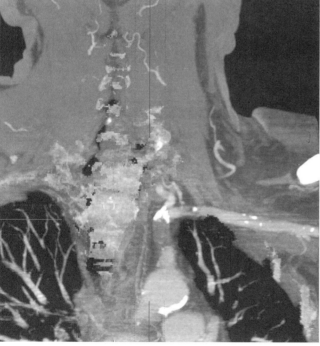

1. Where is the lesion in this entity?

2. Describe the findings on gadolinium-enhanced MRI.

3. Describe the features on three-dimensional time-of-flight (TOF) nonenhanced MRI.

4. Describe clinical symptoms.

Subclavian Steal

1. The proximal subclavian artery before the origin of the vertebral artery.

2. Both vertebral arteries and the stenosis are seen.

3. Only one vertebral artery and the stump of the subclavian artery are seen.

4. Early arm fatigue, ataxia, vertigo, and dizziness, all worse with arm exercise. Focal sensory or motor loss, dysphasia, and unilateral visual disturbances rarely may occur.

Reference

Shadman R, Criqui MH, Bundens WP, et al: Subclavian artery stenosis: prevalence, risk factors, and association with cardiovascular diseases, *J Am Coll Cardiol* 44:618–623, 2004.

Cross-Reference

Neuroradiology: THE REQUISITES, pp 180–183.

Comment

The risk of subclavian stenosis and steal phenomenon is increased in subjects with smoking history, hypertension, hypercholesterolemia, and peripheral artery disease in the legs. The prevalence of subclavian stenosis ranges from 1.9% to 7.1% in adults.

Staging of subclavian steal ranges from reduced antegrade vertebral flow (stage I), to reversal of flow during reactive hyperemia testing of the arm (stage II), to permanent retrograde vertebral flow (stage III) without exercise inducement.

One can explain the difference in the appearances of subclavian steal between the gadolinium-enhanced MRI pulse sequence and unenhanced TOF MRI by virtue of the flow saturation pulses typically applied (or not applied) in the two sequences. In TOF MRI without contrast administration (whether two-dimensional or three-dimensional), a superior flow saturation pulse is applied, eliminating venous downward flow. In the case of subclavian steal, one also saturates and eliminates the downward flowing vertebral artery as it goes to supply the distal upper extremity. For gadolinium-enhanced MRI, one relies on the temporal resolution for seeing the contrast in the vessels, and no saturation pulses are applied. In this scenario, one may see the affected vertebral artery and its (downward) flow potentially at the same time as the other arteries or more commonly delayed compared with the first arterial sample, even into the venous phase.

This is a diagnosis requiring some careful analysis of MRA images/techniques.

Notes

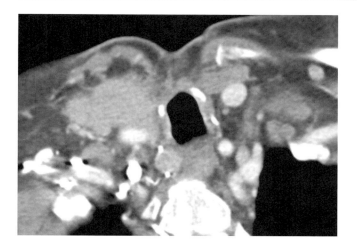
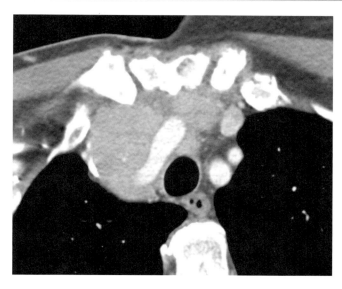

1. Which thyroid cancer is associated with multiple endocrine neoplasia type IIb?
2. Which thyroid cancer can cause high signal intensity lymph nodes on T1W images?
3. What T stage is a 3-cm papillary carcinoma?
4. Which differentiated thyroid cancer has the highest rate of distant metastases?

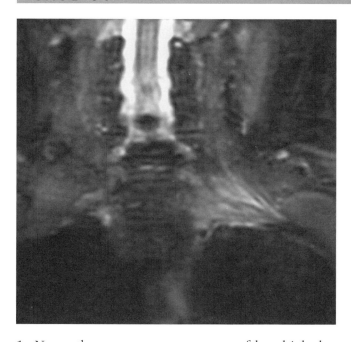
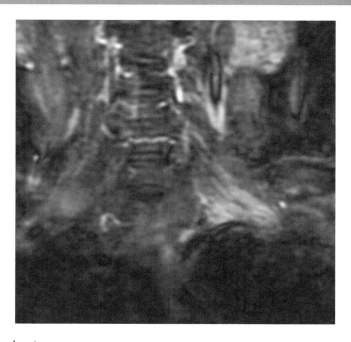

1. Name the most common cause of brachial plexopathy in a neonate.
2. What does it mean if the intrinsic muscles of the hand are weak?
3. What does it mean if there is deltoid weakness?
4. How does chronic inflammatory demyelinating polyneuropathy manifest in the brachial plexus?

CASE 60

Papillary Carcinoma of the Thyroid Gland

1. Medullary carcinoma.

2. Papillary (ones with colloid production).

3. T2 (T1 is <1 cm, T2 is 2 to 4 cm, T3 is >4 cm).

4. Follicular carcinoma.

Reference

Iwata M, Kasagi K, Misaki T, et al: Comparison of whole-body 18F-FDG PET, 99mTc-MIBI SPET, and post-therapeutic 131I-Na scintigraphy in the detection of metastatic thyroid cancer, *Eur J Nucl Med Mol Imaging* 31:491–498, 2004.

Cross-Reference

Neuroradiology: THE REQUISITES, pp 740–745.

Comment

Papillary carcinoma of the thyroid gland has many different manifestations, primarily in the thyroid gland and with respect to its metastases. This tumor may show adenopathy, which is bright on T1W scans because of the presence of colloid in the lymph node or because of hemorrhage. In addition, cystic, hypervascular, and calcified lymph nodes may be seen with papillary carcinoma in the thyroid gland.

The primary tumor may show the psammomatous calcifications represented as microcalcifications in the lesion, or it may show more chunky calcifications. Another primary manifestation of papillary carcinoma is a nodule within a cyst in the thyroid gland; this nodule also may show small calcifications.

Hematogenous metastases from papillary carcinoma may be hemorrhagic or cystic. Micrometastases in a papillary fashion in the lungs also have been described. Fluorodeoxyglucose positron emission tomography has been shown to be superior to technetium-99m MIBI and iodine-131 scintigraphy in detecting metastases of follicular and papillary carcinomas of the thyroid gland.

Notes

CASE 61

Brachial Plexitis

1. Shoulder dystocia delivery leading to root avulsions.

2. Lower cervical nerve root injury (C7-T1).

3. Upper C5-6 injury.

4. Enlarged nerve roots, bright on T2W scan and most often enhancing.

Reference

Zhou L, Yousem DM, Chaudhry V: Role of magnetic resonance neurography in brachial plexus lesions, *Muscle Nerve* 30:305–309, 2004.

Cross-Reference

Neuroradiology: THE REQUISITES, pp 734–736.

Comment

Use the mnemonic "*r*ad *t*echs *d*rink *c*old *b*eer" to identify the levels of the brachial plexus from the *r*oots, *t*runks, *c*ords, *d*ivisions, and *b*ranches. The brachial plexus is derived from the C5 through T1 nerve roots. In general, the roots and upper, middle, and lower trunks are seen from the midportion of the anterior scalene muscle back to the vertebrae.

From the midportion of the scalene muscle to the clavicle, one sees the anterior and posterior divisions of the brachial plexus. At the clavicular level, one begins to identify the lateral, posterior, and middle cords. Beyond the clavicle, one usually is dealing with the branches of the nerves to the arm.

The brachial plexus in infants usually is injured secondary to birth trauma and shoulder dystocia, leading to either Erb palsy or Klumpke palsy. Trauma from yanking on a child's arm also may lead to brachial plexus injury.

In adults, the most common etiology for brachial plexus pathology is a viral plexitis. In older adults with neoplasms, one should consider a Pancoast tumor, breast cancer, lymphadenopathy from neoplasms, or radiation plexitis.

The University of Washington has optimized visualization of brachial plexus pathology through the use of custom-made surface coils, high-resolution imaging, and inversion recovery fast spin echo scanning of the anatomy. In general, brachial plexus pathology shows high signal intensity on the inversion recovery fast spin echo T2W scan and, in certain instances, also shows contrast enhancement. High signal intensity is less commonly seen in viral and radiation-induced plexitis as opposed to chronic idiopathic demyelinating polyneuropathy.

Notes

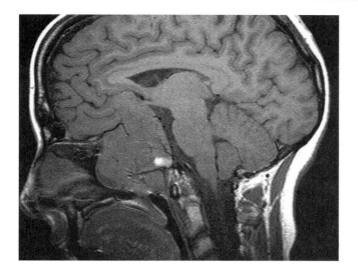

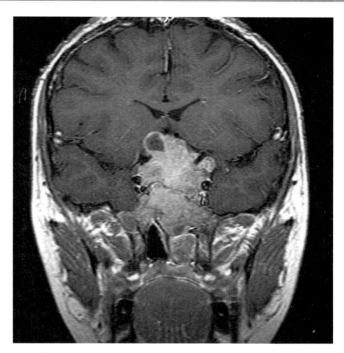

1. At which percentage of encasement of the carotid wall is cavernous sinus invasion suggested?

2. What is the implication if the carotid sulcus venous compartment (inferomedial to the cavernous internal carotid artery) is not visualized?

3. *True or False:* There is a higher rate of postoperative CSF leak in a patient with a pituitary adenoma with cavernous sinus invasion versus one without invasion.

4. What percentage of pituitary adenomas invade the cavernous sinus?

Pituitary Adenoma

1. >67% of the internal carotid artery wall encased.

2. Cavernous sinus invasion.

3. True.

4. 6% to 10%.

Reference

Cottier JP, Destrieux C, Brunereau L, et al: Cavernous sinus invasion by pituitary adenoma: MR imaging, *Radiology* 215:463–469, 2000.

Cross-Reference

Neuroradiology: THE REQUISITES, pp 532–534.

Comment

Cavernous sinus invasion by pituitary adenomas is important from the standpoint of marked elevation of hormonal levels when the tumor has access to the venous system of the cavernous sinus. In addition, it makes surgical extirpation much more difficult and unlikely via a transsphenoidal approach. In many cases, the surgeon simply decompresses the tumor mass in the midline, then tries to deal with the adenoma hormonally or via radiation therapy if there is cavernous sinus disease.

The best criteria for showing cavernous sinus involvement are predicated on drawing lines along the medial-most margin of the turns of the carotid artery in the cavernous sinus, the midpoint of the carotid artery within the two turns of the cavernous carotid artery, and the lateral wall of the carotid artery within the cavernous sinus loops. Tumor that is lateral to the lateral wall margin line of the cavernous carotid artery is said to be infiltrating the cavernous sinus 100% of the time. Tumor that is between the midpoint of the cavernous carotid artery and the lateral wall infiltrates the cavernous sinus approximately 54% of the time. Tumor that is medial to the midpoint of the cavernous lumen in general is not infiltrating the cavernous sinus. If tumor is identified inferior and medial to the inferiormost loop of the carotid artery in the cavernous sinus, in the carotid sulcus venous compartment, this generally suggests there is involvement of the cavernous sinus. This inferior extension is the exception to the aforementioned marginal criteria.

If the carotid artery is narrowed by the neoplasm that is growing into the cavernous sinus, one should consider another pathologic entity besides pituitary adenoma: most often a meningioma. Nonetheless, if the pituitary adenoma has been histologically proven, and this narrowing is seen, one should assume that cavernous sinus invasion has occurred.

Besides the cavernous sinus, the impact of sellar tumors on the optic nerves and optic chiasms should be discussed in any report on a mass in this location.

Notes

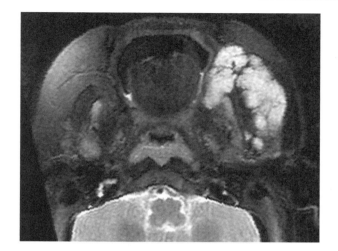

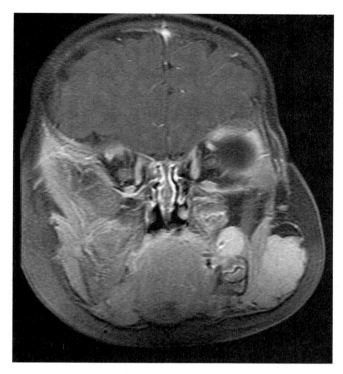

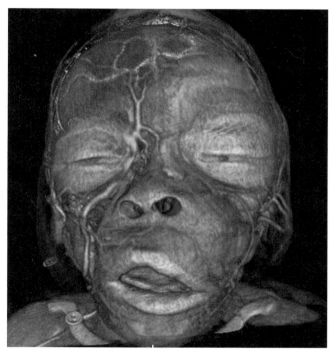

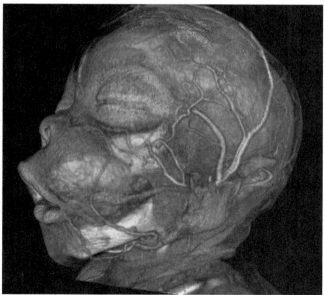

1. What is the differential diagnosis?

2. Which lesion regresses with age, a capillary hemangioma or a low-flow venous malformation?

3. Which lesion has increased endothelial turnover, a capillary hemangioma or a low-flow vascular malformation?

4. Identify the indications for treatment of head and neck low-flow vascular malformations.

Low-Flow Vascular Malformation

1. Venous vascular malformation, schwannoma, neurofibroma, and fibromatosis.

2. A capillary hemangioma.

3. A capillary hemangioma.

4. Pain, recurrent bleeding, malocclusion, airway obstruction, cosmetic deformity, speech impediment, and dysphagia.

Reference

Boll DT, Merkle EM, Lewin JS: Low-flow vascular malformations: MR-guided percutaneous sclerotherapy in qualitative and quantitative assessment of therapy and outcome, *Radiology* 233:376–384, 2004.

Cross-Reference

Neuroradiology: THE REQUISITES, pp 232–234.

Comment

The description of arteriovenous malformations of the soft tissues of the face has undergone a revision of nomenclature. The lesions are separated on the basis of involvement of the arterial, venous, capillary, or lymphatic system, or are classified in terms of low-flow versus high-flow vascular malformations. In most cases, capillary and venous vascular malformations are low-flow lesions, whereas true arterial venous malformations or arterial venous fistulas are high-flow states.

In the common vernacular, people generally use the term *hemangioma* for nearly all nonlymphatic vascular malformations of the soft tissues of the head and neck. Nonetheless, most students of the topic now use the term *capillary hemangioma* to refer to the lesion that is present at birth and that generally regresses through adolescence or maturity or with the prodding of steroids or laser therapy. These lesions include the "stork bite" of infancy or other red-hued lesions of the skin and soft tissues that resolve with age. The other lesion that was referred to as a hemangioma (e.g., in the orbit) has been reclassified as a *venous vascular malformation.* This is a low-flow vascular lesion with venous channels. One might identify small calcifications representing phleboliths within a venous vascular malformation. Phleboliths would be unusual in a capillary hemangioma. Venous vascular malformations are found in the head and neck and have several associations with various congenital syndromes.

The treatment of high-flow vascular malformations of the head and neck usually requires coils, balloons, or other embolizing agents. Protection may be afforded by traps placed in the internal carotid artery to prevent distal embolizations. For low-flow vascular malformations, another strategy is required. In most cases, sclerotherapy is an option. Using sclerosing agents, such as ethanol-based products, makes sense because there is prolonged exposure of the epithelium of a low-flow malformation to the point where thrombosis and fibrosis can occur rather than rapid wash-through as in a high-flow state. Because of the potential complications of tissue necrosis and distal embolizations, careful monitoring of the effectiveness of this therapy is required.

Heretofore fluoroscopy has been the mainstay of the monitoring modality for sclerotherapy. MRI has the advantage over fluoroscopy of being able to see the vascular lesion in cross-section and can be used for guiding and monitoring the treatment. Although one might assume that the MRI-guided procedure would be a lengthy one, these usually can be performed successfully within a 90-minute time slot on the scanner. Swelling adjacent to the carotid sheath can be monitored closely by MRI and can be one factor used to decide when to terminate a sclerosing session. Often lesions require many therapeutic sessions, and recurrence is common.

Intralesional steroid injections, laser therapy, cytokine injections, cryosurgery, and surgical excision are other treatment options.

Notes

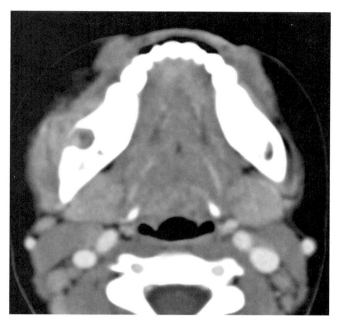

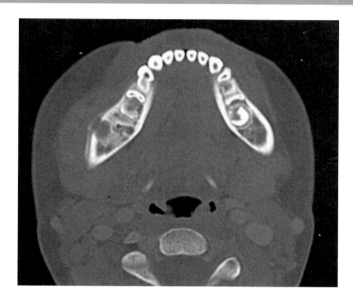

1. In which condition does noninfectious osteomyelitis occur at multiple sites?

2. What are the demographics of this condition?

3. What are the Munson criteria for chronic recurrent multifocal osteomyelitis?

4. What is the most common cause of osteomyelitis of the mandible?

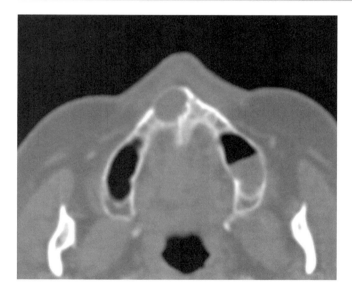

1. What is the differential diagnosis?

2. What is the etiology?

3. Identify synonyms for this entity.

4. What is the usual presentation?

CASE 64

Osteomyelitis of the Mandible

1. Chronic recurrent multifocal osteomyelitis.

2. Children age 4 to 14; girls affected five times more frequently than boys.

3. (1) Two radiographically confirmed bone lesions, (2) at least 6 months of remissions and exacerbations of signs and symptoms, (3) radiographic and bone scan evidence of osteomyelitis, (4) lack of response to antimicrobial therapy at least 1 month in duration, and (5) lack of an identifiable cause.

4. Dental caries > trauma > surgery.

Reference

Schuknecht B, Valavanis A: Osteomyelitis of the mandible, *Neuroimaging Clin N Am* 13:605–618, 2003.

Cross-Reference

Neuroradiology: THE REQUISITES, pp 796–798.

Comment

The imaging findings of osteomyelitis of the mandible include periosteal reaction, erosion, and sclerosis. Sclerosing osteomyelitis of Garre is an entity that has been described specifically in the case of mandibular osteomyelitis. Most commonly, the etiologic agent is dental caries with extension through the root of the tooth into the adjacent mandible. The spread of inflammation may be along the vascular channels, which enter the teeth from branches of the external carotid artery (internal maxillary artery, lingual artery, facial artery). The presence of a sequestrum or involucrum in cases of osteomyelitis of the mandible has a higher incidence of occurrence here than in other facial bone locations.

Another inflammatory mass is called *Kuttner tumor,* which is a chronic sclerosing sialadenitis of the submandibular gland. The Kuttner tumor resembles a submandibular gland malignant neoplasm clinically because of its presentation as a hard mass. This presents as a soft tissue mass below the mandible usually associated with inflammatory odontogenic disease.

Notes

CASE 65

Nasopalatine Cyst

1. Radicular cyst and globulomaxillary cyst.

2. Congenital resulting from epithelial rests causing cyst.

3. Incisive canal cyst, medial palatal cyst, and medial alveolar cyst.

4. Discovered incidentally.

Reference

Elliott KA, Franzese CB, Pitman KT: Diagnosis and surgical management of nasopalatine duct cysts, *Laryngoscope* 114:1336–1340, 2004.

Cross-Reference

Neuroradiology: THE REQUISITES, pp 660–661.

Comment

A nasopalatine cyst is the most common congenital cyst of the maxilla, occurring in 1% of the population and in males more commonly than females. Nasopalatine cysts are considered nonodontogenic congenital fissural cysts. They usually are found at the nasopalatine foramen, a hole that transmits branches of the maxillary nerve to the incisor teeth—hence the other term for this lesion, *incisive canal cyst.* The cyst is most often asymptomatic. Occasionally it grows large enough to present as a painless mass or with displacement of maxillary teeth. In such cases, enucleation of the cyst is warranted.

On MRI, these cysts are usually bright on T1W scans, thought to be due to keratin debris or high protein content. On CT, they are ovoid lesions that may assume a valentine shape when bilateral. Rarely they perforate anteriorly through the maxilla.

Globulomaxillary cysts arise between the lateral incisor and the canine teeth. Nasopalatine cysts arise between the two incisors. Globulomaxillary cysts splay the teeth apart more commonly than nasopalatine cysts. Median palatal cysts arise along the line of fusion between the two palatal processes or shelves of the maxilla and usually arise posterior to the typical locations of nasopalatine cysts. Nasolabial (nasoalveolar) cysts arise along the fusion line of the maxillary process, lateral nasal process, and globular process.

Notes

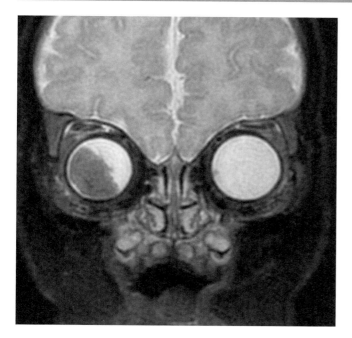

1. Name the classic clinical finding in a child with this disorder.
2. What are the genetics of this disease?
3. What is the unique finding of this tumor on CT?
4. Explain the significance of multifocality.

Bilateral Retinoblastoma

1. Leukokoria.

2. It is due to the deletion of the *Rb* gene on chromosome 13, which normally suppresses tumors. This is autosomal dominant.

3. Calcification in 90%.

4. It means that the patient has the gene, and the condition is harder to treat because bilateral enucleation is likely not an option.

Reference

Provenzale JM, Gururangan S, Klintworth G: Trilateral retinoblastoma: clinical and radiologic progression, *AJR Am J Roentgenol* 183:505–511, 2004.

Cross-Reference

Neuroradiology: THE REQUISITES, pp 479–483.

Comment

Retinoblastomas are the most common ocular malignancies of infancy. Most patients present before the age of 2 with leukokoria, the presence of a white pupillary reflex. The mean age of onset is 4.5 months. In 90% of cases, calcification occurs within the neoplasm. One third of cases of retinoblastoma are genetic in origin, and these cases may be bilateral.

The genetic defect associated with retinoblastoma is the deletion of the *Rb* gene, a tumor-suppressor gene found on chromosome 13. The *Rb* gene seems to regulate normal cell division. The absence of this gene accounts for the presence of an increased incidence of sarcoma in patients with familial retinoblastoma and the predilection for other primitive neuroectodermal tumors, including pineoblastomas. The mean age of diagnosis of the intracranial tumor is 26 months. Subarachnoid seeding is an issue.

As opposed to other entities that are associated with calcification in a small globe (phthisis bulbi, retinopathy of prematurity, and Coats disease), the globe in retinoblastoma is normal sized.

Contrast-enhanced fat-suppressed MRI of the orbit is the most sensitive imaging technique for detecting retinoblastomas of the globe. With the exception of von Hippel–Lindau disease and multiple hemangioblastomas, it would be unusual to see multiple ocular lesions in a child.

Radiation therapy and enucleation are the mainstays of treatment for retinoblastoma. The use of radiation therapy adds to the risk of subsequent sarcoma development, however.

Notes

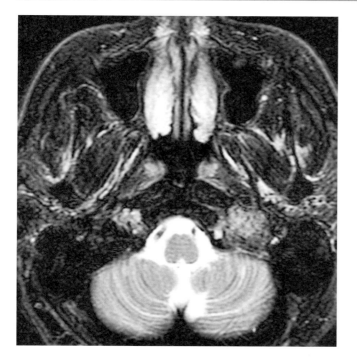 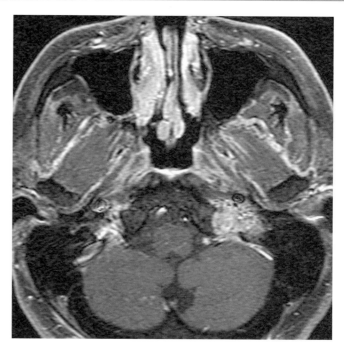

1. How often are paragangliomas multiple in sporadic cases?

2. How often are paragangliomas multiple in familial cases?

3. How does succinate dehydrogenase relate to paragangliomas?

4. What percentage of paragangliomas of the head and neck are inherited?

CASE 67

Paraganglioma; Glomus Jugulare

1. 3% to 5%.

2. 20% to 30%.

3. The gene encoding succinate dehydrogenase subunit D on chromosome 11 predisposes to multiple paragangliomas.

4. 35%.

Reference

Macdonald AJ, Salzman KL, Harnsberger HR, et al: Primary jugular foramen meningioma: imaging appearance and differentiating features, *AJR Am J Roentgenol* 182:373–377, 2004.

Cross-Reference

Neuroradiology: THE REQUISITES, pp 584–588.

Comment

The four major types of paraganglioma are glomus tympanicum, glomus jugulare, glomus vagale, and carotid body tumor. Of these, glomus jugulare and carotid body tumor are the most common lesions. As evident by their name, glomus jugulare tumors arise from paraganglia tissue in the jugular foramen region. These tumors occasionally grow to be extremely large and extend into the middle ear cavity, at which point they often are termed *glomus jugulotympanicum tumors*. Alternatively, they may extend inferiorly into the neck, growing around or within the jugular vein. The carotid body tumors occur at the carotid bifurcation and tend to splay the internal carotid artery and the external carotid artery apart. These lesions are noted for their speckled appearance partly because of potential flow voids from blood vessels and stroma from the tumor.

Glomus vagale tumors are unusual lesions that most commonly occur at the skull base or at the upper neck along the carotid sheath. They may be located in a similar position as vagus schwannomas. They may cause vagal nerve deficits, including vocal cord paralysis. When discovered, glomus vagale tumors are usually quite large. Because of the tinnitus associated with them, glomus jugulare and glomus tympanticum tumors may be caught earlier than glomus vagale and carotid body tumors.

A carotid body tumor is a hypervascular process, which splays the internal carotid artery and external carotid artery apart as it grows. The vasculature is fed by predominantly external carotid artery branches. Occasionally, one sees internal carotid artery unnamed branches in the proximal internal artery segment also supplying these tumors; because of this, preoperative embolization is recommended.

Rarely these tumors secrete epinephrine/norepinephrine–like substances that are vasoactive; this could result in patients' having hypertensive episodes precipitated by the injection of iodinated contrast material. For that reason, it has been recommended that vasoactive compounds be searched for in the urine collected before angiography or that the angiographer be prepared to treat a hypertensive episode acutely in the angiography suite with α-adrenergic blockers.

The differential diagnosis of a jugular foramen mass is limited; however, one should consider meningiomas; metastases from thyroid carcinoma, renal cell carcinoma, and melanoma; nasopharyngeal carcinoma; and schwannomas. A centrifugal infiltration of the skull base, a permeative-sclerotic appearance to the bony margins of the jugular foramen, prominent dural tails, and absence of flow voids distinguish primary jugular foramen meningioma from paraganglioma.

Notes

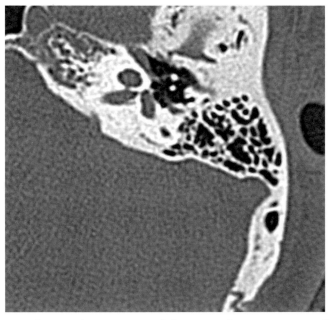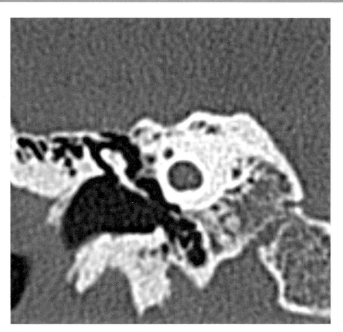

1. What is the term used for complete agenesis of the inner ear structures?

2. How many turns should a normal cochlea have?

3. Name the common congenital condition associated with inadequate spiralization of the cochlea.

4. Is the hearing loss in a Mondini malformation usually gradual or sudden?

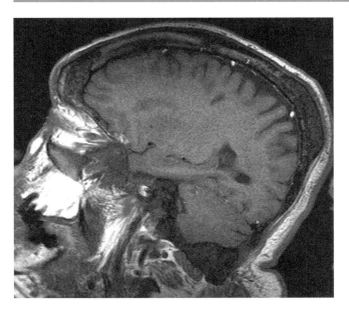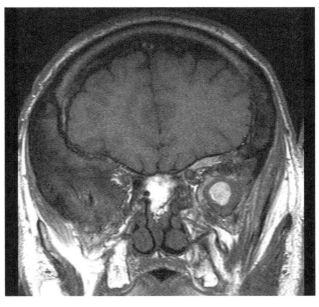

1. What percentage of polyostotic disease has hormonal abnormalities of precocious puberty and McCune-Albright syndrome?

2. What percentage of cases of fibrous dysplasia present with monostotic disease?

3. In what percentage of cases of McCune-Albright syndrome does sarcomatous degeneration develop?

4. How does resorption or displacement of the teeth help to make the diagnosis of cementoossifying fibroma?

Mondini Malformation

1. Michel deformity.

2. ≥2.5.

3. Enlarged vestibular aqueduct syndrome.

4. Sudden.

Reference

Naganawa S, Ito T, Iwayama E, et al: MR imaging of the cochlear modiolus: area measurement in healthy subjects and in patients with a large endolymphatic duct and sac, *Radiology* 213:819–823, 1999.

Cross-Reference

Neuroradiology: THE REQUISITES, pp 592–593.

Comment

Mondini malformation refers to incomplete spiralization of the modiolus of the cochlear. Normally there are 2.5 turns to the cochlea with reference to the basal, middle, and apical turns. The basal hair cells are responsible for the high-frequency sounds, whereas the apical hair cells transmit the lower frequency sounds.

Mondini malformation is associated with a defect generally occurring at 8 to 10 weeks of gestational age. Arrest of the spiralization of the cochlea occurs at this time. There may be associated dilation of the endolymphatic sac and vestibular aqueduct secondary to a defect at a similar time in gestation. Earlier in gestation, an arrest of development might result in a common cavity in the cochlea and the vestibule. This cavity often assumes a figure-of-eight conformation. Even earlier, one may have complete cochlear aplasia, in which the cochlea does not form. In these examples of abnormal development, one always should be cognizant of the potential of having an absent cochlear nerve, evaluated best on high-resolution MRI. For this determination, one should perform sagittal high-resolution T2W thin-section images through the internal auditory canal perpendicular to the plane of orientation of the cranial nerves. One is looking for the absence of the cochleal nerve in the anteroinferior portion of the internal auditory canal. The importance of an absent nerve is that surgical repair of the associated ossicular defects or implantation of a cochlear device to augment hearing would be ineffective without a nerve leading to the cochlea.

Notes

Fibrous Dysplasia; McCune-Albright Syndrome

1. 3%.

2. 75%.

3. 3%.

4. Cementoossifying fibroma resorbs or displaces the teeth; fibrous dysplasia does not.

Reference

MacDonald-Jankowski DS: Fibro-osseous lesions of the face and jaws, *Clin Radiol* 59:11–25, 2004.

Cross-Reference

Neuroradiology: THE REQUISITES, p 713.

Comment

McCune-Albright syndrome refers to polyostotic fibrous dysplasia with multiple café-au-lait spots and precocious puberty. Precocious puberty is defined as puberty occurring before 8 years of age in girls and 9.5 years of age in boys. This syndrome may be caused by hormonally active ovarian cysts in girls; 85% of girls with McCune-Albright syndrome have menstruation before 12 years of age. The syndrome is seen more commonly in girls than boys. The fibrous dysplasia of the facial bones most commonly affects the mandible and maxilla, but all facial bones may be affected. If involvement is diffuse and involves the upper skull and face, one may have the entity known as *leontiasis ossea*. In general, McCune-Albright syndrome is followed with bone scans to ascertain activity of disease. This syndrome also may be associated with soft tissue asymmetry and hemihypertrophy. McCune-Albright syndrome may be associated with multinodular goiter, acromegaly, and soft tissue myxomas (Mazabraud syndrome). The genetic defect is thought to be from the *GNAS1* gene, but the entity is a sporadic one without familial transmission. Seventy-five percent of cases of fibrous dysplasia are monostotic, and 25% are polyostotic.

McCune-Albright syndrome may be confused with neurofibromatosis, which also may have associated café-au-lait spots (which in McCune-Albright syndrome are irregular ["coast of Maine"] in shape and in neurofibromatosis are smooth ["coast of California"] in shape) and unilateral hypertrophy.

Notes

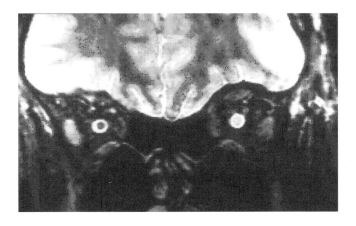
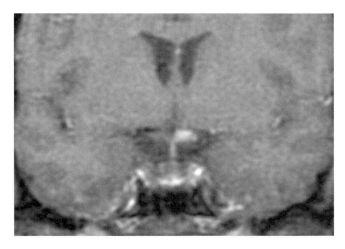

1. What percentage of patients with this diagnosis and a brain lesion develop multiple sclerosis (MS) in 10 years?

2. What pulse sequence shows demyelination in the optic nerves the earliest?

3. Name other sources of optic neuritis.

4. What are the Barkof criteria for MS?

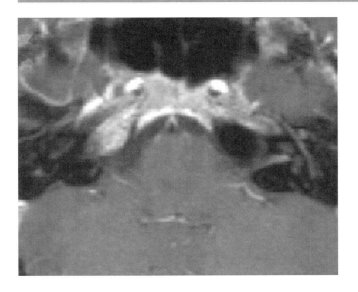
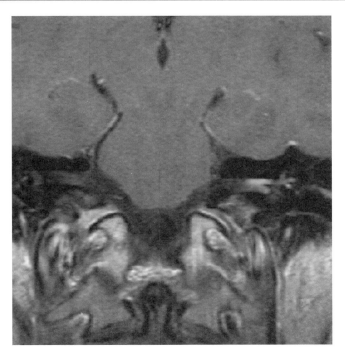

1. What is the eponym for herpes zoster oticus?

2. How would this patient present?

3. What are the structures that may be enhanced with this entity?

4. Is intraparotid facial nerve enhancement associated with this entity?

Optic Neuritis

1. 60%.

2. Gadolinium-enhanced fat-suppressed T1W scans.

3. Ischemia, virus, acute disseminated encephalomyelitis, sarcoidosis, compressive lesions, radiation therapy, Lyme disease, lupus, syphilis, and toxin.

4. The criteria of Barkof require 1 infratentorial lesion, 1 juxtacortical lesion, 3 periventricular lesions, and either 1 gadolinium-enhanced lesion or >9 lesions on T2W scans.

Reference

Jackson A, Sheppard S, Laitt RD, et al: Optic neuritis: MR imaging with combined fat- and water-suppression techniques, *Radiology* 206:57–63, 1998.

Cross-Reference

Neuroradiology: THE REQUISITES, pp 492–493.

Comment

Optic neuritis is a common manifestation of MS. It has been shown that >80% of individuals who have MS at some point over the course of their disease have an episode of optic neuritis. This episode usually is manifested by monocular visual blurring. With the animal model of MS, experimental allergic encephalomyelitis, the earliest feature of optic neuritis is contrast enhancement of the optic nerve rather than high signal intensity on T2W scan. Some have advocated using scans that have fat suppression and water suppression to identify the best optic neuritis within the optic nerve sheath complex on T2W/flair sequences.

If one evaluates isolated optic neuritis in a patient, the likelihood that the patient will develop MS within 5 years is approximately 50%. This percentage is increased significantly if the patient also has white matter lesions in the brain (although clinically silent). The combination of optic neuritis and transverse myelitis of the spinal cord is termed *Devic syndrome*, which typically has a more fulminant course than MS and which may be monophasic. This entity usually has a spinal cord abnormality that extends over many spinal segments, larger than typical MS plaques of the cord, which is solitary segment disease.

Variants of MS include the following:

Baló concentric sclerosis—concentric bands of demyelination and remyelination, seen in Asians
Devic syndrome—neuromyelitis optica
Marburg disease—acute fulminant MS
Schilder disease—childhood onset, cortical blindness secondary to occipital involvement, large bilateral lesions

Notes

Herpes Zoster Infection of the Seventh Cranial Nerve

1. Ramsay Hunt syndrome.

2. Facial nerve palsy, herpetic outbreak with pain around ear, dysequilibrium, tinnitus, and vertigo.

3. Cranial nerves VII and VIII in the internal auditory canal; geniculate ganglion and labyrinthine, tympanic, and mastoid segments of cranial nerve VII; cochlea; vestibule; and semicircular canals.

4. No.

Reference

Sartoretti-Schefer S, Kollias S, Valavanis A: Ramsay Hunt syndrome associated with brain stem enhancement, *AJNR Am J Neuroradiol* 20:278–280, 1999.

Cross-Reference

Neuroradiology: THE REQUISITES, p 290.

Comment

Ramsey Hunt syndrome refers to reactivation of shingles (varicella-zoster infection) involving cranial nerve VII. In this case, one sees clinically herpetic vesicles around the external ear region. These vesicles are exquisitely painful and may be distributed along the sensory distribution of cranial nerve VII, which affects portions of the external auditory canal and tympanic membrane. Intracranially, one may see enhancement of cranial nerve VII within the internal auditory canal and the labyrinthine portion, geniculate ganglion (presumably where the virus lies dormant), tympanic portion, and mastoid portion of cranial nerve VII. The patient may have tinnitus, vertigo, hearing loss, and facial nerve paralysis. Although the tympanic and mastoid portions may enhance normally secondary to the circumneural vascular plexus, the labyrinthine portion and internal auditory canal portion enhancement is decidedly unusual.

Herpes zoster ophthalmicus may affect branches of cranial nerve V within the orbit. Secondary extension to the optic nerve and optic nerve sheath can cause significant visual disturbances and pain within the orbit. Ischemic optic neuritis also may be superimposed.

Notes

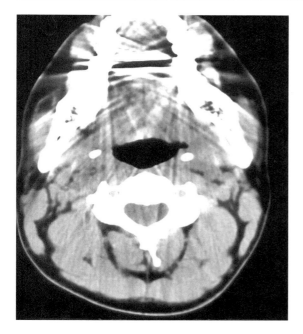

1. Why does this patient have a sticking pain that radiates to the ear when swallowing?
2. What innervates the stylohyoid, styloglossus, and stylopharyngeus muscles?
3. What is the treatment for this process?
4. Identify the clinical examination test that clinches the diagnosis.

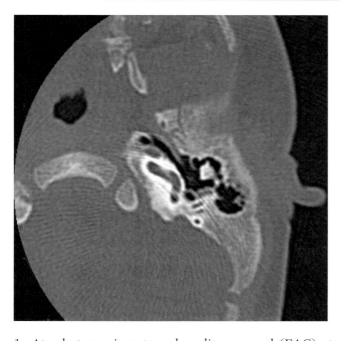
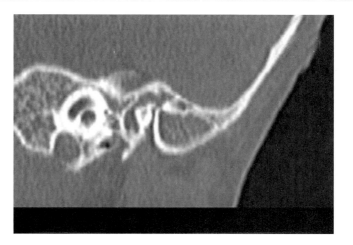

1. At what age is external auditory canal (EAC) atresia surgically treated and why?
2. How often are there concomitant inner ear anomalies?
3. How often are there anomalous locations of vessels with severe EAC dysplasia?
4. How often is the middle ear cavity small in EAC atresia?

CASE 72

Eagle Syndrome

1. The ligaments of the stylohyoid muscle are protruding along the submucosal space.

2. Cranial nerves VII, XII, and IX, respectively.

3. Surgical amputation of the stylohyoid ligament calcification, the styloid process.

4. Manual palpation of the ligament or elongated styloid process through the tonsillar fossa leading to patient's typical pain.

Reference

Mortellaro C, Biancucci P, Picciolo G, Vercellino V: Eagle's syndrome: importance of a corrected diagnosis and adequate surgical treatment, *J Craniofac Surg* 13:755–758, 2002.

Cross-Reference

Neuroradiology: THE REQUISITES, p 653.

Comment

Elongation of the styloid process or stylohyoid ligament ossification or both occur in 33% of women and 29% of men. The pain, sometimes termed *styalgia,* occurs with the head turned and on swallowing. In some cases, the sensation experienced has nothing to do with the styloid process, but in other cases, relief occurs when anesthetics and corticosteroids are injected in the same location.

The styloid process is normally <3 cm in length, but is >3 cm in 4% to 7% of the population. Of these, <10% are symptomatic. All three of the muscles mentioned in question 2 arise from the styloid process. It is unclear whether compression of one of the nerves that innervate the muscles or the trigeminal nerve is the source of the patient's pain.

Notes

CASE 73

External Auditory Canal Atresia

1. Usually at 4 to 5 years old in preparation for school.

2. 13%.

3. 38%.

4. 27% to 63%.

References

Gassner EM, Mallouhi A, Jaschke WR: Preoperative evaluation of external auditory canal atresia on high-resolution CT, *AJR Am J Roentgenol* 182:1305–1312, 2004.

Mayer TE, Brueckmann H, Siegert R, et al: High-resolution CT of the temporal bone in dysplasia of the auricle and external auditory canal, *AJNR Am J Neuroradiol* 18:53–65, 1997.

Cross-Reference

Neuroradiology: THE REQUISITES, pp 565–567.

Comment

EAC atresia is a defect related to the first branchial apparatus. The first branchial cleft creates the EAC. The branchial pouch endoderm creates the eustachian tube and tympanic cavity. The first branchial arch helps to create the mandible, malleus, incus, muscles of mastication, mylohyoid, tensor veli palatini, and tensor tympani muscle. The nerve that is associated with the first branchial apparatus is cranial nerve V; mandible abnormalities frequently coexist with ear abnormalities (e.g., Treacher Collins syndrome and Pierre Robin syndrome).

EAC atresia occurs bilaterally in approximately 30% of cases. It is a more common phenomenon than EAC stenosis, in which the lumen of the EAC is merely narrowed. Ossicular anomalies occur in most cases of EAC atresia. Inner ear anomalies arise only in 10% to 20%. The temporomandibular joint is often anomalous in association with auditory canal atresia.

When evaluating a patient with EAC atresia, it is important to mark the location of the internal carotid artery, jugular vein, and facial nerve to assist the otologist in appropriate presurgical planning.

Notes

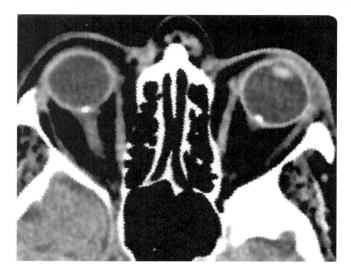

1. How often is this entity bilateral?

2. How is this entity distinguished from retinoblastoma?

3. What are the symptoms?

4. What is the treatment?

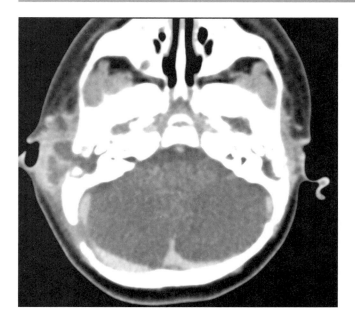 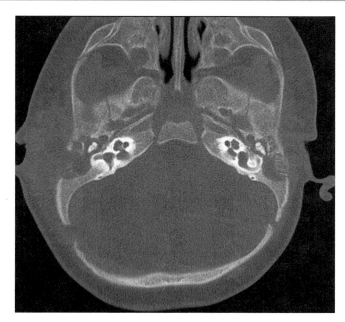

1. What finding suggests an aggressive infection in this individual?

2. What site is the usual source of coalescent mastoiditis?

3. Name the most common pathogen.

4. Name three sites that are most commonly eroded in coalescent mastoiditis.

CASE 74

Optic Nerve Drusen

1. 70%.

2. Retinoblastoma occurs in children; optic nerve head drusen occur in later life.

3. Usually asymptomatic; rarely, visual acuity diminution is present.

4. There is no treatment.

Reference

Ramirez H, Blatt ES, Hibri NS: Computed tomographic identification of calcified optic nerve drusen, *Radiology* 148:137–139, 1983.

Cross-Reference

Neuroradiology: THE REQUISITES, pp 491–492.

Comment

Optic nerve drusen are tiny calcifications at the optic nerve head insertion of the globe. These represent senescent hyaline deposits or calcifications or both that usually have no clinical significance. When prominent, they create the appearance on ophthalmoscopy of papilledema because the optic nerve head insertion may be raised. This appearance might suggest to the clinician the presence of increased intracranial pressure. On the contrary, the patient's intracranial pressure is normal, and this is an example of pseudopapilledema. Occasionally, drusen may be associated with macular degeneration, which is one of the most common causes of blindness in the elderly. These drusen are not depicted at the optic nerve head and may be seen as a patchy area of blanching of the normal retinal pigment.

Other senescent calcifications associated with the globe include calcifications at the insertion sites of the rectus muscles and at the superior oblique tendinous trochlea.

Notes

CASE 75

Coalescent Mastoiditis

1. Bony septae destruction implying coalescent mastoiditis soft tissue mass.

2. Otitis media.

3. *Streptococcus pneumoniae.*

4. (1) The cortical plate overlying the sigmoid sinus, (2) the air cell septa, and (3) the lateral wall of the mastoid air cells.

Reference

Vazquez E, Castellote A, Piqueras J, et al: Imaging of complications of acute mastoiditis in children, *Radiographics* 23:359–372, 2003.

Cross-Reference

Neuroradiology: THE REQUISITES, pp 575–583.

Comment

Although otomastoiditis is a relatively benign entity common in children and thought to be due in part to eustachian tube obstruction secondary to adenoidal tissue in children, in some cases it may be due to a defect in the mucociliary clearance down the eustachian tube as well. Otomastoiditis is a condition readily treatable with conservative measures and decongestants and antibiotics.

With coalescent mastoiditis, one sees loss of the septations of the mastoid air cells, and consequently sclerosis is seen in the septations of the mastoid air cells that remain; this indicates the presence of subtle osteomyelitis of the mastoid air cells. This becomes a difficult infection to eradicate and often requires intravenous antibiotics. Complications of coalescent mastoiditis include thrombophlebitis, thrombosis of venous sinuses, and development of epidural abscess formation.

The imaging findings that suggest coalescent mastoiditis are the loss of the septations and the sclerosis of the bone. How does one distinguish between a cholesteatoma affecting the mastoid bowl versus coalescent mastoiditis? In general, patients with coalescent mastoiditis are much sicker and have acute infection, whereas patients with cholesteatoma present with hearing loss and a chronic indolent course. The middle ear is not enlarged with coalescent mastoiditis, although it is often completely opacified.

Notes

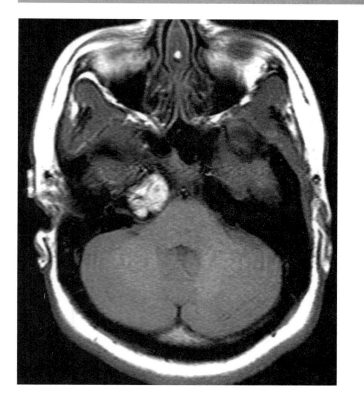
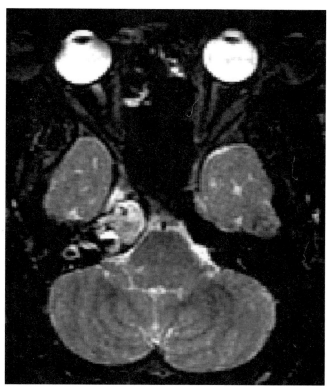
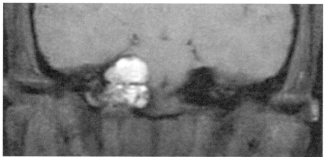
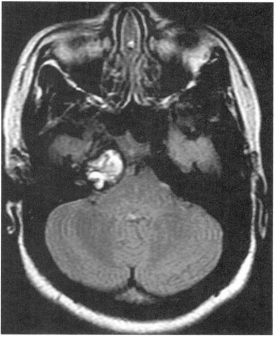

1. What is the differential diagnosis for this lesion?

2. Identify the mechanism of development of a cholesterol granuloma.

3. Where do cholesterol granulomas occur most frequently?

4. What is Gradenigo syndrome?

Petrous Apex Cholesterol Granuloma

1. Cholesterol granuloma, mucocele, aneurysm with clot, hemorrhagic metastasis, and epidermoid.

2. A hemorrhagic foreign body reaction.

3. Middle ear > petrous apex > dental.

4. Otitis/otorrhea, facial pain, and cranial nerve VI palsy.

Reference

Warakaulle DR, Anslow P: Differential diagnosis of intracranial lesions with high signal on T1 or low signal on T2-weighted MRI, *Clin Radiol* 58:922–933, 2003.

Cross-Reference

Neuroradiology: THE REQUISITES, pp 600–602.

Comment

One of the classic imaging diagnoses is that of a petrous apex cholesterol granuloma. This lesion is due to recurrent hemorrhage and foreign body reaction within the aerated petrous apex. Considering that only one third of individuals normally have aeration of the petrous apex, cholesterol granuloma is infrequently diagnosed. Most commonly, the difficulty arises in patients who have T1W scans and non–fat-suppressed spin echo T2W scans, at which time a fatty replaced petrous apex that is bright on T1W scans and bright on T2W scans might simulate the subacute blood products seen with cholesterol granuloma, which is also bright on T1W scans and bright on T2W scans. For this reason, we advocate performing fat-saturated T2W fast spin echo scans through the brain so as to depress the fat and eliminate the confusion.

In general, cholesterol granulomas expand the bone and thin the walls of the petrous apex. They may come in contiguity with the petrous portion of the internal carotid artery, and the differential diagnosis then includes a pseudoaneurysm with thrombosis of the petrous internal carotid artery.

Patients' symptoms generally include hearing loss, tinnitus, and headache. It is possible in some patients to drain the cholesterol granuloma through the sphenoid sinus with an endoscopic approach.

Notes

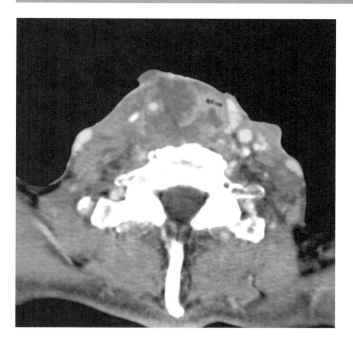

1. What is the implication of the encasement of the carotid artery with the mass in this case?
2. If this patient already has been irradiated, what is the additional risk?
3. What is the most common tumor to encase the internal carotid artery?
4. Identify the best criterion to determine carotid encasement that cannot be cured surgically.

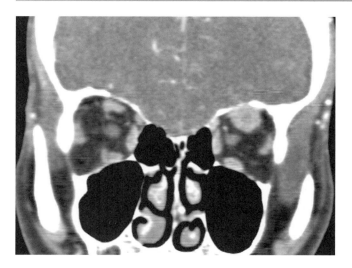

1. Name the causes of superior rectus enlargement.
2. What muscle is most commonly affected by Horner syndrome?
3. What primary tumor goes to the orbit most frequently?
4. Where do most breast metastases to the orbit lodge?

Carotid Encasement

1. The carotid artery must be sacrificed for cure.

2. Carotid blowout with hemorrhage into the neck.

3. Pituitary adenoma.

4. 270 degrees of circumferential involvement.

Reference

Yousem DM, Hatabu H, Hurst RW, et al: Carotid artery invasion by head and neck masses: prediction with MR imaging, *Radiology* 195:715–720, 1995.

Cross-Reference

Neuroradiology: THE REQUISITES, pp 689, 728–729.

Comment

When a patient has a neoplastic process that is encasing the carotid artery, the surgeon asks: Can this lesion be resected from the carotid artery, and can clean margins be obtained? By clean margins, the surgeon generally means no evidence of macroscopic disease.

To address these questions, one might use criteria that include intraluminal neoplasms in the vessel wall or look for irregularity in the wall of the blood vessel or enhancement of the blood vessel. These findings are either insensitive (intraluminal tumor) or nonspecific (enhancement of the wall in the artery). It has been shown that circumferential involvement of the carotid artery of >270 degrees is a reliable predictor of whether or not the surgeon would be able to resect the tumor off the carotid artery in a curative peel. With tumor involving >270 degrees of the carotid circumference, this is virtually impossible to do, and the carotid artery is thought to be infiltrated. Such is the case with most carcinomas. In patients who have mucoid lesions, such as chordomas, presumably the surgeon can suck the tumor off of the vessel wall and still have clean margins.

Notes

Breast Metastasis to the Orbit

1. Thyroid eye disease, pseudotumor, vascular congestion, lymphoma, sarcoidosis, and metastasis.

2. Levator palpebrae muscle.

3. Breast.

4. The choroid of the globe.

References

Dieing A, Schulz CO, Schmid P, et al: Orbital metastases in breast cancer: report of two cases and review of the literature, *J Cancer Res Clin Oncol* 130:745–748, 2004 (Epub Sept 7, 2004).

Shields JA, Shields CL, Scartozzi R: Survey of 1264 patients with orbital tumors and simulating lesions: the 2002 Montgomery Lecture, part 1, *Ophthalmology* 111: 997–1008, 2004.

Cross-Reference

Neuroradiology: THE REQUISITES, pp 501–503, 512–513.

Comment

In a survey of 1264 orbital masses, the listing included 64% benign causes and 36% malignant causes. Vascular lesions (including hemangiomas and venous vascular malformations) accounted for 17% of the total; inflammatory lesions, 11%; lymphoma and leukemia, 10%; lacrimal gland lesions, 9%; optic nerve lesions, 8%; and metastases, 7%. Rhabdomyosarcoma was the most common malignancy in children, and lymphoma was the most common in adults.

Most orbital metastases from breast cancers lodge in the choroid of the globe followed by the anterior chamber. These metastases may cause blurred vision or glaucoma; both may cause orbital pain. When choroidal metastases are found, they are bilateral in 20% to 40% of patients. Only 3% to 10% occur outside the globe. On autopsy specimens, 10% to 30% of patients dying from breast cancer have orbital/ocular metastases, but few of these metastases manifest clinically. The ones that do usually also have brain or bone metastases or both.

One should always think of breast cancer if enophthalmos and an orbital mass are present. The scirrhous variety is causative.

Treatment is with local radiotherapy of 32 to 50 Gy. Median survival time in a patient with breast cancer and clinically evident ocular metastases is 5 to 17 months.

Notes

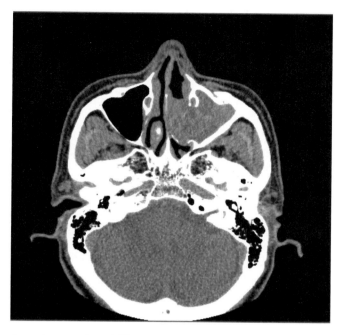

1. What is the differential diagnosis?

2. What percentage of polyps are antrochoanal?

3. What is the characteristic shape?

4. What would solid nodular enhancement imply?

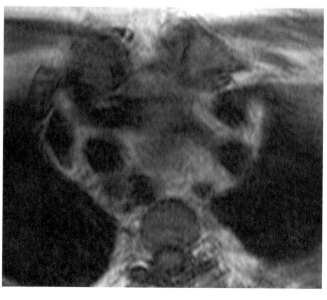 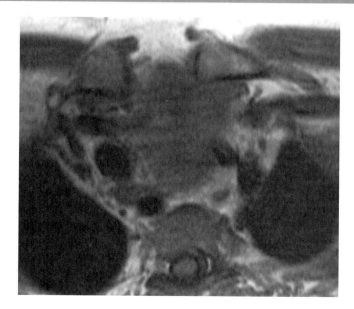

1. What is the cause of this patient's dysphagia?

2. What is the usual presentation for this phenomenon?

3. Which vascular loop is at fault?

4. What is the most common variation in the branches of the aortic arch?

CASE 79

Antrochoanal Polyp

1. Mucocele, inverted papilloma, and cephalocele.

2. 3% to 6% of all polyps.

3. Dumbbell.

4. More likely a neoplasm.

Reference

De Vuysere S, Hermans R, Marchal G: Sinochoanal polyp and its variant, the angiomatous polyp: MRI findings, *Eur Radiol* 11:55–58, 2001.

Cross-Reference

Neuroradiology: THE REQUISITES, pp 629–631.

Comment

An antrochoanal polyp is a unique polyp, which is often seen causing complete opacification of the maxillary antrum. This polyp extends into the nasal cavity and even into the nasopharynx through either the accessory maxillary sinus ostium or the maxillary ostium itself. It usually expands that opening and causes displacement of bony walls. There is a grading system of description for the antrochoanal polyp, which describes its limitations to the maxillary sinus, the nasal cavity, or the nasopharynx. These lesions are rarely bilateral and need not be associated with sinonasal polyps or sinusitis. An antrochoanal polyp may arise as an isolated lesion within the sinonasal cavity. In a similar fashion, one may have ethmochoanal or sphenochoanal polyps.

Angiomatous polyps (which enhance diffusely) may coexist with nonenhancing antrochoanal polyps.

On MRI, antrochoanal polyps usually are quite bright on T2W scans and show peripheral enhancement characteristics that differentiate them from an inverted papilloma.

Notes

CASE 80

Aberrant Subclavian Artery

1. Aberrant right subclavian artery.

2. It usually is discovered incidentally.

3. Right fourth dorsal aorta vascular loop regression.

4. "Bovine origin" of the left common carotid artery from the innominate artery.

Reference

Donnelly LF, Fleck RJ, Pacharn P, et al: Aberrant subclavian arteries: cross-sectional imaging findings in infants and children referred for evaluation of extrinsic airway compression, *AJR Am J Roentgenol* 178:1269–1274, 2002.

Cross-Reference

Neuroradiology: THE REQUISITES, pp 180–183.

Comment

Aberrant right subclavian artery refers to a right subclavian artery that passes behind the esophagus from the distal aortic arch to reach the right axilla. This looping around the esophagus and behind the trachea is derived from a persistence of one of the six aortic arches that are created as part of the branchial system of development. Involution of the right fourth vascular loop from the right dorsal aorta (which normally would form the right subclavian artery from the innominate artery) leads to the seventh intersegmental artery assuming this supply from the descending aorta. Aberrant right subclavian arteries occur in 0.5% to 1.8% of the general population. They are more common in patients with Down syndrome.

Aberrant subclavian arteries can cause dysphagia lusoria (dysphagia by a freak of nature) secondary to the compression of the posterior wall of the esophagus. Occasionally, there is a diverticulum (of Kommerell) that may lead to more prominent swallowing symptoms.

Notes

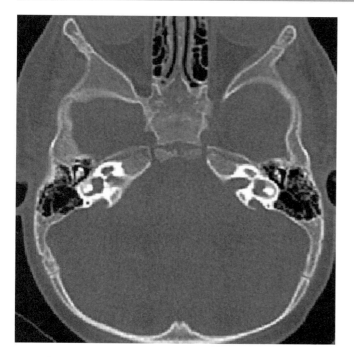

1. What is the upper limit of size allowable for the vestibular aqueduct?

2. What is the incidence of concurrent cochlear anomaly?

3. How commonly is this finding encountered bilaterally?

4. What are the ramifications of a calcified mass associated with the vestibular aqueduct?

Enlarged Vestibular Aqueduct

1. 1.5 mm.

2. 100%.

3. 90%.

4. Consider endolymphatic sac tumor.

Reference

Yuen HY, Ahuja AT, Wong KT, et al: Computed tomography of common congenital lesions of the temporal bone, *Clin Radiol* 58:687–693, 2003.

Cross-Reference

Neuroradiology: THE REQUISITES, pp 594–595.

Comment

The terms *large endolymphatic sac anomaly* and *large vestibular aqueduct syndrome* refer to the same entity. One can assess for this entity either by measuring the transverse width of the vestibular aqueduct or by comparing the size of the aqueduct with that of the lateral semicircular canal (it should be equal to or smaller than the lateral semicircular canal). On high-resolution MRI, a visible sac in the posterior fossa usually implies abnormality. The presence of cochlear dysplasia with incomplete partition occurs at a high rate with enlarged vestibular aqueducts; this affects the apical turn most frequently.

This entity occurs as a result of an embryologic anomaly in week 7 of gestation at the same time that cochlear development is occurring. It is considered the most common form of congenital hearing loss, but the hearing loss is usually from the concurrent cochlear malformation rather than the vestibular aqueduct. The hearing loss deteriorates over time, often with traumatic episodes.

Pendred syndrome may be related to large vestibular aqueduct syndrome in that it is the most common cause of syndromic bilateral sensorineural deafness, accounting for >5% of all autosomal recessive hearing loss cases. It is characterized by the coexistence of goitrous thyroid glands with or without hypothyroidism.

Notes

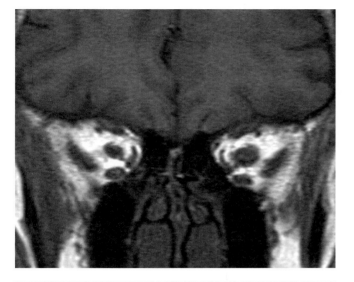

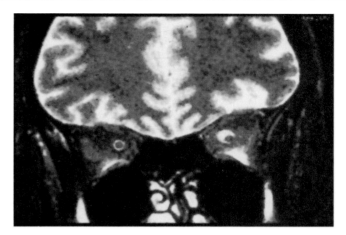

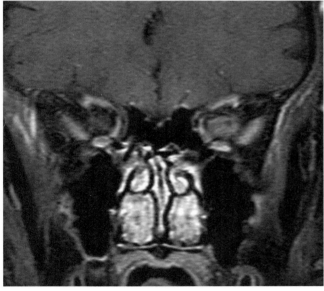

1. Which is more common, optic sheath meningioma or optic nerve glioma?

2. What is the ratio of benign to malignant neoplasms of the orbit?

3. How often is calcification seen in optic nerve sheath meningiomas?

4. What does the Simpson grade refer to?

Optic Nerve Meningioma

1. Optic sheath meningiomas.

2. 2:1 in favor of benign.

3. 30%.

4. Degree of resection:

   Grade I—macroscopically complete removal of dura, bone
   Grade II—macroscopically complete removal, dural coagulation
   Grade III—complete tumor resection, dura not coagulated
   Grade IV—partial removal
   Grade V—simple decompression

Reference

Shields JA, Shields CL, Scartozzi R: Survey of 1264 patients with orbital tumors and simulating lesions: the 2002 Montgomery Lecture, part 1, *Ophthalmology* 111:997–1008, 2004.

Cross-Reference

Neuroradiology: THE REQUISITES, pp 496–497.

Comment

Visual loss occurs earlier with optic nerve meningioma than it does with optic nerve gliomas. One might think that a lesion of the nerve itself would cause greater deficits than a lesion that affects the sheath but not the nerve. This paradox can be explained by several factors, not least of which is that the optic nerve glioma is a very low grade astrocytoma that does not disrupt the intrinsic architecture of the nerve until relatively late in the course, allowing function to be maintained. The optic nerve meningioma is a lesion that compromises the arterial supply and venous outflow of the vasculature to the optic nerve. The meningioma itself is not intrinsically affecting or disrupting the nerve. The deficits that occur with an optic nerve meningioma are based more on an ischemic optic neuropathy than on a neoplastic etiology. This is even more so if the optic nerve meningioma affects the nerve at the orbital apex, where the ability to accommodate the additional volume of the meningioma is limited.

With respect to associations within the orbit, the optic nerve glioma is associated with neurofibromatosis 1. The presence of multiple meningiomas may be a manifestation of neurofibromatosis 2, however.

The lower the Simpson grade, the lower the chance of recurrence.

Notes

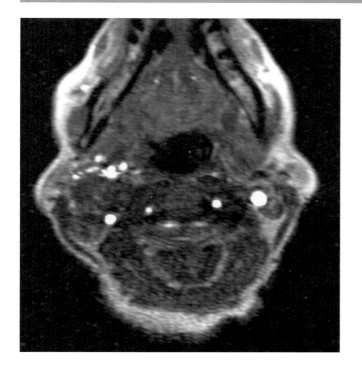
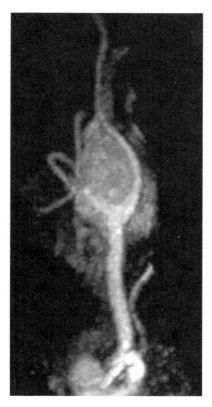

1. Identify the cell of origin of this tumor.

2. What other lesions can arise at the bifurcation of the carotid arteries?

3. Can paragangliomas metastasize?

4. What is the most common site of head and neck paragangliomas?

Carotid Body Tumor

1. Neuroendocrine cells from paraganglia.

2. Aneurysms, pseudoaneurysms, nodal metastases, Bailey type 3 branchial cleft cysts, and schwannomas.

3. Yes.

4. Carotid bifurcation.

Reference

Pellitteri PK, Rinaldo A, Myssiorek D, et al: Paragangliomas of the head and neck, *Oral Oncol* 40:563–575, 2004.

Cross-Reference

Neuroradiology: THE REQUISITES, pp 727–728.

Comment

A carotid body tumor is one of the tumors identified as a paraganglioma. This lesion is a hypervascular process, which splays apart the internal and external carotid arteries as it grows. The vasculature is fed by predominantly external carotid artery branches. Occasionally, one sees internal carotid artery unnamed branches in the proximal internal artery segment also supplying these tumors. Because of this, preoperative embolization is recommended.

Rarely these tumors secrete vasoactive epinephrine/norepinephrine–like substances. This secretion could result in patients having hypertensive episodes precipitated by the injection of iodinated contrast material. For that reason, it has been recommended that vasoactive compounds be searched for in the urine collected before angiography or that the angiographer be prepared to treat a hypertensive episode acutely in the angiography suite with α-adrenergic blockers.

Differential diagnosis is limited; however, one should consider hypervascular lymph nodes from thyroid carcinoma, renal cell carcinoma, and melanoma and schwannomas in the differential diagnosis.

Surgery is curative when complete excision is performed. Rarely the carotid artery must be patched or even resected with the tumor.

Notes

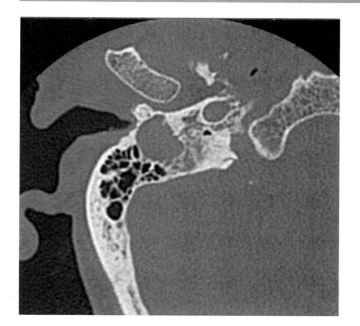

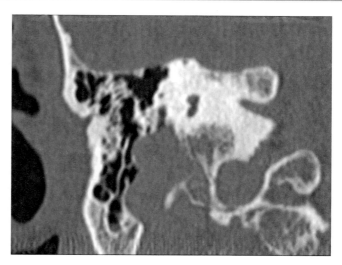

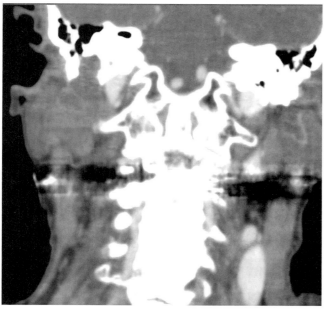

1. Where is this lesion located?

2. Given its location, what are possible diagnoses?

3. How often do schwannomas not enhance?

4. Would you expect lacrimation to be affected in this case?

Facial Nerve Schwannoma

1. Descending portion of the facial nerve canal.

2. Facial nerve schwannoma (neurogenic tumors), perineural spread of malignancy, neurofibroma, hemangioma, and meningioma.

3. 10% of cases.

4. No.

Reference

Jee WH, Oh SN, McCauley T, et al: Extraaxial neurofibromas versus neurilemmomas: discrimination with MRI, *AJR Am J Roentgenol* 183:629–633, 2004.

Cross-Reference

Neuroradiology: THE REQUISITES, pp 107–108, 725–728.

Comment

Facial nerve branches in the temporal bone include branches from the greater superficial petrosal nerve to lacrimation (from the geniculate ganglion), to the stapedius muscle (at the second genu), to the chorda tympani for taste (at the stylomastoid foramen), and to the muscles of the face (throughout but branching within the parotid gland). A lesion of the descending portion of the facial nerve would affect taste and muscle function but not lacrimation or hyperacusis.

Rarely one sees schwannomas that do not enhance at all. One may see schwannomas that have nonenhancing cystic degeneration and a solid enhancing component, but complete lack of enhancement is uncommon. This tends to occur in the periphery much more so than in the CNS, where nonenhancing schwannomas are rare. Neurofibromas are more likely to be nonenhancing than schwannomas, but given the overall prevalence of the two, schwannomas still should be thought of as the leading diagnosis.

According to Jee et al, the points listed in the table may help discriminate between schwannomas and neurofibromas.

Feature	Schwannoma	Neurofibroma
Target sign on T2W	15%	58%
Central enhancement	8%	75%
Fascicular appearance	63%	25%
Thin hyperintense rim	58%	8%
Diffuse enhancement	67%	13%
Cystic area	64%	38%

The classic immunostain for schwannomas is the S-100 protein, which is a neural crest marker.

Notes

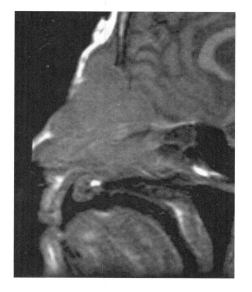
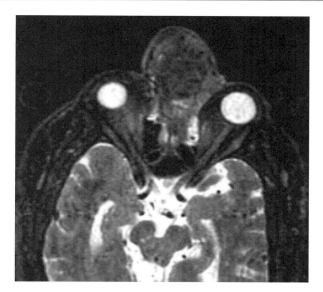
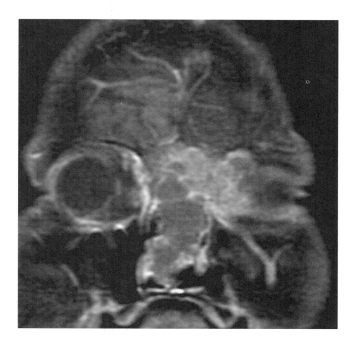
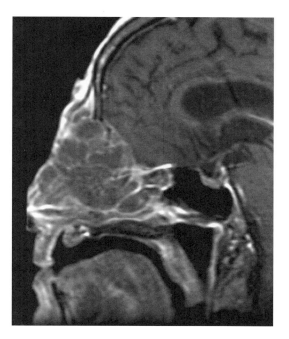

1. Identify the peak age groups for this tumor.

2. Name the cell of origin for the tumor.

3. What is the differential diagnosis?

4. What imaging feature is said to be characteristic of olfactory neuroblastomas?

Olfactory Neuroblastoma

1. 11 to 20 and 51 to 60.

2. Neural crest cells.

3. Squamous cell carcinoma, adenocarcinoma, small cell tumor, adenoid cystic carcinoma, metastasis, and sinonasal undifferentiated carcinoma.

4. An intracranial peripheral cyst associated with a solid mass in the nasal cavity.

Reference

Som PM, Lidov M, Brandwein M, et al: Sinonasal esthesioneuroblastoma with intracranial extension: marginal tumor cysts as a diagnostic MR finding, *AJNR Am J Neuroradiol* 15:1259–1262, 1994.

Cross-Reference

Neuroradiology: THE REQUISITES, pp 635–637.

Comment

Also called an *esthesioneuroblastoma,* olfactory neuroblastomas are staged using the Kadish system for extent (see table).

Stage	Location	5-Year Survival (%)
A	Disease confined to nasal cavity	75
B	Disease confined to nasal cavity and paranasal sinuses	68
C	Local or distant spread beyond nasal cavity or sinuses	41

A TNM classification also has been suggested:

T1—tumor involving the nasal cavity or paranasal sinuses (excluding sphenoid) or both, sparing the most superior ethmoidal cells

T2—tumor involving the nasal cavity or paranasal sinuses (including the sphenoid) or both, with extension to or erosion of the cribriform plate

T3—tumor extending into the orbit or protruding into the anterior cranial fossa, without dural invasion

T4—tumor involving the brain

N0—no cervical lymph node metastasis

N1—any form of cervical lymph node metastasis

M0—no metastasis

M1—distant metastasis

Nodal metastases occur in 22% of cases, and distant metastases occur in 16%.

A sinonasal mass with intracranial marginal cysts is an olfactory neuroblastoma until proved otherwise. Although this finding occurs in less than 10% of olfactory neuroblastomas, it has not been reported at any substantive rate with the other entities listed in the differential diagnosis.

Notes

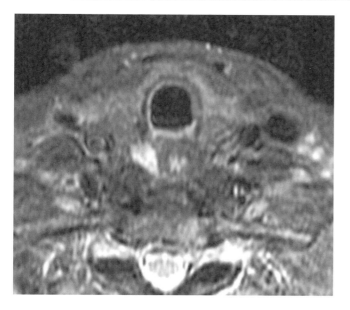 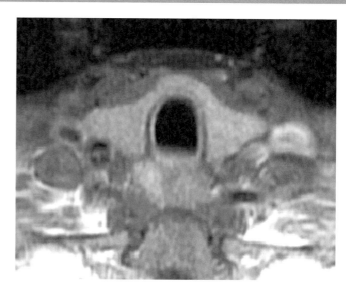

1. What is the differential diagnosis?

2. What is the best imaging study to identify this entity and distinguish among differential diagnoses?

3. What is the rate of carcinoma?

4. Describe the appearance on MRI.

C A S E 8 6

Parathyroid Adenoma

1. Lymph node, thyroid nodule, and schwannoma.

2. Technetium-99m sestamibi scan.

3. 1%.

4. Dark on T1W scan, bright on T2W scan, enhancing.

Reference

Civelek AC, Ozalp E, Donovan P, Udelsman R: Prospective evaluation of delayed technetium 99m sestamibi SPECT scintigraphy for preoperative localization of primary hyperparathyroidism, *Surgery* 131:149–157, 2002.

Cross-Reference

Neuroradiology: THE REQUISITES, pp 743–745.

Comment

Parathyroid adenomas are the most common cause of primary hyperparathyroidism, accounting for >80% of cases. Parathyroid hyperplasia and parathyroid carcinoma are less common causes. Secondary hyperparathyroidism from chronic renal failure is another cause of the bone, gastrointestinal, psychiatric, and renal manifestations of hyperparathyroidism (remember the symptoms of hypercalcemia described as bones [fractures and bone pain], moans [psychiatric disorders], groans [gastrointestinal discomfort], and stones [renal calculi]).

Sestamibi scanning offers the power of a functional imaging test that does well with localization to the point that it decreases the time for operative removal of the lesion. The one *bête noir* of primary hyperparathyroidism and of sestamibi scanning is parathyroid gland hyperplasia, an entity that is hard to diagnose preoperatively (although some authors are now advocating the use of positron emission tomography for this). Sestamibi single-photon emission computed tomography scanning shows accuracy rates of 94% for all parathyroid lesions, including unexplored and reoperated cases (87% to 92%); 96% for solitary adenomas; 83% for multiple adenomas; but just 45% for parathyroid hyperplasia.

Parathyroid hyperplasia may be seen in patients with the multiple endocrine neoplasia syndromes.

Technetium pertechnetate sestamibi scanning is the most cost-effective means for identifying parathyroid adenomas. This functional study readily distinguishes between lymph nodes in the neck and parathyroid adenomas, which is a difficult distinction to make by ultrasound, CT, and MRI. Technetium sestamibi scanning also is capable of evaluating the substernal and mediastinal locations, which is the Achilles heel for ultrasound.

The exact mechanism by which sestamibi scanning works is unclear. It may be related to the mitochondrial activity and potassium influx into the cells associated with parathyroid adenomas.

Most parathyroid adenomas are identified in a perithyroidal location. Nonetheless, in approximately 10% to 20% of cases, the parathyroid adenoma may be in an ectopic location, which may include the paratracheal, paraesophageal, upper cervical, and mediastinal regions.

Notes

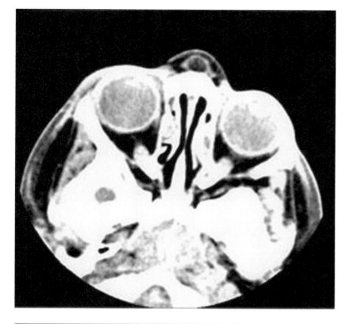

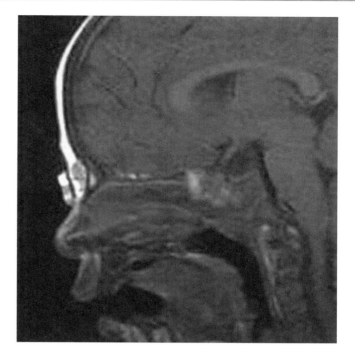

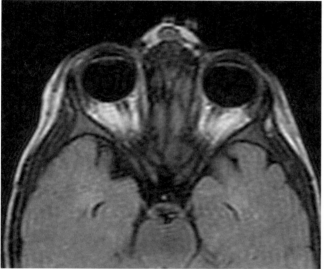

1. What would be the significance of a bifid crista galli and a large foramen cecum in this case?

2. Explain the significance of fluid density versus fat density in this lesion.

3. What percentage of nasal dermoids have an intracranial tract?

4. What is the differential diagnosis?

Nasal Epidermoid

1. It would imply a sinus tract extending intracranially.

2. Fluid implies epidermoid; fat implies dermoid.

3. 20%.

4. Nasal/extranasal glioma, nasofrontal encephalocele, and venous/lymphatic vascular malformation.

Reference

Huisman TA, Schneider JF, Kellenberger CJ, et al: Developmental nasal midline masses in children: neuroradiological evaluation, *Eur Radiol* 14:243–249, 2004.

Cross-Reference

Neuroradiology: THE REQUISITES, pp 615–616.

Comment

When the clinician encounters a small dimple on the top of the nose in the midline, the differential diagnosis includes nasal epidermoid versus dermal sinus tract. The dermoid sinus tract may have a connection to the intracranial space or may end blindly. If the dermal sinus tract extends to the intracranial space, one usually sees widening of the perpendicular plate of the nasal septum and enlargement and patency of the foramen cecum through the cribriform plate, leading ultimately to the meninges of the anterior cranial fossa. Chemical meningitis from fat within the subarachnoid space in the anterior cranial fossa could be present, or there could be spread of an infection from the nasal site into the intracranial compartment leading to meningitis. In most cases, the dermoid sinus tract does not extend intracranially but closes shortly after entering the nasal cavity.

Despite the fact that they are called *dermoids,* implying fat within the lesion, many dermoids do not have such skin appendages and are seen merely as a cyst at the dorsum of the nose.

MRI is probably the study of choice in these lesions to exclude intracranial extension and to keep the radiation exposure in children (most lesions occur in children <5 years old) at a minimum.

Notes

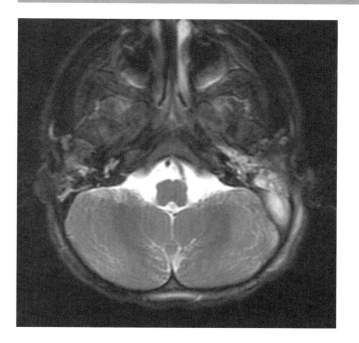
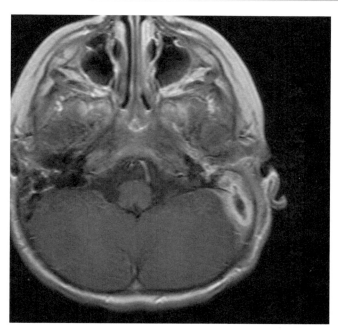

1. Identify the primary disease and its secondary complication.

2. What is the abscess called that occurs below the mastoid tip into the sternocleidomastoid muscle?

3. Where is Macewen's triangle, and what is its importance?

4. What is the dreaded complication of sinus thrombosis?

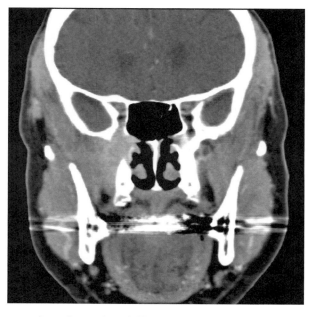
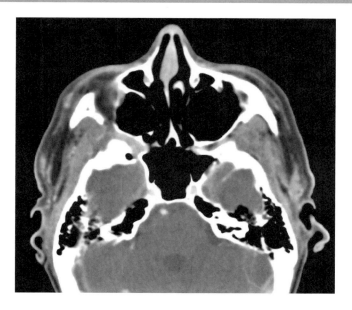

1. What does the differential diagnosis include?

2. Name the cranial nerve that is associated with the pterygopalatine fossa.

3. Identify the type of lymphoma typically seen in an extranodal location in the head and neck.

4. What is the risk of a fatal contrast dye reaction during an enhanced CT scan?

CASE 88

Sigmoid Sinus Thrombosis from Otomastoiditis

1. Otomastoiditis with secondary sigmoid sinus thrombosis.

2. Bezold abscess.

3. A small triangular depression at the junction of the posterior and superior borders of the external auditory canal, posterior to the suprameatal spine; this is the site of surgical entry to the mastoid antrum, but also a weak point where infection can collect in the postauricular area.

4. Acute intracranial hypertension leading to ischemia and herniation.

Reference
van den Bosch MA, Vos JA, de Letter MA, et al: MRI findings in a child with sigmoid sinus thrombosis following mastoiditis, *Pediatr Radiol* 33:877–879, 2003.

Cross-Reference
Neuroradiology: THE REQUISITES, pp 575–584.

Comment
Sinus thrombosis after otomastoiditis may be due to direct extension or to venous infiltration via emissary veins. Propagation more centrally can lead to major increases in intracranial pressure. Hemorrhagic infarction may ensue, and the prognosis worsens. Clinical findings include papilledema. CT venography may be coupled with thin-section temporal bone CT to create the best study to define the disease. MRI and magnetic resonance venography are equally useful.

Notes

CASE 89

Lymphoma of the Pterygopalatine Fossa

1. Lymphoma, sarcoma, minor salivary gland tumor, plasmacytoma, and posttransplantation lymphoproliferative disorder.

2. The maxillary nerve (second division of cranial nerve V).

3. Non-Hodgkin B cell lymphoma—diffuse immunoblastic or large cell.

4. 1:130,000.

Reference
Bettmann MA: Frequently asked questions: contrast agents, *Radiographics* 24:3–10, 2004.

Cross-Reference
Neuroradiology: THE REQUISITES, pp 25–28.

Comment
The risk of contrast agent complications is manifold. Contrast agent–induced nephropathy occurs in patients who have preexisting renal dysfunction. Usually the risk factors are long-standing diabetes, dehydration, and coexistent medications. Acetylcysteine (Mucomyst) has helped to prevent contrast agent–induced renal dysfunction. Acetylcysteine is given in four doses twice daily starting on the day before contrast agent injection or intravenously 30 minutes before the injection. Coupled with acetylcysteine administration, patients should be receiving hydration.

According to one publication, the risk of death from iodinated contrast agents is approximately 1:130,000. If one has had a prior reaction to iodinated contrast material, the likelihood of a recurrent reaction with a subsequent injection is approximately 8% to 25%; it is appropriate to use a different contrast agent in these individuals. A history of other severe allergies and asthma increases the risk of an adverse event, but only to a small degree. The association of an allergy to shellfish with iodinated contrast allergy seems to be false.

If a patient has high blood levels of metformin (Glucophage or Glucovance), he or she is at risk for developing lactic acidosis after the study, which, although exceedingly rare, may be fatal 50% of the time. Metformin use should be stopped at the time of an iodinated contrast agent injection, and the patient should wait 48 hours before resuming metformin. At that time, the patient should be reevaluated clinically, and, if necessary, creatine levels should be obtained to determine if there is renal dysfunction.

Iodixanol (Visipaque) has been shown to be effective for preventing contrast agent nephropathy.

Notes

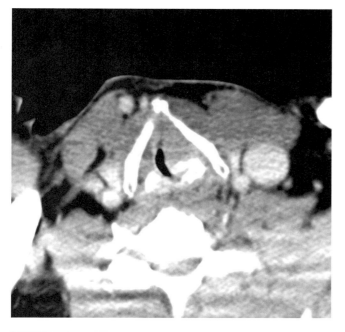

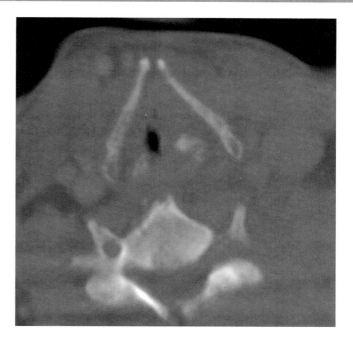

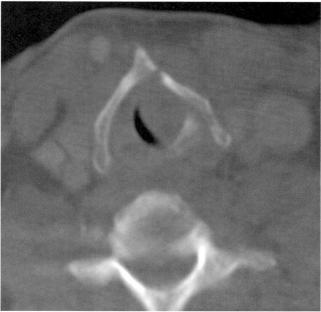

1. What is the 5-year survival rate of patients with T1 glottic carcinoma?

2. Name the CT criterion that is most specific for cartilage invasion.

3. Name the MRI criterion that is most specific for cartilage invasion.

4, Why do patients with supraglottic cancers do worse than those with glottic cancers?

Cartilage Invasion

1. 90%.

2. Tumor on both sides of the cartilage.

3. Enhancement of the cartilage on fat-suppressed T1W postgadolinium scans.

4. Supraglottic cancers have earlier and more widespread lymph node spread and manifest later.

References

Becker M, Zbaren P, Delavelle J, et al: Neoplastic invasion of the laryngeal cartilage: reassessment of criteria for diagnosis at CT, *Radiology* 203:521–532, 1997.

Yousem DM, Tufano RP: Laryngeal imaging, *MRI Clin North Am* 10:451–465, 2002.

Cross-Reference

Neuroradiology: THE REQUISITES, pp 672–681.

Comment

Because the thyroid cartilage may be either chondrified or ossified, it is the most difficult cartilage of the larynx to evaluate for tumor erosion. Nonossified cartilage is of similar CT density and MRI intensity as squamous cell cartilage. Becker et al looked at several CT findings, including sclerosis of cartilage, erosion of cartilage, lysis of cartilage, irregular border of cartilage, extralaryngeal tumor beyond the cartilage, and cartilage expansion, to determine which of these factors had the highest degree of reliability in evaluating the thyroid, cricoid, and arytenoid cartilage. Although sclerosis is the most sensitive (83%) criterion in all of the cartilages, histopathologically it often corresponds to reactive inflammation, particularly in the thyroid cartilage (specificity 40%). Becker et al found that extralaryngeal tumor and erosion or lysis of cartilage yielded the highest specificity (83% specificity with sensitivity of 71%) for thyroid cartilage invasion. Identifying tumor adjacent to nonossified cartilage, a serpiginous contour and obliteration of marrow space also were relatively specific (86% to 95%) findings for arytenoid and cricoid cartilage invasion (but not for the thyroid cartilage at 41% to 55% specificity). A combination of extralaryngeal tumor, sclerosis, and lysis provided the highest degree of accuracy, approximately 80% for the thyroid cartilage.

From the standpoint of MRI findings, high signal intensity within the cartilage on fat-suppressed fast spin echo T2W scans and cartilaginous enhancement on fat-suppressed T1W scans seem to be the most accurate criteria. A metaanalysis of the major studies comparing MRI versus CT for cartilage invasion reveals that MRI is the more accurate test, although at a loss of specificity because of false-positive cases. The inflammatory and reactive changes associated with adjacent neoplasm may yield high signal intensity on T2W scan and even contrast enhancement into the cartilage. CT, by virtue of its lack of sensitivity, could lead to residual tumor being left behind and recurrence after conservation surgery. Combining the two modalities (e.g., when MRI is positive for cartilage invasion, a corroborating CT scan is performed) may be the most effective strategy for evaluating a patient with laryngeal carcinoma.

Notes

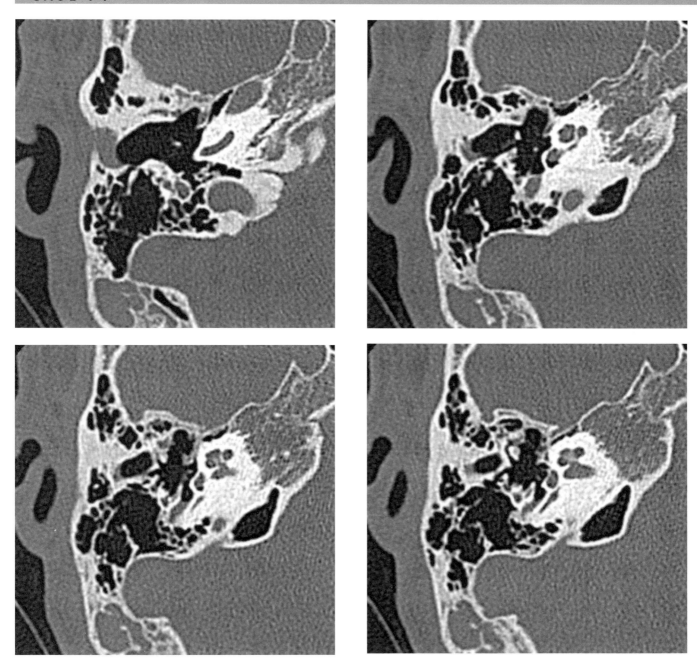

1. What is missing on these images?
2. From which branchial arch is this structure derived?
3. What is the likely symptom?
4. What are the causes of ossicular erosions?

Absent Incus

1. The incus

2. The second arch predominantly; portions from the first arch

3. Conductive hearing loss

4. Acute otitis media, cholesteatoma, trauma, epidermoid, CHARGE syndrome, avascular necrosis

Reference

Khan I, Jan AM, Shahzad F: Middle-ear reconstruction. a review of 150 cases. *J Laryngol Otol* 116: 435–439, 2002.

Cross-Reference

Neuroradiology: THE REQUISITES, pp 574–584.

Comment

This patient shows absence of the incus on a congenital basis. This is usually due to a second branchial arch anomaly, as opposed to the first arch anomaly that commonly results in external auditory canal atresia with fusion of the malleus and incus.

When the incus is eroded or absent, a sculpted autologous incus replacement (interposition) prosthesis may be employed in the reconstruction. This will attach the handle of the malleus with the head of the stapes. Sometimes homologous grafts of cartilage from the rib or knee are used.

If both the malleus and the incus are involved, a partial ossicular prosthesis that can extend from the tympanic membrane to the head of the stapes is used. Sometimes cartilage is placed between the PORP and the eardrum to reduce the rate of rejection. If the incus and the stapes are eroded, a total ossicular replacement prosthesis (TORP) is used between the tympanic membrane and the footplate of the stapes.

The success rate of middle ear reconstructions is approximately 80% in experienced hands. Failures of ORPs may be due to adhesions, resorption, malposition, recurrent disease, extrusion of the graft, incorrect sizing, cartilaginous necrosis, and retraction of the tympanic membrane leading to extraction of the prosthesis.

CHARGE (coloboma, heart defect, atresia of choanae, retarded growth, genital hypoplasia, and ear anomalies) syndrome is associated with hypoplastic incus and semicircular canal agenesis.

Notes

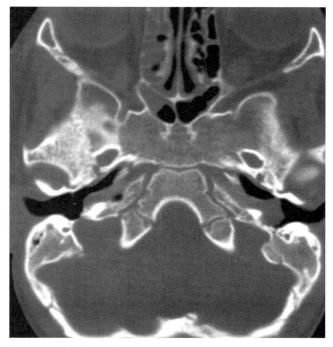

1. Explain the difference between an aberrant internal carotid artery (ICA) and a lateralized ICA.

2. What causes the tinnitus of an aberrant ICA?

3. How often does an aberrant ICA have a persistent stapedial artery with it?

4. What is the implication of an absent foramen spinosum?

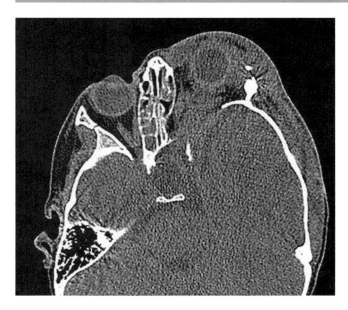

1. What phakomatosis does this finding suggest?

2. What is the most common neurocutaneous disorder?

3. What percentage of patients with neurofibromatosis 1 have a cranial bony dysplasia?

4. Name other orbital manifestations of neurofibromatosis 1.

Aberrant Internal Carotid Arteries

1. The aberrant ICA enters via the enlarged inferior tympanic canaliculus; the lateralized ICA just has a dehiscent lateral wall in its petrous portion. The aberrant ICA is more laterally located.

2. Usually there is a stenosis of the vessel at the junction between the vertical segment and the horizontal segment of the artery.

3. 30% of the time.

4. No middle meningeal artery and high likelihood of persistent stapedial artery.

Reference

Zahneisenl G, Kimmich T, Arnold W: Radiology quiz case 1: aberrant internal carotid artery (ICA) of the right middle ear, *Arch Otolaryngol Head Neck Surg* 130:1120–1124, 2004.

Cross-Reference

Neuroradiology: THE REQUISITES, pp 588–589.

Comment

When faced with a retrotympanic red vascular mask, one should always consider an aberrant ICA. This is a diagnosis that is easy to identify if one pays attention to the posterolateral wall of the ICA in its carotid canal within the petrious portion of the carotid artery. In cases of aberrant ICA, there is dehiscence in this area, and one can identify the carotid artery extending too far posteriorly and too far laterally along the cochlear promontory. In this location, the aberrant ICA simulates a glomus tympanic tumor.

Aberrancey of the ICA is related in some ways to persistence of the hyoid artery and the vascular loop that extends to and enlarges the inferior tympanic caniculus. The vascular loop then courses anteriorly to join the horizontally oriented petrous carotid artery.

Aberrancey of the ICA may be associated with a persistent stapedial artery, which is suggested by the absence of a foramen spinosum for the middle meningeal artery. The persistent stapedial artery also tracks along the cochlear promontory to a position adjacent to the facial nerve and its tympanic portion. A persistent stapedial artery may be another cause of a retrotympanic mass along with glomus tympanicum, glomus jugulare, jugular diverticulum, jugular dehiscence, and cholesteatoma.

Notes

Sphenoid Wing Dysplasia

1. Neurofibromatosis 1.

2. Neurofibromatosis 1.

3. 5%.

4. Optic nerve glioma, cranial nerve V plexiform neurofibroma, ocular Lisch nodule, enlarged foramina, and buphthalmos.

Reference

Farmer JP, Khan S, Khan A, et al: Neurofibromatosis type 1 and the pediatric neurosurgeon: a 20-year institutional review, *Pediatr Neurosurg* 37:122–136, 2002.

Cross-Reference

Neuroradiology: THE REQUISITES, pp 449–453.

Comment

One of the seven basic criteria for neurofibromatosis 1 is a bony dysplasia. In some cases, this dysplasia may affect the tibia, but in others it may be a sphenoid wing dysplasia. In this example, the sphenoid bone's greater and lesser wings have not developed appropriately, which leads to transmission of CSF pulsations from the middle cranial fossa temporal lobe to the orbit. Hence the patient may show a pulsatile exophthalmos.

The other six criteria for neurofibromatosis 1 include six or more café-au-lait spots, three or more Lisch nodules, optic pathway glioma, axillary freckling, first-degree family relative with neurofibromatosis, and plexiform neurofibroma. Several of these criteria occur in the head and neck regions.

The gene for neurofibromatosis 1 is located on chromosome 17, and the gene protein is neurofibromin, a growth suppressor.

Notes

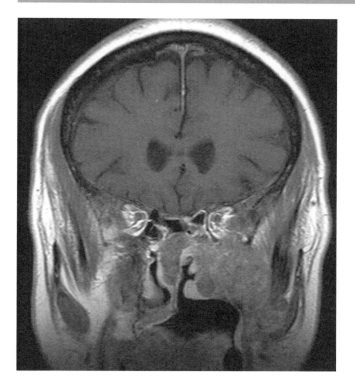
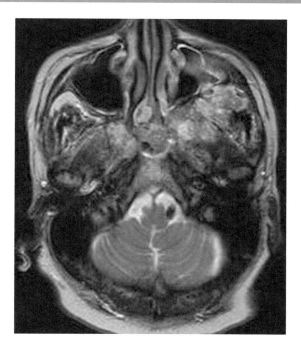

1. What are the usual histologies of sinus malignancies?

2. What is the implication of sinonasal undifferentiated carcinoma?

3. What T stage of cancer would you call this lesion?

4. Identify the "premalignant" lesions of the paranasal sinuses.

Sinus Squamous Cell Carcinoma

1. Squamous cell carcinoma, adenocarcinoma, melanoma, sinonasal undifferentiated carcinoma, adenoid cystic carcinoma, lymphoma, and sarcoma.

2. Sinonasal undifferentiated carcinoma has a poor prognosis with an aggressive life cycle of the cancer.

3. T3.

4. Inverted papilloma and posttransplant lymphoproliferative disorder.

Reference

Loevner LA, Sonners AI: Imaging of neoplasms of the paranasal sinuses, *MRI Clin North Am* 10:467–493, 2002.

Cross-Reference

Neuroradiology: THE REQUISITES, pp 634–635.

Comment

The staging of maxillary sinus squamous cell carcinoma is as follows:

> T1—tumor limited to maxillary sinus mucosa with no erosion or destruction of bone
>
> T2—tumor causing bone erosion or destruction, including extension into the hard palate or middle nasal meatus or both except for extension to posterior wall of maxillary sinus and pterygoid plates
>
> T3—tumor invades bone of the posterior wall of maxillary sinus, floor or medial wall of orbit, pterygoid fossa, or ethmoid sinuses
>
> T4a—tumor invades anterior orbital contents, skin of cheek, pterygoid plates, infratemporal fossa, cribriform plate, or sphenoid or frontal sinuses
>
> T4b—tumor invades orbital apex, dura, brain, middle cranial fossa, cranial nerves other than V2, nasopharynx, or clivus

There usually is no way to differentiate on imaging among the various malignancies of the maxillary sinus other than a few unreliable hints, as follows:

> If bright on T1W scan, favor melanoma
>
> If homogeneous on T2W scan and dark, favor lymphoma.
>
> If growing aggressively and showing dural metastases, favor sinonasal undifferentiated carcinoma.
>
> If associated with necrotic lymph nodes, favor squamous cell carcinoma.
>
> If in a woodworker and more ethmoid than maxillary, favor adenocarcinoma.
>
> If showing perineural spread, favor adenoid cystic carcinoma.
>
> If in a child, favor rhabdomyosarcoma.

Notes

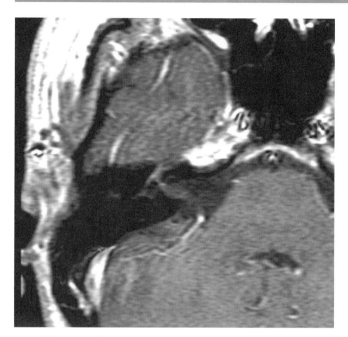

1. Where is the most common site for cranial nerve VII to enhance (pathologically) with Bell's palsy?

2. What percentage of unilateral facial nerve paralysis is due to Bell's palsy?

3. What is the differential diagnosis of enhancing facial nerve?

4. If the brain is negative for cranial nerve VII abnormality, where is the next place to look for a cause of the illness?

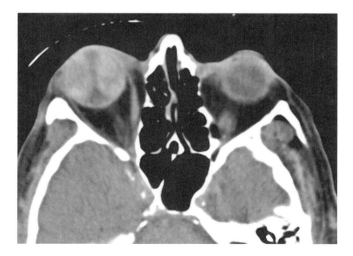

1. What type of ocular detachment is this?

2. Where is the fluid accumulating?

3. Name the most common causes of choroidal detachment.

4. What is the significance in the difference between serous and hemorrhagic choroidal detachment?

CASE 95

Bell's Palsy

1. At the junction between the fundus of the internal auditory canal and the labyrinthine portion of the facial nerve.

2. 60% to 75%.

3. Lyme disease, lymphoma, leukemia, subarachnoid seeding, Ramsay Hunt syndrome secondary to varicella-zoster infection, amyloidosis, acute disseminated encephalomyelitis, diabetic neuropathy, cytomegalovirus infection, and Guillain-Barré syndrome.

4. The parotid gland.

Reference

Gilden DH: Bell's palsy, *N Engl J Med* 351:1323–1331, 2004.

Cross-Reference

Neuroradiology: THE REQUISITES, pp 591–592.

Comment

Bell's palsy is a disease that can affect all age groups, but individuals >70 years old are affected the most frequently. Most people (71% to 84%) have complete resolution of Bell's palsy, but a few have long-lasting effects. The older the patient and the more complete the paralysis, the higher the rate of permanent effects.

The illness is caused by herpes simplex virus. The damage may be caused by the swelling of the nerve with neurovascular compromise at the tightest point of its course—going into the temporal bone from the internal auditory canal. This swelling has been observed in cases treated with surgical decompression of the nerve. Electromyography has confirmed conduction blocks at this segment of the nerve.

Treatment with steroid or antiviral medications or both may be warranted for patients with persistent disease at the end of 1 week. If decompression is to be performed, it is most effective within the first 2 to 3 weeks of onset.

Imaging generally is not indicated acutely but is reserved for patients with persistent paralysis.

Notes

CASE 96

Choroidal Detachment

1. Choroidal detachment.

2. In the suprachoroidal space.

3. Trauma, postoperative, global hypotony, inflammation, corneal erosions, and retinal photocoagulation.

4. Long-term prognosis is worse with hemorrhagic choroidal detachments (40% permanent visual loss).

Reference

Mafee MF, Peyman GA: Retinal and choroidal detachments: role of magnetic resonance imaging and computed tomography, *Radiol Clin North Am* 25: 487–507, 1987.

Cross-Reference

Neuroradiology: THE REQUISITES, pp 485–487.

Comment

The differentiation between retinal detachment and choroidal detachment is fundamental. The retinal detachment by and large appears as elliptical densities that have at their apex the optic nerve insertion to the globe. Retinal detachments do not extend anteriorly beyond the level of the ora serrata. The ora serrata is generally seen at 10 o'clock and 2 o'clock on the globe and is proximal to the uveal apparatus. The retinal detachment is due to fluid in the subretinal layer of the retinal pigment and is limited to the extent to which one has retinal-pigmented epithelium, which is confined to the region outlined by the ora serrata.

Choroidal attachments may occur in multiple locations along the globe. They are defined by the attachment of the choroid at the ciliary body of the uveal tract, which means that they can extend further anteriorly than the retinal detachment. Choroidal attachments tend to be confined by optociliary vessels that lead to a biconvex location, which does not involve the optic nerve insertion to the globe.

In both cases, the collection may include either blood or proteinaceous material. Choroidal or retinal detachments may occur from trauma, surgery, neoplasms such as melanoma or retinoblastomas, or diabetic retinopathy. Cytomegalovirus infection in patients who are HIV positive is another potential cause of detachment of the scleral membranes.

Notes

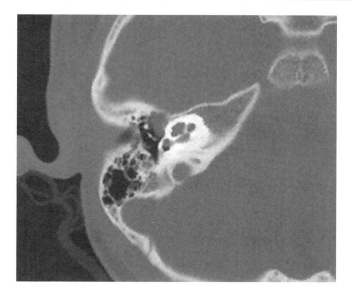

1. In this location, what does the differential diagnosis include?
2. With stippled calcification, what would be the best diagnosis?
3. Would this patient present with hyperacusis?
4. What is the best way to distinguish between a schwannoma and paraganglioma?

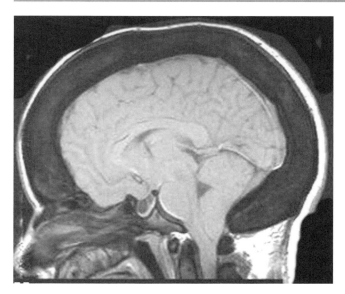 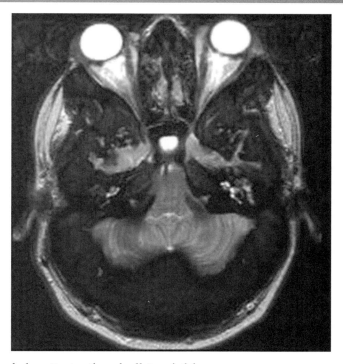

1. Name at least three entities that may cause increased density to the skull in children.
2. Name at least three entities that may cause decreased density to the skull in children.
3. What entity frequently is represented by the presence of bones with increased density, anemia, and optic atrophy?
4. Which form of osteopetrosis manifests at birth?

Schwannoma versus Paraganglioma

1. Schwannoma, paraganglioma, hemangioma, meningioma, epidermoid, and metastasis.

2. Facial nerve hemangioma.

3. Yes. The cranial nerve VII fibers to the stapedius are distal to this level, and may be affected.

4. Dynamic scanning (see explanation in Comment section).

Reference

Vogl TJ, Mack MG, Juergens M, et al: Skull base tumors: gadodiamide injection-enhanced MR imaging—drop-out effect in the early enhancement pattern of paragangliomas versus different tumors, *Radiology* 188:339–346, 1993.

Cross-Reference

Neuroradiology: THE REQUISITES, pp 725–728.

Comment

Several findings distinguish between a paraganglioma and a schwannoma. For schwannomas, one should look for heterogeneity of the signal intensity indicative of the variable distribution of the Antoni A and Antoni B tissue, cystic degeneration, oblong shape, distribution along a cranial or peripheral nerve, and enhancement. Paragangliomas have flow voids when they are larger; intense enhancement; a more homogeneous, although speckled signal intensity; and characteristic locations along the carotid sheath, vagus nerve, carotid bifurcation, skull base, and inner ear. Nonetheless, there are many instances when a small schwannoma that is uniformly enhancing and a small paraganglioma that is uniformly enhancing and has not developed the flow voids owing to its small size look alike. In these instances, one can employ dynamic scanning at a single location within the mass to determine its contrast uptake. With gadolinium or iodine-based contrast dye, the paraganglioma should show an early downward dip at approximately the 30- to 45-second mark, whereas schwannomas do not have a similar downward dip. The slope of the uptake of the contrast dye also is more vertical with paragangliomas than it is with schwannomas. In the end, there are still cases when a fine-needle aspiration or a conventional arteriogram, which shows the blush of the paraganglioma, is required. Embolotherapy can help the surgeon reduce blood loss at the time of removal.

Notes

Osteopetrosis

1. Osteopetrosis, pyknodysostosis, craniodiaphyseal dysplasia, thalassemia, and sickle cell anemia.

2. Osteogenesis imperfecta, achondrogenesis, hypophosphatasia, Menkes syndrome, and rickets.

3. Osteopetrosis (the optic atrophy may be due to encroachment on the optic canals).

4. The autosomal recessive form, which is due to a defect in acidification at the bone-osteoclast interface, presents at birth, whereas the autosomal dominant form presents in the first decade of life.

Reference

Glass RB, Fernbach SK, Norton KI, et al: The infant skull: a vault of information, *Radiographics* 24:507–522, 2004.

Cross-Reference

Neuroradiology: THE REQUISITES, pp 440–441.

Comment

Osteopetrosis, also known as Albers-Schönberg disease, is a hereditary autosomal recessive disorder in which the bone is "marbleized." Despite the fact that there may be increased thickness and increased density to the bone on CT scan, this bone is less rigid than the normal bone and bone marrow. It is more susceptible to fractures. For some reason, these bones are also more susceptible to infection.

The neurologic manifestations may run the gamut owing to compression of cranial nerves VIII, VII, and V; the arteries; and the veins. Hydrocephalus may be due to venous outflow obstruction (less common) or from skull base CSF egress issues.

On MRI, the absence of the normal marrow signal in most of the bones is notable when the osteopetrosis is of the diffuse infantile type. The differential diagnosis includes fibrous dysplasia and Paget disease on MRI; however, these are distinguished easily on CT scan because osteopetrosis does not have the ground-glass appearance of fibrous dysplasia and does not show the lytic pattern of osteoporosis circumscripta of Paget disease. Osteopetrosis also may have findings of a small foramen magnum and associated Chiari I malformation (as seen here).

Notes

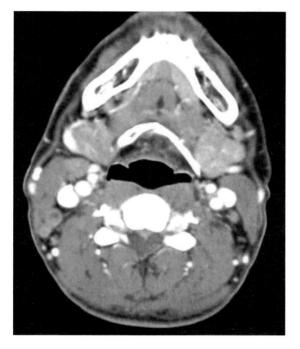

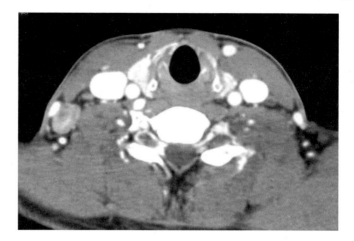

1. Describe the classic features of tuberculous adenitis.

2. Which mycobacteria affect children more than adults?

3. What is the most common manifestation of tuberculous infection in the head and neck?

4. How does nontuberculous mycobacterial infection present on CT compared with tuberculous adenitis?

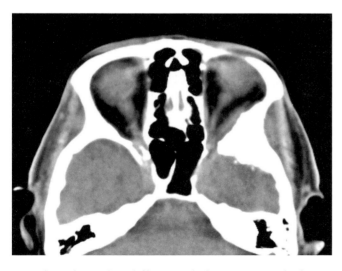

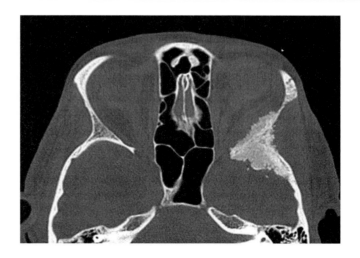

1. What does the differential diagnosis include?

2. Define SAPHO syndrome.

3. What is the most common site for osteomyelitis in the head and neck?

4. What resides in the osteoblastic bone of meningiomas?

CASE 99

Tuberculous Adenitis

1. (1) Multiloculated or multichambered (conglomerate nodal) mass, (2) central necrosis, (3) thick rims of enhancement, (4) minimal infiltration of the fat and fascia, and (5) posterior triangle predilection.

2. *Mycobacterium scrofulaceum* and *Mycobacterium avium*.

3. Cervical adenitis.

4. Same with periparotid or submandibular predilection.

Reference

Bagla S, Tunkel D, Kraut MA: Nontuberculous mycobacterial lymphadenitis of the head and neck: radiologic observations and clinical context, *Pediatr Radiol* 33:402–406, 2003.

Cross-Reference

Neuroradiology: THE REQUISITES, pp 683–685.

Comment

Calcified lymph nodes with confluence, necrosis, and extracapsular inflammation are the sine qua non of tuberculosis adenitis. Tuberculous adenitis most commonly is caused by mycobacterial infection. Concomitant pulmonary tuberculosis is present in approximately 90% of the cases. Alternatively, tuberculous adenitis may be due to *M. avium*; this is associated with HIV infection and an immunocompromised host.

Previously, *M. scrofulaceum* and *M. bovis* were the causative agents, usually resulting from contaminated milk products. These infections occur less often now in the modern era with good sterilization of milk products.

Patients often present with pain, fever, and a fluctuant mass in the neck. The pulmonary mycobacterial infection may not be clinically obvious, and the neck mass may be the presenting symptom. This is a difficult infection to eradicate with antibiotics and may require a long course of therapy and occasionally surgical resection of the nodal mass.

Notes

CASE 100

Sphenoid Wing Meningioma

1. Meningioma, osteomyelitis, metastasis, Paget's disease, osteosarcoma, and SAPHO syndrome.

2. *S*ynovitis, *a*cne, *p*ustulosis, *h*yperostosis, and *o*steitis.

3. The mandible.

4. In some cases, it is meningioma; in some cases, merely reactive change.

Reference

Abdel-Aziz KM, Froelich SC, Dagnew E, et al: Large sphenoid wing meningiomas involving the cavernous sinus: conservative surgical strategies for better functional outcomes, *Neurosurgery* 54:1375–1384, 2004.

Cross-Reference

Neuroradiology: THE REQUISITES, pp 512–513.

Comment

The issues that are critical to the description of sphenoid wing meningioma revolve around the extent of disease. Extension to the cavernous sinus is one critical determinant in this regard. Cases with involvement of the lateral wall of the cavernous sinus can be completely resected with microdissection. If extension to the medial cavernous sinus occurs or the internal carotid artery is encased, resection is nearly impossible. If the carotid artery is also narrowed, the likelihood of successful treatment is low. Infiltration of the superior orbital fissure and the optic canal is another feature of sphenoid wing meningiomas that must be scrutinized. Cranial nerve deficits also portend unresectability.

Sex, histologic grade, and tumor location are associated with meningioma recurrence. The recurrence rate is 19% for men and 12% for women ($P < .05$) and >65% for anaplastic and hemangiopericytic meningiomas. Tumors in poorly accessible surgical sites have a high recurrence rate.

Notes

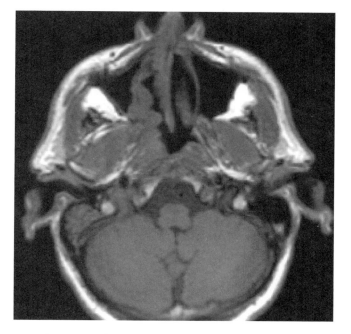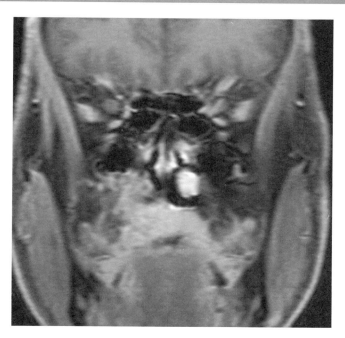

1. What is included in the differential diagnosis of sinonasal masses?
2. What percentage of time do squamous cell carcinoma and inverted papilloma coexist?
3. Name the most common primary tumor to metastasize to the sinus.
4. What is the recurrence rate of inverted papilloma?

Inverted Papilloma

1. Squamous cell carcinoma, adenocarcinoma, minor salivary gland carcinoma, melanoma, lymphoma, olfactory neuroblastoma (esthesioneuroblastoma) metastasis, inverted papilloma, and polyp.

2. 11%.

3. Kidney.

4. 15%.

Reference

Yousem DM, Fellows DW, Kennedy DW, et al: Inverted papilloma: evaluation with MR imaging, *Radiology* 185:501–505, 1992.

Cross-Reference

Neuroradiology: THE REQUISITES, pp 632–633.

Comment

Inverted papillomas straddle the fence between benign and malignant lesions. They have a high rate of coexistent squamous cell carcinoma and are treated aggressively by head and neck surgeons. They also have growth patterns that may lead to skull base and orbital infiltration. The quandary becomes whether to perform orbital exenterations or craniofacial surgeries for what, in most cases, is benign disease. There is no way to distinguish between squamous cell carcinoma and inverted papilloma on imaging.

Krouse recommended the following staging system for inverted papillomas:

T1—tumor confined to the nasal cavity
T2—tumor limited to medial or superior portions of the maxillary sinus or involving the ethmoid sinus
T3—tumor involving lateral, inferior, anterior, or posterior walls of the maxillary sinus, the sphenoid sinus, or the frontal sinus
T4—tumor outside the sinonasal cavity

T1 and T2 tumors can be treated endoscopically. T3 tumors usually are treated with open surgery, and T4 tumors require an extranasal approach.

The most common site of occurrence is the lateral nasal wall, followed by the nasal septum. The lesion is dark on T2W scans, making an easy distinction from other polyps but looking similar to squamous cell carcinoma, lymphoma, and esthesioneuroblastoma.

The enhancement pattern of inverted papilloma has been described as crenated or cerebriform in that there is usually linear streakiness to it within the pattern of solid gyriform enhancement. There must be central enhancement to distinguish inverted papilloma from obstructed secretions or mucoceles, which have peripheral rim enhancement.

Notes

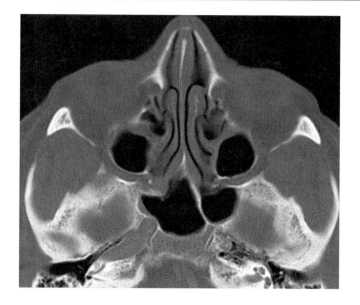
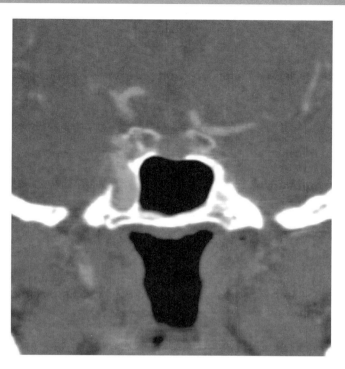

1. What is the major finding in this case?
2. How often is this entity seen?
3. What syndrome is associated with this entity?
4. What are typical symptoms?

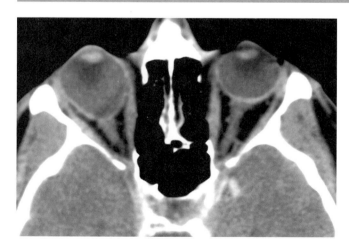

1. Of the various causes of a big eye, which is this one and why?
2. What is the most common cause of an elongated eye?
3. What is the most common cause of a congenital large eye?
4. Name at least four entities associated with buphthalmos.

CASE 102

Absent Internal Carotid Artery

1. Absence of the internal carotid artery (ICA) on the left.

2. <0.1%.

3. Neurofibromatosis.

4. Asymptomatic. Because this is a congenital anomaly, collaterals develop early in life, and the circle of Willis is protective.

Reference

Tasar M, Yetiser S, Tasar A, et al: Congenital absence or hypoplasia of the carotid artery: radioclinical issues, *Am J Otolaryngol* 25:339–349, 2004.

Cross-Reference

Neuroradiology: THE REQUISITES, pp 588–589.

Comment

The absence of the ICA as seen in the skull base as an absent carotid canal may be due to anomalous development of the primitive vascular arches associated with the branchial system. Amniotic bands are another source of unilateral ICA agenesis. The left carotid artery is affected more commonly than the right. Bilateral involvement occurs in 10% of cases. Usually, by virtue of the development of this anomaly in utero, the patient is asymptomatic. In adulthood, as atherosclerosis may develop in the remaining cervical vessels, the agenesis may be discovered as part of a transient ischemic attack or stroke workup.

By virtue of greater flow that is likely in the contralateral carotid artery, there may be an increased association with aneurysm formation on the side opposite the agenesis.

This patient was being evaluated for sinusitis, and the finding was incidental.

Notes

CASE 103

Axial Myopia

1. Staphyloma because there is thinning of the posterior scleral margins.

2. Nearsightedness.

3. Coloboma.

4. Neurofibromatosis 1, Proteus syndrome, Sturge-Weber syndrome, Lowe syndrome, Marfan syndrome, homocystinuria, and glaucoma.

Reference

Smith M, Castillo M: Imaging and differential diagnosis of the large eye, *Radiographics* 14:721–728, 1994.

Cross-Reference

Neuroradiology: THE REQUISITES, pp 469–475.

Comment

There are numerous causes for elongation of the globe. The most common is nearsightedness, in which axial myopia is present in individuals who have difficulty seeing at far distances. When this condition gets severe enough, tension can build up on the scleral membranes such that retinal detachments can occur. This process also may be associated with macular degeneration.

Buphthalmos is an entity in which there is congenital glaucoma and enlargement of the eye in the shape of a cow's eye—hence the term *buphthalmos*. This entity is due to a congenital weakness in the formation of the sclera.

Another cause of elongation of the eye is a staphyloma. Staphyloma refers to thinning of the scleral membranes often secondary to inflammatory processes. This thinning and bulging of the globe may be off-centered as opposed to most axial myopia due to nearsightedness, in which the globe remains symmetric. These examples of elongation of the globe are to be distinguished from colobomas, in which there is a defect in the choroidal fissure, with a more focal outpouching of the globe usually occurring around the optic nerve insertion. Colobomas can occur anywhere throughout the globe.

Enlargement of the globe also may be seen in patients with neurofibromatosis or Proteus syndrome.

Oculocerebral renal syndrome, also known as Lowe syndrome, comprises the triad of congenital cataracts, neonatal or infantile hypotonia with subsequent mental retardation, and renal tubular dysfunction. Fanconi anemia has been included in this syndrome. Affected children (X-linked and mostly boys) may have large eyes secondary to congenital glaucoma.

Notes

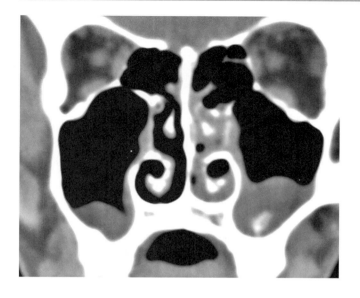
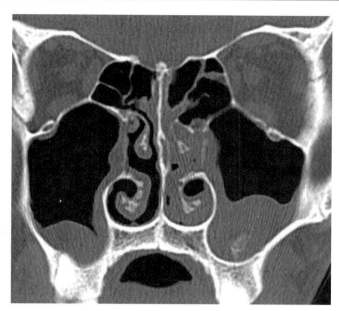

1. What is a Caldwell-Luc procedure?

2. What is FESS?

3. What is the egress from the sphenoid sinus called?

4. What is the differential diagnosis of a calcified mass in the sinus?

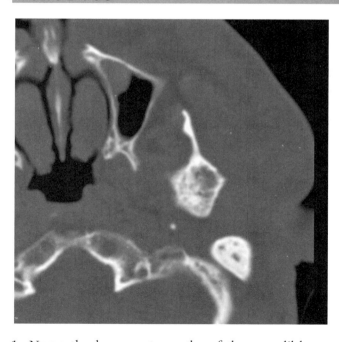
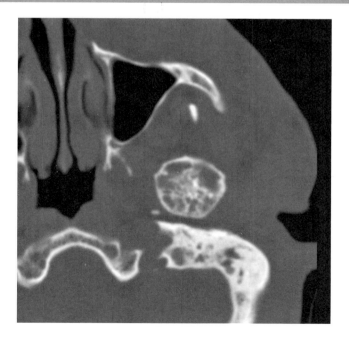

1. Name the bony outgrowths of the mandible.

2. From what part of the mandible do osteochondromas typically arise?

3. How often do patients with hereditary multiple exostoses develop malignancies?

4. What features on MRI suggest malignant degeneration?

CASE 104

Sinusitis

1. A maxillary sinus surgical procedure performed intraorally with a lip incision leading to a medial antrostomy (nasal-antral window). The mucosa is stripped free.

2. Functional endoscopic sinus surgery.

3. Sphenoethmoidal recess.

4. Sinolith, fungus ball, fungus sinusitis, osteoma, fibrous dysplasia, fracture fragment, inverted papilloma, olfactory neuroblastoma, and osteosarcoma.

Reference

Yoon JH, Na DG, Byun HS, et al: Calcification in chronic maxillary sinusitis: comparison of CT findings with histopathologic results, *AJNR Am J Neuroradiol* 20: 571–574, 1999.

Cross-Reference

Neuroradiology: THE REQUISITES, pp 620–627.

Comment

Sinonasal disease is classified into several anatomic patterns. The sporadic pattern shows no clear relationship to the primary drainage routes of the ostiomeatal complex. The maxillary infundibular pattern is the classic pattern with obstruction of the maxillary sinus ostium and the channel lateral to the uncinate process, the infundibulum. The frontal recess pattern occludes the drainage of the frontal and far anterior ethmoid air cells. The ostiomeatal unit pattern is associated with obstruction of the channel posteromedial to the uncinate process, which leads ultimately to obstructed anterior ethmoid sinuses. The maxillary antra also may become opacified. Finally the sphenoethmoidal recess pattern is associated with posterior ethmoid and sphenoid sinus disease. A related entity is the sinonasal polyposis pattern, in which polypoid mucosal thickening exists throughout the sinuses associated with cystic fibrosis or the aspirin allergy syndrome or both.

The pattern of intrasinus calcification may help distinguish a fungal sinusitis from a nonfungal type. Fungal sinusitis more commonly has irregularly marginated, fine punctate, linear, and nodular calcification patterns. It virtually never has smooth-margined, round, or eggshell calcification. In patients with fungal sinusitis, all calcifications seen have irregular margins. Aspergillus sinusitis has calcifications in nearly two thirds of cases within the necrotic mycelia.

Notes

CASE 105

Mandibular Osteochondroma

1. Osteomas, chondromas, osteoblastomas, osteochondromas (exostoses), chondroblastomas, and sarcomas.

2. The anteromedial surface of the condyle near the tendinous attachment of the pterygoids.

3. 25%.

4. Interval growth of the exostosis after adolescence, widening of the cartilaginous cap > 1.5 cm or interval growth, and enhancement of the cap.

Reference

Vanhoenacker FM, Van Hul W, Wuyts W, et al: Hereditary multiple exostoses: from genetics to clinical syndrome and complications, *Eur J Radiol* 40:208–217, 2001.

Cross-Reference

Neuroradiology: THE REQUISITES, pp 631–632.

Comment

Mandibular osteochondromas are unusual bony excrescences from the mandible. The most common bony excrescence seen associated with the mandible is the torus mandibularis. Similar to its benign maxilla counterpart, the torus palatinus, this represents hyperostotic bone that may be felt by the tongue along the lateral margin of the mandible protruding into the oral cavity. True osteochondromas are bony neoplasms, which may project more toward the buccal rather than the lingual surface of the mandible. Presumably, osteochondromas have a cartilaginous basis to their development. Multiple osteochondromas may be seen with Ollier syndrome. This syndrome has a significant rate of malignant transformation, and the osteochondromas that the patient experiences by and large have a mushroom shape, which may be differentiated from the appearance of an osteoma or exostoses or broad-based torus mandibularis.

Herditary multiple exostoses show benign cartilage capped bony excrescences. Three genetic loci for the disease have been isolated on chromosomes 8, 11, and 19 with a heterogeneous expression. Osteochondromas typically arise perpendicular to the epiphyseal growth plate. Presentation is usually in the first decade of life with multiple painless masses near the joints. Symptomatic bursitis also may lead to the discovery of the diagnosis.

Notes

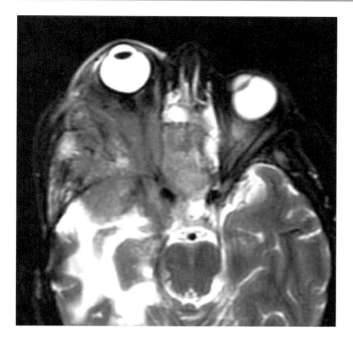
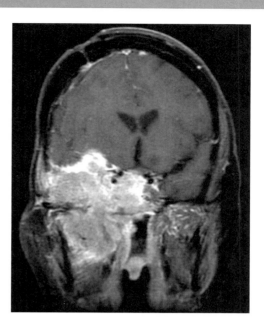

1. List the three most common head and neck sites for extracranial meningiomas.
2. What percentage of meningiomas are extracranial?
3. Name the most common temporal bone site of extracranial meningiomas.
4. What are the World Health Organization characteristics that make a meningioma malignant?

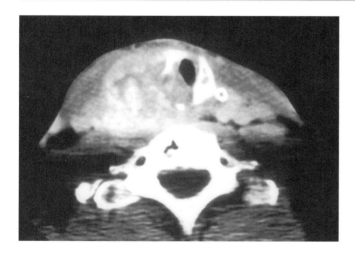

1. Which histology of thyroid cancers has the worse prognosis?
2. What is its 5-year prognosis?
3. Which histologic subtypes are iodine avid?
4. What is the staging classification of anaplastic carcinoma of the thyroid gland?

CASE 106

Atypical Meningioma

1. Orbit, sinonasal, and temporal bone.

2. 2%.

3. The middle ear.

4. ≥20 mitoses/10 high-power fields, anaplasia, rhabdoid subtype, or papillary subtype.

Reference

Thompson LD, Bouffard JP, Sandberg GD, Mena H: Primary ear and temporal bone meningiomas: a clinicopathologic study of 36 cases with a review of the literature, *Mod Pathol* 16:236–245, 2003.

Cross-Reference

Neuroradiology: THE REQUISITES, pp 102–104, 633.

Comment

Many different histologic types of meningioma are classified by the World Health Organization. Most are graded type I, which is the benign form of meningioma; this includes the histologic subtypes of fibroblastic, transitional, meningothelial, secretory, microcystic, psammomatous, angiomatous, and metaplastic varieties. Type II meningiomas are classified as atypical and are considered transitional lesions to type III meningiomas, which are more aggressive. Histologic subtypes classified as type II include chordoid, clear cell, and atypical. Type III malignant meningiomas have three subtypes: rhabdoid, papillary, and anaplastic.

Two entities that initially were considered malignant meningiomas have been separated into classifications of their own. Hemangiopericytoma has been shown to arise from different cell lines than meningioma and is no longer staged as meningioma. Similarly, angiosarcoma is staged separately from meningioma.

The pleomorphism of meningiomas is perplexing, and hemangiomas can undergo extensive calcification, cystic change, and fatty degeneration. Meningiomas adjacent to the calvaria may cause osteoblastic perforation and extensive bony changes. Nonetheless, most neuropathologists, on viewing the bone specimens associated with meningiomas, say that there are meningiomatous cells and tissue within the bone and that it is not exclusively reactive change. In certain circumstances, meningiomas simply can grow through the bone and into the soft tissue.

Notes

CASE 107

Anaplastic Carcinoma of the Thyroid Gland

1. Anaplastic carcinoma.

2. <10%.

3. Papillary and follicular.

4. It is automatically T4.

Reference

Takashima S, Morimoto S, Ikezoe J, et al: CT evaluation of anaplastic thyroid carcinoma, *AJR Am J Roentgenol* 154:1079–1085, 1990.

Cross-Reference

Neuroradiology: THE REQUISITES, pp 742–743.

Comment

Anaplastic carcinoma of the thyroid gland has a very poor prognosis. At the time of diagnosis, the lesion often has spread outside the thyroid capsule. Local invasion is usually the cause of death with airway compromise and spread into the anterior mediastinum.

The T staging of thyroid carcinoma is as follows:

T1—tumor ≤2 cm in greatest dimension

T2—tumor >2 cm but <4 cm in greatest dimension

T3—tumor >4 cm in greatest dimension limited to the thyroid or with minimal extrathyroid extension (extension to sternothyroid muscle or perithyroid soft tissues)

T4a—tumor of any size extending beyond the thyroid capsule to invade subcutaneous soft tissues, larynx, trachea, esophagus, or recurrent laryngeal nerve

T4b—tumor invading prevertebral fascia or encasing carotid artery or mediastinal vessels

All anaplastic carcinomas are considered T4 tumors:

T4a—intrathyroidal anaplastic carcinoma

T4b—extrathyroidal anaplastic carcinoma

Nodal staging of thyroid cancer is as follows:

N0—no regional lymph node metastasis

N1—regional lymph node metastasis

N1a—metastasis to level VI (pretracheal, paratracheal, and prelaryngeal/Delphian nodes)

N1b—metastasis to unilateral, bilateral, or contralateral cervical or superior mediastinal lymph nodes

Anaplastic carcinoma has a high rate (>50%) of intratumoral calcification, necrosis, and heterogeneity. Local direct spread to the carotid sheath, trachea, esophagus, and larynx seems to be inevitable.

Notes

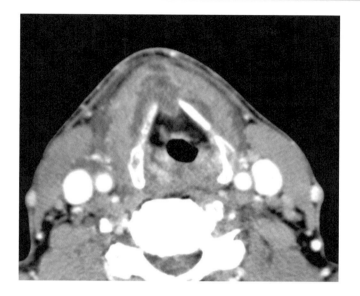

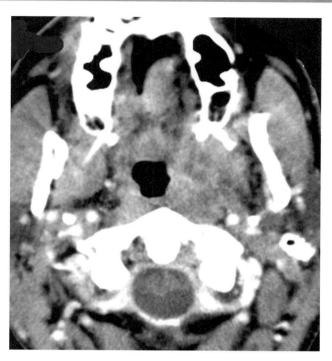

1. What is the congenital lesion to be considered in this location?
2. What is the typical presentation of that congenital lesion?
3. Could this be an abscess?
4. Name two foramina cecums in the head and neck.

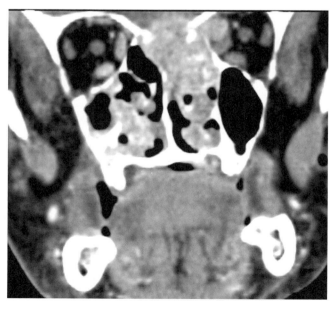

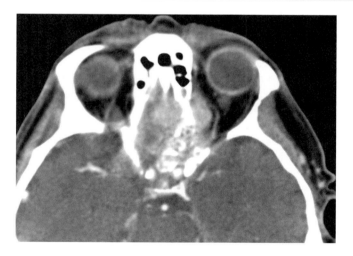

1. Which histologic subtype is the most common nasal cavity cancer?
2. What percentage of sinonasal carcinomas arise in the nasal cavity?
3. What is the major risk factor for nasal cancer?
4. What is the American Joint Commission for Cancer's staging of nasal cavity cancer?

Anterior Neck Phlegmon

1. Thyroglossal duct cyst.

2. Incidentally found neck mass.

3. Given the lack of enhancement, unlikely.

4. In the base of the tongue and in the cribriform plate.

Reference

Branstetter BF 4th, Weissman JL: Infection of the facial area, oral cavity, oropharynx, and retropharynx, *Neuroimaging Clin N Am* 13:393–410, 2003.

Cross-Reference

Neuroradiology: THE REQUISITES, pp 730–731.

Comment

Most clinicians use the term *phlegmon* to represent an inflammatory process that is not so well defined as to be called an abscess but that is more defined than simple cellulitis. Usually this inflammatory process manifests, as in this case, as a collection that does not show a peripheral rim of enhancement or thickened walls. It is often low density. The implication of distinguishing an abscess from a phlegmon is that the latter is not easily drainable by surgical or percutaneous intervention. No clear planes in the soft tissue are present. Antibiotics may still be curative. Is this an immature abscess, which, with time, would consolidate into a well-formed abscess? Perhaps.

Whenever a lesion is embedded in the strap muscles, a thyroglossal duct cyst should be considered. In this case, the patient had a tonsillar/peritonsillar infection that had spread into the anterior neck.

The false-negative rate for CT in suggesting abscess is 13%, and the false-positive rate is 10%. Scalloping of the abscess wall may predict more accurately a pus collection rather than a phlegmon in 64%. Some people use the term *phlegmon* whenever dealing with retropharyngeal cellulitis.

Notes

Nasal Carcinoma

1. Squamous cell carcinoma.

2. 30%.

3. Wood dust exposure.

4. Nasal cavity and ethmoid sinus. Primary tumor (T):

TX—primary tumor cannot be assessed
T0—no evidence of primary tumor
Tis—carcinoma in situ
T1—tumor restricted to any one subsite, with or without bony invasion
T2—tumor invading two subsites in a single region or extending to involve an adjacent region within the nasoethmoidal complex, with or without bony invasion
T3—tumor extends to invade the medial wall or floor of the orbit, maxillary sinus, palate, or cribriform plate
T4a—tumor invades any of the following: anterior orbital contents, skin of nose or cheek, minimal extension to anterior cranial fossa, pterygoid plates, or sphenoid or frontal sinuses
T4b—tumor invades any of the following: orbital apex, dura, brain, middle cranial fossa, cranial nerves other than cranial nerve V_2, nasopharynx, or clivus

Reference

Loevner LA, Sonners AI: Imaging of neoplasms of the paranasal sinuses, *Neuroimaging Clin N Am* 14:625–646, 2004.

Cross-Reference

Neuroradiology: THE REQUISITES, pp 629–631.

Comment

Nasal cancers, similar to cancers of the paranasal sinuses, are overwhelmingly squamous cell carcinomas in their histologies. Although other histologies also may affect this region, including melanoma, minor salivary gland tumors, lymphoma, and sarcomas, there are no definite imaging characteristics to distinguish among these lesions other than potentially the MRI findings that can be seen with melanoma, in which signal intensity may be bright on T1W scans. If one has a chondrosarcoma of the nasal septum, the whorled calcified appearance that is typical for chondroid lesions is seen.

Benign nasal cavity tumors include hemangiomas, inverted papillomas, and enchondromas. Hemangiomas may be characterized by their hypervascularity and their avid enhancement, and enchondromas have a cartilaginous appearance to them. Sinonasal polyposis is probably the most common mass to be seen in the nasal cavity and paranasal sinuses.

Notes

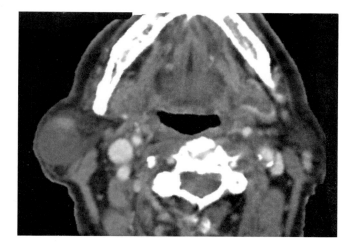

1. What is the second most common benign tumor of the parotid gland?

2. How often is it multiple in location?

3. Identify a risk factor for Warthin tumors.

4. What percentage is extraparotid?

Warthin Tumor

1. Warthin tumor.

2. 30%.

3. Eight times increased risk in smokers.

4. 8%, but not believed to be metastatic disease; may be primary disease or multifocal.

Reference

Ikeda M, Motoori K, Hanazawa T, et al: Warthin tumor of the parotid gland: diagnostic value of MR imaging with histopathologic correlation, *AJNR Am J Neuroradiol* 25:1256–1262, 2004.

Cross-Reference

Neuroradiology: THE REQUISITES, p 708.

Comment

Warthin tumor (cystadenoma lymphomatosum) is a common benign tumor of the parotid gland. It tends to occur in elderly men as opposed to middle-aged women, who tend to have pleomorphic adenomas. Warthin tumors have a predilection for the tail of the parotid gland, and some reports of extraparotid Warthin tumors have been published. Warthin tumor has no malignant potential. It can be observed over time rather than needing to be immediately resected.

Warthin tumors and another benign tumor of the parotid gland, oncocytoma, are avid on technetium pertechnetate nuclear medicine scintigraphy. Rarely, malignancies of the parotid gland occur that also might take up the technetium pertechnetate, which is why this imaging study is rarely performed in the evaluation of parotid masses.

If one sees a mass in the tail of the parotid gland in an elderly man, the first diagnosis should be a Warthin tumor. This tumor is usually hypointense and heterogeneous in signal intensity on T2W scans, making it among the few benign tumors that are not bright on T2W scans.

The average washout ratio of Warthin tumors (at 44%) is higher than that of malignant parotid tumors (at 12%). Apparent diffusion coefficient values are generally lower in Warthin tumors than in malignancies.

Notes

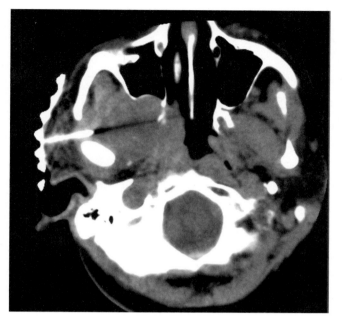 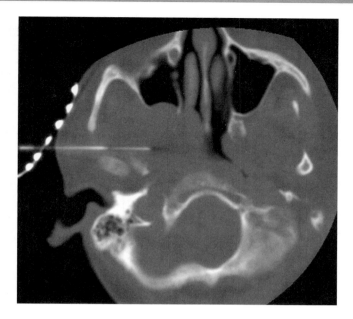

1. How large a needle can be used for biopsies before worrying about seeding along the biopsy tract?

2. What are the average results for nondiagnostic samples with a cytologist on site assessing the specimen?

3. Which primary sites warrant routine use of 25G needles for aspirations?

4. Which tumor requires separate sampling for flow cytometry?

Fine-Needle Aspiration of a Rhabdomyosarcoma

1. 16G.

2. 10% to 15%.

3. Thyroid gland lesions.

4. Lymphoma.

Reference
Sherman PM, Yousem DM, Loevner LA: CT-guided aspirations in the head and neck: assessment of the first 216 cases, *AJNR Am J Neuroradiol* 25:1603–1607, 2004.

Cross-Reference
Neuroradiology: THE REQUISITES, pp 721–723.

Comment
Fine-needle aspiration (FNA) is an effective means for diagnosing most head and neck lesions. The value of FNA includes its low invasiveness, use of small needles in an area where several vascular structures are present, and the lack of a telltale scar from the procedure. The pain associated with FNA is usually minimal when adequate local anesthetic is used. Neither sedation nor general anesthesia is required.

Image-guided FNA can evaluate nonpalpable lesions accurately, particularly lesions in a poorly accessible or deep location in the head and neck. Ultrasound-guided FNA is an established technique for lesion localization, particularly in evaluation of the thyroid gland and superficial cervical lymph nodes. Lesions deep to the bony structures of the face and air-containing spaces are not well localized by ultrasound but can be localized and aspirated accurately under CT guidance.

Typical series from experienced investigators obtain a diagnostic sample in 85% to 90% of cases, and a correct diagnosis is made in 83% to 88% of cases. On-site cytology is crucial. It has been shown that blind aspiration of a mass without a cytologist there is rarely diagnostic with a single FNA pass. In part, this is because the cytologist often wants aspirations of different portions of the lesions to reduce sampling error. It also may be that initial passes through the lesions have a greater amount of contamination with adjacent tissue than subsequent passes where a track already has cleared a path of the underlying subcutaneous fat and deep muscle. A 20% increase in obtaining diagnostic specimens when a cytopathologist is present has been reported in some series.

Notes

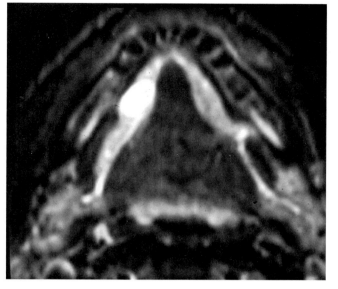
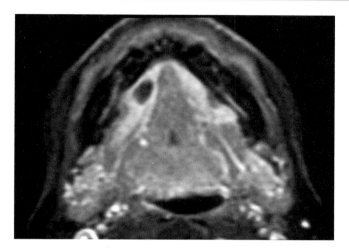
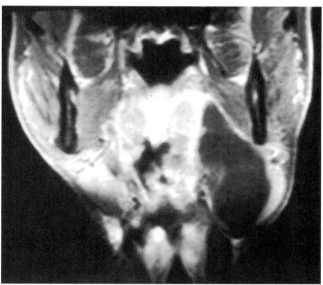

1. List the various names for this entity.
2. What is the critical anatomic structure to consider in assessing this lesion?
3. Are these lesions more a phenomenon of the sublingual gland or submandibular gland?
4. What is the ratio of simple to plunging ranulas?

Ranula

1. Ranula, mucous escape reaction, mucous escape cyst, and anterior lingual mucocele.

2. The mylohyoid muscle to distinguish a simple ranula (above) from a plunging ranula (which goes below the mylohyoid muscle).

3. Sublingual gland.

4. 3:1 in favor of simple ranula.

Reference

Zhao YF, Jia Y, Chen XM, Zhang WF: Clinical review of 580 ranulas, *Oral Surg Oral Med Oral Pathol Oral Radiol Endod* 98:281–287, 2004.

Cross-Reference

Neuroradiology: THE REQUISITES, pp 660–661, 705–706.

Comment

A ranula is due to an obstruction, trauma, or extravasation from the sublingual duct system or the minor salivary glands within the sublingual space. Ranulas are separated into simple, plunging type, or mixed varieties. A simple ranula remains above the floor of the mouth confined by the layer of the mylohyoid muscle. A plunging ranula usually extends more posteriorly and perforates through a weak area of the mylohyoid muscular sling and may present as a focal neck mass below the mandible. Simple ranulas are approached via a transoral incision with marsupialization or excision, whereas plunging ranulas must be approached via an incision under the mandible and delivered through the neck.

The differential diagnosis of ranulas in the floor of the mouth includes mere mucous retention cysts and abscesses. Ranulas show little contrast enhancement and should not infiltrate the adjacent soft tissues with inflammation the way one would expect an abscess to. When a ranula presents below the mandible, one might consider a dermoid cyst, thyroglossal duct cyst, and branchial cleft cyst. Usually dermoid cysts and thyroglossal cysts are midline lesions, whereas ranulas are typically off midline, lying as it were along the plane of the floor of the mouth. Branchial cleft cysts are located more posteriorly in the neck behind the submandibular gland and do not have an attachment to the floor of the mouth.

Ranulas are slightly more common in women and usually present by the 20s. Excision of the sublingual gland results in the lowest rate of recurrence.

Notes

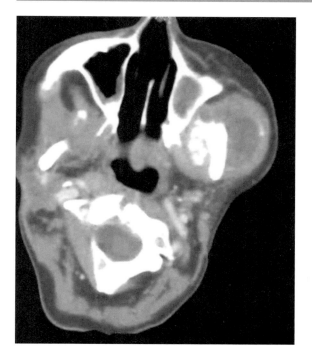 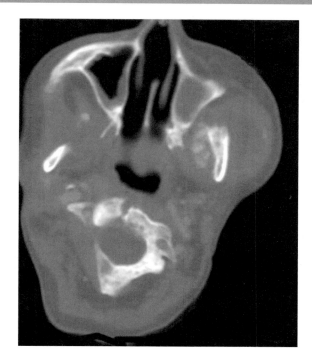

1. Identify the primary malignancies of the mandible.
2. What is the secondary finding on the study?
3. Name entities that predispose to osteosarcomas.
4. What cranial nerve runs through the mandible?

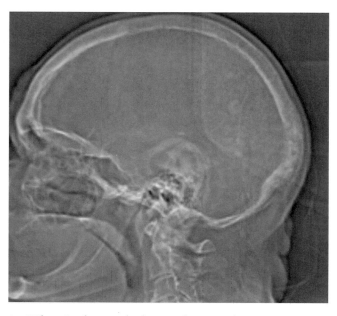 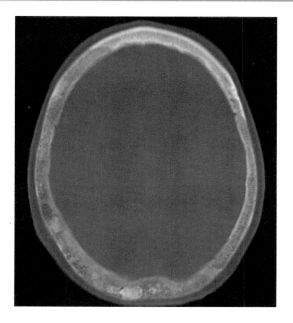

1. What is the underlying abnormality?
2. What percentage of patients with this disorder show calvarial changes?
3. What findings may be noted on a plain film of the skull with chronic renal failure?
4. Is the bone scan generally hot or cold in a skull with secondary hyperparathyroidism?

CASE 113

Osteosarcoma of the Mandible

1. Osteosarcoma, Ewing sarcoma, and lymphoma.

2. A blastic metastasis to the cervical spine.

3. Paget disease, retinoblastoma gene, and radiation.

4. V3.

Reference

Yamaguchi S, Nagasawa H, Suzuki T, et al: Sarcomas of the oral and maxillofacial region: a review of 32 cases in 25 years, *Clin Oral Invest* 8:52–55, 2004.

Cross-Reference

Neuroradiology: THE REQUISITES, pp 662–665.

Comment

Among primary bone tumors in the mandible, ameloblastoma, which has benign and malignant features, needs to be considered. This tumor may develop in a preexisting odontogenic lesion. Nonodontogenic benign lesions include aneurysmal bone cysts, simple unicameral cysts, and giant cell lesions.

Malignant mandibular masses include metastases, multiple myeloma, plasmacytoma, and lymphoma. These systemic disorders outnumber isolated mandibular primary bone tumors, including osteosarcomas and Ewing sarcoma. The latter two often show the typical sunburst pattern of periosteal reaction or onion skinning.

Sarcomas of the maxillofacial region are slightly more common in the mandible than the maxilla. Osteosarcomas outnumber malignant fibrous histiocytomas and rhabdomyosarcomas. Most are osteoblastic and present in patients in their 30s and 40s. Metastatic disease is common; the 5-year prognosis is approximately 60%. The prognosis is better in this location than in the long bones.

Notes

CASE 114

Chronic Renal Failure of the Skull

1. Secondary hyperparathyroidism from chronic renal failure.

2. 15%.

3. Basilar invagination, soft tissue calcinosis, florid dural calcification, resorption of lamina dura of the teeth, Brown tumors, salt and pepper skull, osteomalacia, and calcifications in dental pulp.

4. Hot.

Reference

Collins WO, Buchman CA: Radiology quiz case 2: metastatic calcifications of the middle and external ear and osteitis fibrosa of the temporal bones as a result of secondary hyperparathyroidism, *Arch Otolaryngol Head Neck Surg* 128:457, 459–460, 2002.

Cross-Reference

Neuroradiology: THE REQUISITES, pp 558–563.

Comment

Secondary hyperparathyroidism creates a unique pattern in the skull. The skull looks as though it has been moth-eaten, with tiny dots of lysis and sclerosis. The differential diagnosis includes multiple myeloma.

Other findings of secondary hyperparathyroidism that one may see in the head and neck include lysis of the lamina dura of the teeth such that there is an appearance of demineralization around the roots of the teeth.

A Brown tumor, osteoclastoma, is another manifestation of chronic renal failure in secondary hyperparathyroidism. One may see a large lytic lesion in the bones of the head and neck, most commonly the mandible. The differential diagnosis includes many of the other bubbly bone lesions (e.g., giant cell tumor, osteoblastoma, aneurysmal bone cyst, reparative granuloma, ameloblastoma).

Parathyroid hyperplasia is another head and neck manifestation of renal failure; this is due to a secondary reaction to the calcium-phosphorus dysmetabolism associated with renal failure.

Acceleration of atherosclerosis is another manifestation of renal failure. Atherosclerotic change in the superficial temporal arteries outside the calvaria is a good marker for long-standing chronic renal failure or diabetes with severe arteriolosclerosis.

Notes

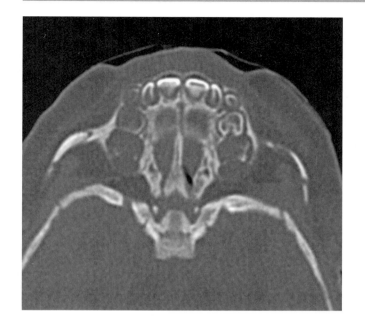
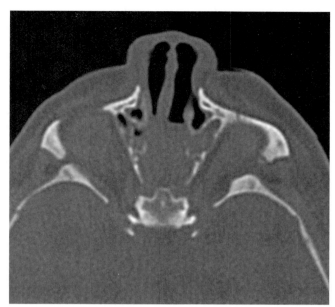
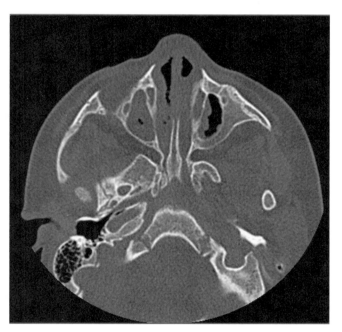

1. What is the minimum posterior choanal width in normal children < 2 years old?

2. What bone is widened in choanal atresia?

3. Which side is more commonly atretic?

4. How often is it bilateral?

Choanal Atresia

1. 0.34 cm.

2. Vomer.

3. Right.

4. One third of the time.

Reference

Black CM, Dungan D, Fram E, et al: Potential pitfalls in work-up and diagnosis of choanal atresia, *AJNR Am J Neurorad* 19:326–329, 1998.

Cross-Reference

Neuroradiology: THE REQUISITES, pp 615–616.

Comment

Choanal atresia usually is diagnosed clinically when a neonate is unable to breathe easily through the nose. Because neonates are obligate nose breathers, the presence of choanal atresia, particularly if it is bilateral, causes respiratory distress. When the clinician attempts to pass a small nasogastric tube, he or she finds that it is unable to pass through the nose. The infant must breathe through the mouth.

Choanal atresia may be membranous or bony. The degree of stenosis and the length of the block in an anteroposterior dimension may vary. In some cases, there is a complete bony block of the entire nasal channel, whereas in other cases there may be a thin membrane that separates the nasal cavity from the nasopharynx. The job of the radiologist is to determine the length of the stenosis or atretic plate, the width of the nasal passageway, and whether the blockage is due to bone or soft tissue. Treatment for a short membrane choanal stenosis differs from treatment for a thick bony atretic plate because the former can be managed endoscopically.

CHARGE syndrome consists of *c*olobomas, *h*eart defect, *a*tresia of choanae, *r*etardation mentally or physically or both, *g*enitourinary malformations, and *e*ar anomalies. Medial bowing and thickening of the lateral wall of the nasal cavity, widening of the vomer, and fusion of these two structures are often seen.

Notes

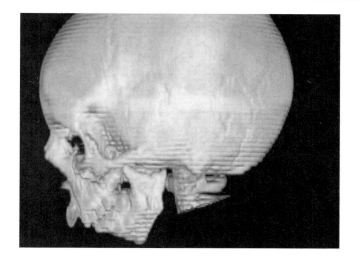

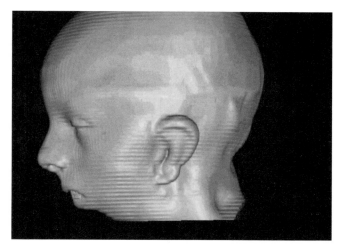

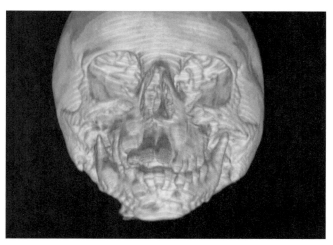

1. Name at least five syndromes that include a small jaw.

2. What is the classic triad of Pierre Robin syndrome?

3. Identify the two main risks of micrognathia.

4. Which branchial apparatus is responsible for development of the mandible?

Micrognathia: Pierre Robin Syndrome

1. Treacher Collins, Goldenhar, Miller, Pierre Robin, Stickler, pyknodysostosis, trisomy 13, trisomy 18, and Turner.

2. Micrognathia, U-shaped cleft palate, and relative macroglossia.

3. Inadequate feeding and relative macroglossia resulting in airway obstruction.

4. First.

Reference

Cademartiri F, Luccichenti G, Lagana F, et al: Effective clinical outcome of a mandibular distraction device using three-dimensional CT with volume rendering in Pierre-Robin sequence, *Acta Biomed Ateneo Parmense* 75:122–125, 2004.

Cross-Reference

Neuroradiology: THE REQUISITES, p 709.

Comment

Innumerable syndromes are associated with micrognathia. Pierre Robin syndrome constitutes the triad of micrognathia, cleft palate, and ptotic tongue. This is an autosomal recessive syndrome, and its central feature is the maldevelopment of the mandible, which leads secondarily to the cleft palate. Ear anomalies include otitis media and ossicular dysplasia. Ocular anomalies constitute congenital glaucoma, axial myopia, retinal detachment, and, less commonly, microphthalmia. Syndactyly and polydactyly occur frequently.

Treatment of mandibular hypoplasia is by distraction osteogenesis, which progressively lengthens the mandible by surgically fracturing it, then progressively distracting the pieces. This treatment approach obviates the need for bone grafting by letting the body's own callus formation create the new bone necessary to lengthen the mandible.

Notes

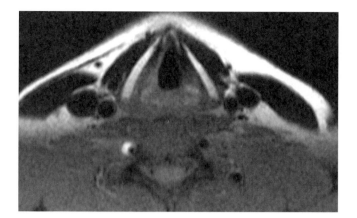

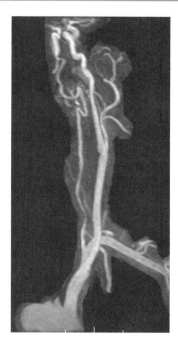

1. What percentage of patients with arterial dissections in the neck develop or present with a stroke?
2. How often do intracranial arterial dissections cause subarachnoid hemorrhage?
3. How often do patients have headache or neck pain with vertebral artery dissection?
4. Can pulsatile tinnitus be a sign of arterial dissection?

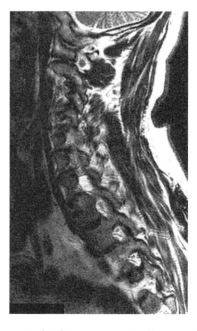

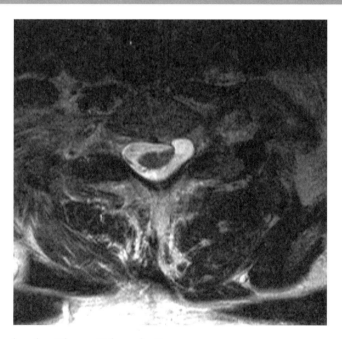

1. Which roots typically are involved with an Erb palsy?
2. Which roots typically are involved with a Klumpke paralysis?
3. What is the significance of the expression "Rad techs drink cold beer"?
4. How does a neuroma affect the brachial plexus?

CASE 117

Vertebral Artery Dissections

1. 50% to 60%.

2. 20%.

3. 50% to 80%.

4. Yes.

Reference

Christian MD, Detsky AS: Clinical problem-solving: a twist of fate? *N Engl J Med* 351:69–73, 2004.

Cross-Reference

Neuroradiology: THE REQUISITES, pp 221–224.

Comment

For the most part, the intravertebral segment of the vertebral artery (V2) is protected from damage leading to arterial dissection. The more vulnerable parts of the vertebral artery include the V1 segment from its origin at the subclavian artery to its entry at the C6 or C7 vertebra. Superiorly, as the vertebral artery passes from the vertebral column to the intracranial compartment (V3), there again is an increased vulnerability to dissection, in part because of the anchoring of the vertebral artery within the vertebral column (V2) and the anchoring of its dural attachment as it enters the intracranial compartment (V4). Chiropractic manipulation of the spinal column potentially also can injure the portion of the vertebral artery in the foramen transversarium.

Symptoms of vertebral artery dissection include neck pain, dizziness, vertigo, and posterior circulation infarction.

On imaging, the best sequence on MRI to identify the dissection is a fat-suppression T1W scan. The fat suppression is useful in being able to distinguish the hyperintense mural clot from the surrounding fat in a vertebral artery at all locations of the neck. The tortuous nature of the vertebral artery may lead to high signal intensity within the blood vessel secondary to turbulent flow. Sometimes one must evaluate the artery in multiple projections to exclude an intramural thrombus. Downward loops, in particular, may be problematic. Magnetic resonance angiography with evaluations of the raw data to assess the luminal configuration also is useful to this evaluation. Stretch injuries to the arteries and spasm are seen better on magnetic resonance angiography than on the spin echo data.

Notes

CASE 118

Nerve Root Avulsions

1. C5-6.

2. C7-T1.

3. It denotes the anatomy of the brachial plexus from medial to lateral with roots, trunks, divisions, cords, and branches.

4. After an avulsion or stretch injury, one may get an enlarged nerve from the trauma or scar as it heals. This does not conduct impulses well and may lead to persistent brachial plexopathy.

Reference

Carvalho GA, Nikkhah G, Matthies C, et al: Diagnosis of root avulsions in traumatic brachial plexus injuries: value of computerized tomography myelography and magnetic resonance imaging, *J Neurosurg* 86:69–76, 1997.

Cross-Reference

Neuroradiology: THE REQUISITES, pp 838–840.

Comment

The setting for nerve root avulsion is divided largely along neonatal versus adult lines. In the neonate, one may see nerve root avulsions during traumatic vaginal deliveries. As the shoulder is vigorously rotated to extract the infant from the vagina, the force may lead to avulsion of the lower cervical nerve roots. Ninety percent of brachial plexopathies in children are due to birth trauma; 80% heal without neurologic sequelae. Erb-Duchenne palsies are much more common than Klumpke paralysis.

In young adults, the source of the nerve root avulsions is a motor vehicle accident with a classic description being that of a motorcyclist thrown from his or her bike landing on outstretched arms.

Radiographically, nerve root avulsion is distinguished by absence of the nerve root within the nerve root sleeve. Often the spinal cord is retracted away from the side of the nerve root avulsion. One also may see outpouchings of the nerve root sleeve or thecal sac of what is termed a *pseudomeningocele*. CT-myelography is more accurate (85%) than MRI (52%) because of confounding factors of partial rootlet avulsion (false-negative), scarring (false-negative), and dural ectasias (false-positive).

Pseudomeningoceles also are part of the spectrum of disease that one might see with neurofibromatosis 1, Marfan disease, and ankylosing spondylitis.

Notes

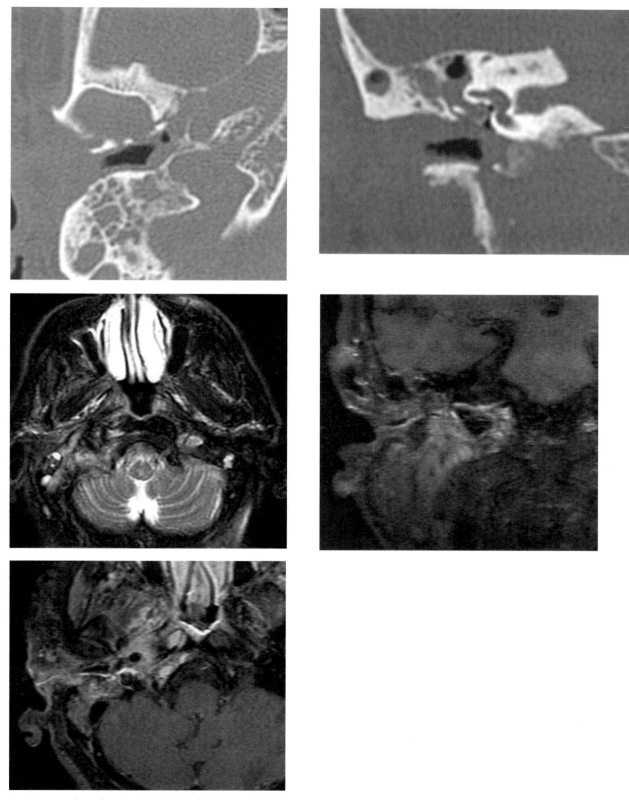

1. Name the classic imaging findings for this entity.

2. What are the clinical symptoms?

3. Why is MRI not useful in monitoring the therapy of malignant otitis externa (MOE)?

4. What are the routes of spread of MOE?

Malignant Otitis Externa

1. External auditory canal opacification, erosion of the canal, and inflammation at the skull base or parapharyngeal space.

2. Otitis externa, otalgia with deep and throbbing pain worse at night, and otorrhea.

3. It typically lags way behind the clinical response and the erythrocyte sedimentation rate decrease.

4. Anteroinferomedially through the fissures of Santorini to the skull base and parapharyngeal space, medially to the jugular foramen and carotid canal, and posteriorly into the mastoid air cells and cortical plate of the sigmoid sinus.

Reference

Ismail H, Hellier WP, Batty V: Use of magnetic resonance imaging as the primary imaging modality in the diagnosis and follow-up of malignant external otitis, *J Laryngol Otol* 118:576–579, 2004.

Cross-Reference

Neuroradiology: THE REQUISITES, pp 567–569.

Comment

MOE represents an aggressive *Pseudomonas* infection, which usually is seen in an elderly diabetic host. Immunosuppressed patients (HIV-positive patients, transplant patients, patients receiving chemotherapy) also may be susceptible hosts. The history may be that of an individual who has an external otitis and whose ear is irrigated by an otorhinolaryngologist. The irrigation under pressure may drive the *Pseudomonas* bacteria through the fissures of Santorini at the junction of the bony and cartilaginous portions of the external auditory canal. The bacteria may cause erosion of the walls of the external auditory canal and an inflammatory process that extends into the parapharyngeal space or the skull base itself, resulting either in an inflammatory mass that obscures the fat planes of the parapharyngeal space or osteitis and reactive bone change at the clivus or skull base itself.

MOE is hard to eradicate, especially because the patient is in part immunocompromised as a result of the diabetes. Intravenous antibiotics typically are required. As with any osteomyelitis, the course of antibiotic therapy must be extended. Even with treatment with antipseudomonal drugs, third-generation cephalosporins, fluoroquinolones, and local débridement, morbidity is 10% to 20%. The risk is that the patient will develop an abscess or vascular complication of the infection, such as thrombophlebitis or an arteritis. Spread also may occur to the temporomandibular joint, where pain on mastication may be the symptom. Cranial nerve VII is the most common nerve affected by MOE.

Notes

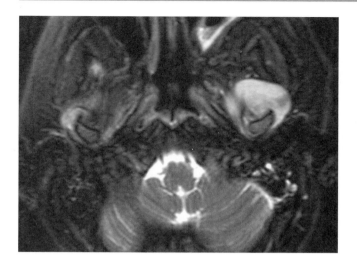 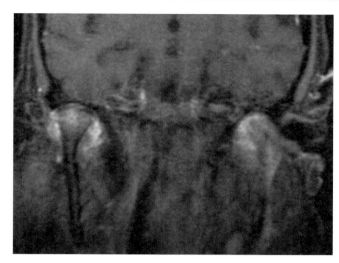

1. Name causes of inflammatory arthritides of the temporomandibular joint (TMJ).

2. At what stage of rheumatoid arthritis (RA) is the TMJ affected?

3. What are the most common findings in RA of the TMJ?

4. Is it more likely to find radiographic TMJ disease without symptoms in patients with RA or symptoms without radiographic abnormalities?

Rheumatoid Arthritis of the Temporomandibular Joint

1. Rheumatoid, lupus, mixed connective tissue disease, gout, pseudogout, septic arthritis, juvenile idiopathic arthritis, psoriatic arthritis, and ankylosing spondylitis.

2. Usually it is late in the course of the disease in individuals with polyarticular disease.

3. Effusion, marginal erosion, synovial proliferation, osteolysis, flattening of the condylar head, and cysts.

4. More likely to have positive imaging findings in the face of no symptoms in the TMJ of patients with RA.

Reference

Melchiorre D, Calderazzi A, Maddali Bongi S, et al: A comparison of ultrasonography and magnetic resonance imaging in the evaluation of temporomandibular joint involvement in rheumatoid arthritis and psoriatic arthritis, *Rheumatology (Oxf)* 42:673–676, 2003.

Cross-Reference

Neuroradiology: THE REQUISITES, p 718.

Comment

Lesions, erosions, and synovial proliferation are findings one may see with RA of the TMJ. TMJ arthritis occurs in approximately 40% to 50% of patients with systemic RA. Patients complain of TMJ pain, stiffness, and decrease in the range of motion.

As opposed to typical cases of internal derangement of the TMJ, the meniscus is not the central/focal point with RA of the TMJ. Instead, one sees erosion of the mandibular condylar head and large joint diffusions. The capsule of the joint is expanded. One also might see signal intensity changes within the marrow signal of the condylar head with replacement of the normal T1W bright fat.

Notes

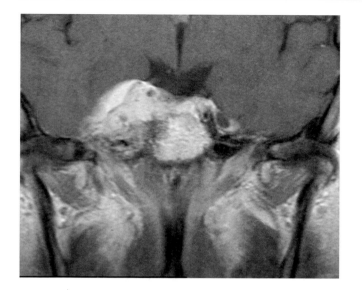
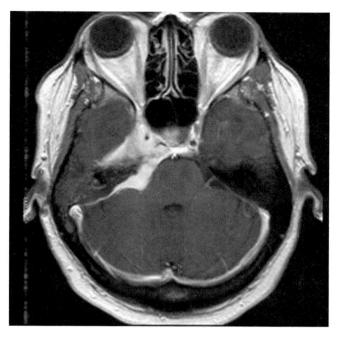

1. What is the eponym for painful ophthalmoplegia secondary to "orbital pseudotumor" of the cavernous sinus?

2. Which cranial nerve is the most closely apposed to the cavernous internal carotid artery?

3. What does the dural tail of a meningioma represent?

4. What would the diagnosis be if this lesion were bright on noncontrast T1W scan?

Cavernous Sinus Meningioma

1. Tolosa-Hunt syndrome.

2. Cranial nerve VI.

3. Either tumor cells or reactive change.

4. Leptomeningeal melanoma.

Reference

Ishikawa M, Nishi S, Aoki T, et al: Predictability of internal carotid artery (ICA) dissectability in cases showing ICA involvement in parasellar meningioma, *J Clin Neurosci* 8(Suppl 1):22–25, 2001.

Cross-Reference

Neuroradiology: THE REQUISITES, pp 102–104.

Comment

As opposed to pituitary adenomas, cavernous sinus and parasellar meningiomas have a predilection for narrowing the carotid artery and encasing the vessel. This stenosis occurs over an extended period, which accounts for the relative lack of vascular and ischemic complications resulting from the carotid stenosis.

The prognosis and surgical success rate when dealing with parasellar meningiomas has less to do with the degree of carotid encasement than it does the involvement of perforating arteries. Surgeons believe that if the tumor is soft and able to be aspirated, complete encasement can be dealt with effectively. If there is long segment disease affecting small perforators, however, the prognosis is worse.

The degree of cavernous carotid artery involvement has been graded using the Hirsch classification (table).

Grade	Tumor Description
1	Touch or partially encircle the cavernous internal carotid artery
2	Completely encircle but do not narrow the lumen of the internal carotid artery
3	Encircle and narrow the lumen of the cavernous internal carotid artery

On unenhanced CT scans, approximately 60% of meningiomas are slightly hyperdense compared with normal brain tissue, and calcification is present in approximately 20% of cases. Meningiomas show avid enhancement.

At the Meckel cave region, the differential diagnosis may include lymphoma, sarcoidosis, plasmacytoma, and subarachnoid seeding.

Notes

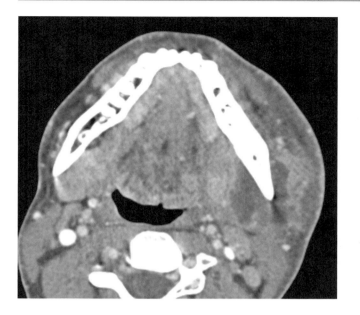 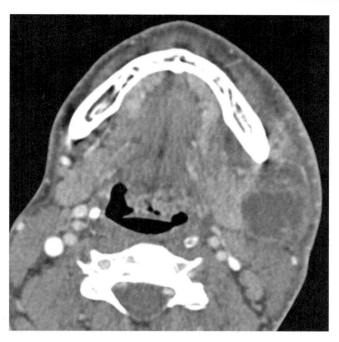

1. What bacteria would you expect to find in this lesion?

2. What is Ludwig angina?

3. Name the part of the tooth that is the most peripheral to the visible surface.

4. What is the tooth's innermost chamber called?

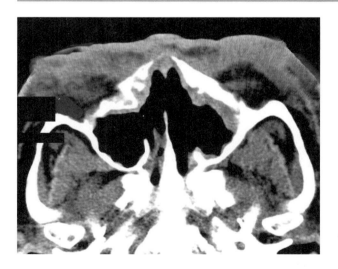 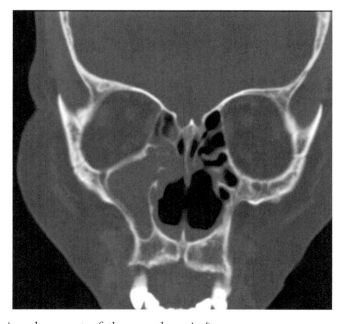

1. What are the most common sites for sarcoidosis involvement of the nasal cavity?

2. Name three infectious causes of nasal septum destruction.

3. How often does sarcoid affect the orbit; head and neck?

4. What are the most common manifestations of sarcoidosis in the head and neck?

Dental Abscess

1. Polymicrobial anaerobes: *Bacteroides, Streptococcus viridans,* and *Fusobacterium.*

2. Infection spread to the floor of the mouth, submandibular region, and upper neck.

3. The root.

4. The pulp.

Reference

Makeieff M, Gresillon N, Berthet JP, et al: Management of descending necrotizing mediastinitis, *Laryngoscope* 114:772–775, 2004.

Cross-Reference

Neuroradiology: THE REQUISITES, pp 660–661.

Comment

Dental inflammation ranks with pharyngitis, sinusitis, and otomastoiditis as one of the most common inflammatory processes to affect the head and neck. Dental caries or gingivitis may lead to infections involving the adjacent soft tissue (cellulitis) or bone (osteomyelitis). Poor oral hygiene, frequent ingestion of sugar-containing foods or alcohol, and infrequent visits to the dentist predispose to these infections.

A periapical abscess originates in the dental pulp and can lead to a cyst, granuloma, or osteomyelitis. Periodontal spread refers to inflammation of the adjacent ligaments and bone.

Spread to the muscles of mastication leads to symptoms of trismus and pain. The parapharyngeal fat may be displaced posteromedially, signifying the presence of a masticator space lesion when the pterygoid muscles are affected. Descending necrotizing mediastinitis may be a lethal complication arising from odontogenic infections.

Notes

Sarcoidosis of the Nasal Septum

1. The septum and the inferior turbinate.

2. Syphilis, leprosy, and tuberculosis. Also klebsiella.

3. 20% to 30%; 15%.

4. Dermatologic findings, cervical adenopathy, and parotitis.

Reference

Schwartzbauer HR, Tami TA: Ear, nose and throat manifestations of sarcoidosis, *Otolaryngol Clin North Am* 36:673–684, 2003.

Cross-Reference

Neuroradiology: THE REQUISITES, pp 624–625.

Comment

There is a broad differential diagnosis for nasal septal perforation. When soft tissue is associated with it, one should consider sarcoidosis, Wegener granulomatosis, and lymphoma. Midline lethal granuloma seems to be a stage of lymphoma of the nasal septum. Systemic lupus erythematosus, antiphospholipid syndrome, cocaine abuse, and cryoglobulinemia are other diagnoses to consider.

Infectious etiologies for nasal septal perforation include *Klebsiella* infection (rhinoscleroma), syphilis (saddle nose deformity), tuberculosis, and leprosy. Cocaine remains the most common source of nasal septal perforation, possibly resulting from a subclinical vasculitis with necrosis of the nasal septum. If one sees a black eschar on the nasal septum, one should consider fungal infection with mucormycosis or nasal septum melanoma. Many of the etiologies for nasal septum perforation and soft tissue mass also are potential causes for orbital infiltration.

Sarcoidosis most often presents in the head and neck with cervical adenopathy (48%), parotid enlargement (6%), or facial nerve palsy. Uveitis (Heerfordt disease, comprising uveitis, facial nerve paralysis, and fever) and diabetes insipidus are other manifestations.

Notes

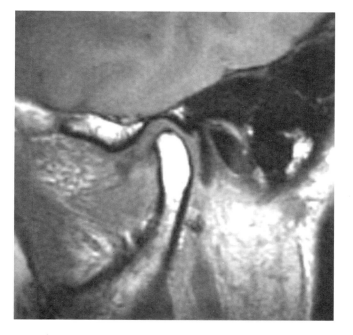
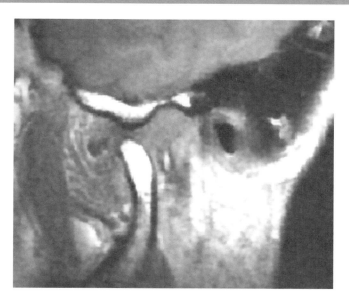

1. What percentage of normal volunteers have internal derangement (of the temporomandibular joint [TMJ])?

2. What percentage of symptomatic patients have internal derangement of the TMJ?

3. What is the difference in the rate of reduction in normal volunteers versus patients?

4. What is the value of coronal imaging of the TMJ?

Anterior Dislocation of the Meniscus

1. 35%.

2. 78%.

3. 100% in normal volunteers; 76% in patients.

4. In approximately 12% of cases, images reveal a meniscal displacement that would not otherwise be evident on the sagittal scans.

Reference

Larheim TA, Westesson P, Sano T: Temporomandibular joint disk displacement: comparison in asymptomatic volunteers and patients, *Radiology* 218:428–432, 2001.

Cross-Reference

Neuroradiology: THE REQUISITES, pp 714–718.

Comment

Typical evaluation of the TMJ includes sagittal T1W or proton density–weighted scans through the plane of the TMJ in the open and closed mouth positions. The closed mouth position is the crucial one because if there is anterior displacement of the meniscus of the TMJ, it is seen reliably on the closed mouth views. The posterior margin of the posterior band of the meniscus should reside at approximately the 11 to 12 o'clock position on the axis of mandibular condyle. If it is anteriorly displaced beyond the 10 o'clock position or beyond 10 degrees from the vertical, it is said to be anteriorly dislocated. This anterior dislocation may "recapture" when one performs an open mouth view; this potentially could result in a sensation or sound of a click when the patient opens the jaw. In more severe disease, the meniscus may remain fixed anteriorly and does not recapture on the open mouth view. Patients may experience limitation of motion on opening of the jaw in such cases; this is termed *anterior displacement without recapture.*

The coronal view is useful because there may be a transverse component to the dislocation in 40% of cases. Medial dislocation in association with an anterior component (rotational dislocation) is more common than isolated lateral dislocation (sideways dislocation). If there is pure sideways displacement, it may be useful to perform an open mouth view in the coronal plane to see if the meniscus recaptures.

Recapturing of the meniscus portends a better prognosis with conservative splinting therapy than does inability to recapture. Individuals without the ability to recapture ultimately may require surgical intervention.

If the meniscus is in a normal position on closed mouth T1W scans, it is extremely likely that the open mouth views will be normal in appearance as well.

In rare cases, the meniscus is "stuck," in which case it does not move at all as it should when one opens the jaw, gliding forward with the mandibular condyle under the articular eminence. Such a stuck disc may be due to fibrotic changes and may be a source of TMJ pain and discomfort.

This is a disease of young women, who are much more conscious of clicking and discomfort in the TMJ than men. Alternatively, anterior dislocation of the meniscus may be a manifestation of ligamentous laxity secondary to the hormonal fluctuations occurring in young women.

Notes

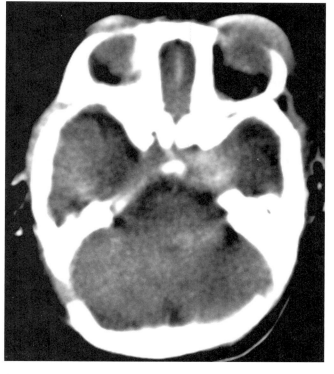

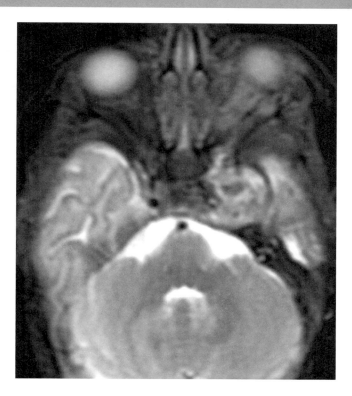

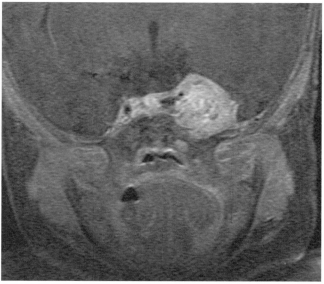

1. Name at least four hyperdense cavernous sinus masses in all age groups.

2. Name at least four predisposing conditions for aneurysm formation in a child.

3. What is the significance of the distinction between an infraclinoid and supraclinoid aneurysm?

4. What treatment should be recommended for this lesion?

C A S E 1 2 5

Cavernous Sinus Aneurysm

1. Aneurysm, hemorrhagic pituitary adenoma, meningioma, cavernous carotid fistula, and cavernous sinus thrombosis.

2. Marfan syndrome, pseudoxanthoma elasticum, Ehlers-Danlos syndrome, mycotic aneurysm from sinusitis, polycystic kidney disease, fibromuscular dysplasia, and dissection.

3. Supraclinoid aneurysms are intracranial and bleed in the subarachnoid space and are more likely to result in death.

4. Trapping with occlusion of the aneurysm.

Reference

Sungarian A, Rogg J, Duncan JA 3rd: Pediatric intracranial aneurysm: a diagnostic dilemma solved with contrast-enhanced MR imaging, *AJNR Am J Neuroradiol* 24: 370–372, 2003.

Cross-Reference

Neuroradiology: THE REQUISITES, pp 538–539.

Comment

This is an unusual case, and it represents a cavernous sinus aneurysm in a neonate. The signal intensity, being bright on T1W scan, suggests the presence of subacute thrombosis; however, turbulent flow also may cause high signal intensity. If this is a partially thrombosed aneurysm, the carotid artery would have a normal appearance, in which case the diagnosis would continue to be obscured. What is in the differential diagnosis? Most cavernous sinus masses would not be expected to be bright on T1W scans. One could consider schwannomas and meningioma; however, they are unusual in an infant. Alternatively, one might think of a teratoma or dermoid's accounting for the high signal intensity; however, by and large these are midline lesions.

The most frequent cause of subarachnoid hemorrhage in a child is trauma or child abuse. More than 75% of children with aneurysms present with subarachnoid hemorrhage. Given 100 aneurysms in each, giant aneurysms (>2.5 cm in size) are more common in children than adults.

Notes

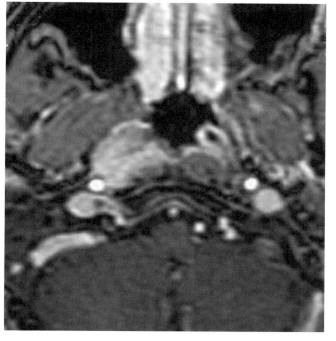

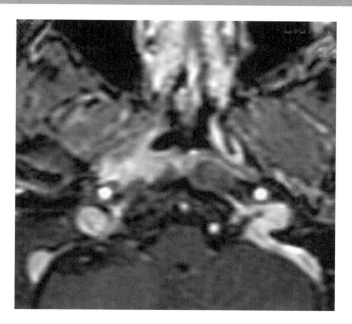

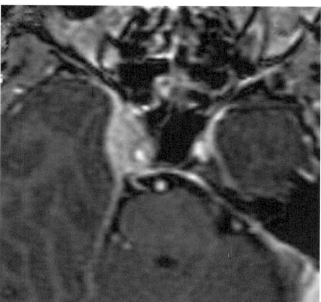

1. What are the most common histologies of nasopharyngeal neoplasms?

2. Name the opening in the fascia that emits the eustachian tube.

3. What are the patterns of spread of nasopharyngeal carcinoma?

4. Describe the stereotypical patient with nasopharyngeal carcinoma.

Nasopharyngeal Carcinoma

1. Squamous cell carcinoma, nonkeratinizing carcinoma, undifferentiated carcinoma, lymphoma, and rhabdomyosarcoma.

2. Sinus of Morgagni.

3. Most commonly into the parapharyngeal space and the retropharynx. The possible routes of spread include along the fifth cranial nerves, along the vidian canal, through the skull, into the cavernous sinus, and laterally into the masticator space.

4. A young Asian patient exposed in the past to Epstein-Barr virus.

Reference

Cheng SH, Tsai SY, Yen KL, et al: Prognostic significance of parapharyngeal space venous plexus and marrow involvement: potential landmarks of dissemination for stage I-III nasopharyngeal carcinoma, *Int J Radiat Oncol Biol Phys* 61:456–465, 2005.

Cross-Reference

Neuroradiology: THE REQUISITES, pp 647–649.

Comment

The staging of nasopharyngeal carcinoma is as follows:

T1—tumor confined to the nasopharynx
T2—tumor extends to soft tissue
    T2a—tumor extends to the oropharynx or nasal cavity or both without parapharyngeal extension
    T2b—with parapharyngeal extension
T3—tumor involves bony structures or paranasal sinuses or both
T4—tumors with intracranial extension or involvement of cranial nerves, infratemporal fossa, hypopharynx, orbit, or masticator space
N0—no regional lymph node metastasis
N1—unilateral metastasis in lymph nodes, ≤6 cm in greatest dimension, above the supraclavicular fossa
N2—bilateral nodes ≤6 cm above supraclavicular fossa
N3—metastasis in lymph nodes >6 cm or to supraclavicular fossa
    N3a—>6 cm in dimension
    N3b—extension to the supraclavicular fossa

Cheng et al have shown that the 5-year recurrence-free survival in cases that do not have parapharyngeal spread is excellent (>95%) when treated with radiation therapy and adjuvant chemotherapy. In cases with parapharyngeal spread or T3 disease, the 5-year recurrence-free survival rate, with and without adjuvant chemotherapy, was 76.8% and 53.2%.

The major risk factors for nasopharyngeal carcinoma are Epstein-Barr virus exposure and Asian ethnicity.

Some clinicians use fluorodeoxyglucose positron emission tomography (FDG PET) for the evaluation of treated nasopharyngeal carcinoma because the appearance of the nasopharynx may be unchanged on MRI and CT despite a good clinical response. The results have shown that the sensitivity and specificity of FDG PET for the detection of recurrent nasopharyngeal carcinoma are >85% for the lymph nodes and >90% for distant metastases. At the primary site, the sensitivity (approximately 90%) exceeds the specificity (approximately 75%).

Notes

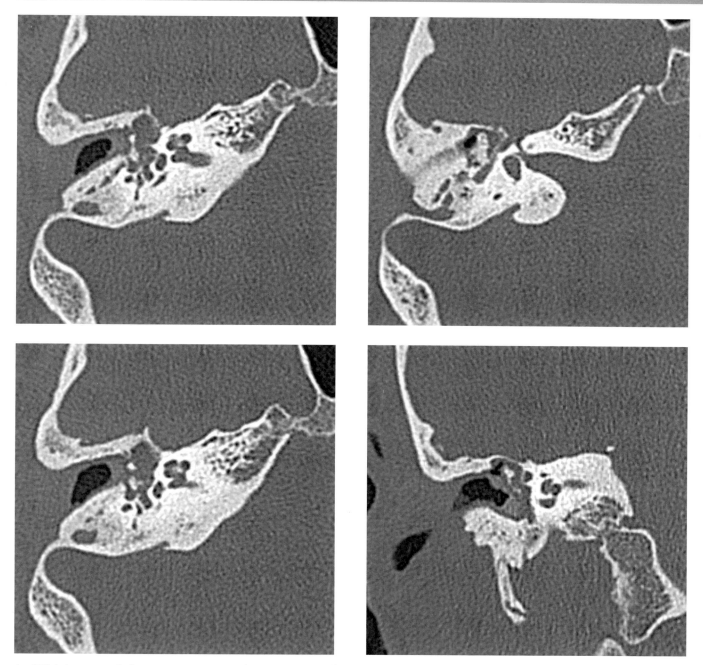

1. Which part of the tympanic membrane is usually perforated in the development of this lesion?

2. What area of dehiscence is shown in this case?

3. What are the most common locations for tympanosclerosis?

4. How often does tympanosclerosis occur with acquired cholesteatoma?

Acquired Cholesteatoma with Tympanosclerosis

1. Pars flaccida.

2. Tympanic portion of the facial canal.

3. Tympanic membrane, ossicles, and ligaments.

4. 2.2% of cases of tympanosclerosis have concomitant cholesteatoma.

Reference

Asiri S, Hasham A, al Anazy F, et al: Tympanosclerosis: review of literature and incidence among patients with middle-ear infection, *J Laryngol Otol* 113: 1076–1080, 1999.

Cross-Reference

Neuroradiology: THE REQUISITES, pp 578–580.

Comment

Cholesteatomas represent squamous epithelial ingrowth through a perforated tympanic membrane. This ingrowth usually occurs through the pars flaccida of the tympanic membrane representing the superioposterior portion of the tympanic membrane. From there, the lesion shows ingrowth into the Prussak space, which is the cavity represented lateral to the scutum and medial to the wall of the tympanic cavity. When it penetrates into the epitympanic space, the cholesteatoma displaces or erodes the middle ear ossicles. It then may grow through the aditus ad antrum to enter the mastoid air cells, where it may displace the bone again and enlarge the mastoid cavity.

Complications of cholesteatoma include dehiscence of the facial nerve canal (usually the horizontal tympanic portion), erosion of the tegmen tympani, or development of a perilymphatic fistula through growth into the lateral semicircular canal.

On MRI, cholesteatomas usually show only peripheral enhancement and are intermediate in signal intensity on T2W scan.

Tympanosclerosis, seen here as extraossific densities associated with the ossicles, represents a reaction to chronic inflammation in the middle ear. It occurs in almost 12% of all patients with chronic suppurative otitis media. Indwelling tympanostomy tubes are associated with a higher incidence of tympanosclerosis. Clinically the fixation of the ossicles by the ligamentous deposits or deposits on the ossicles restrict movement and cause a conductive hearing loss. Treatment may require partial or total replacement of the ossicles.

Notes

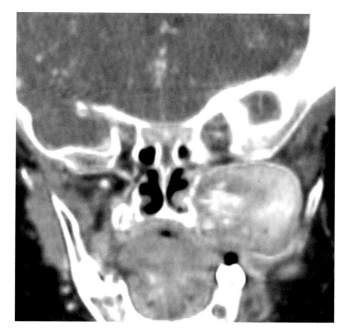 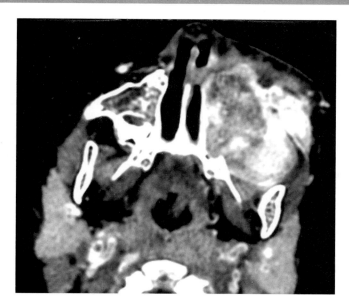

1. Is there malignant potential for this lesion?
2. What is the preferred location for this lesion?
3. What is the expected change in appearance of a central ossifying fibroma with time?
4. What are other names for this entity?

Ossifying Fibroma

1. No.

2. Anterior maxilla, especially incisor/cuspid region.

3. It becomes more and more dense with calcification with time.

4. Cementifying fibroma, cementoossifying fibroma, fibrous osteoma, and osteofibroma.

Reference

Mafee MF, Yang G, Tseng A, et al: Fibro-osseous and giant cell lesions, including brown tumor of the mandible, maxilla, and other craniofacial bones, *Neuroimaging Clin N Am* 13:525–540, 2003.

Cross-Reference

Neuroradiology: THE REQUISITES, p 864.

Comment

Ossifying fibroma is one of the diverse fibroosseous lesions that may affect the head and neck. This lesion is seen more commonly in the long bones than the bones of the face. Nonetheless, when it occurs, it tends to involve the mandible and maxilla and the paranasal sinus. This is a dense lesion that more closely resembles an osteoma than a fibrous dysplasia.

Ossifying fibromas have no potential for malignant degeneration. They usually are seen in young adults in their 20s to 30s. Typical symptoms include pain and facial deformity; however, a substantial proportion are detected incidentally. The ratio of women to men is 3 to 5:1. Although ossifying fibromas are more common in the mandible, the more aggressive form, juvenile active ossifying fibroma, is more common in the maxilla as seen here. It behaves in an aggressive and locally destructive manner but has no malignant or metastatic potential.

Ossifying fibromas of the mandible and maxilla may be confused with sclerosing dense odontogenic lesions, such as cemental dysplasia, odontoma, and Pindborg tumors.

Notes

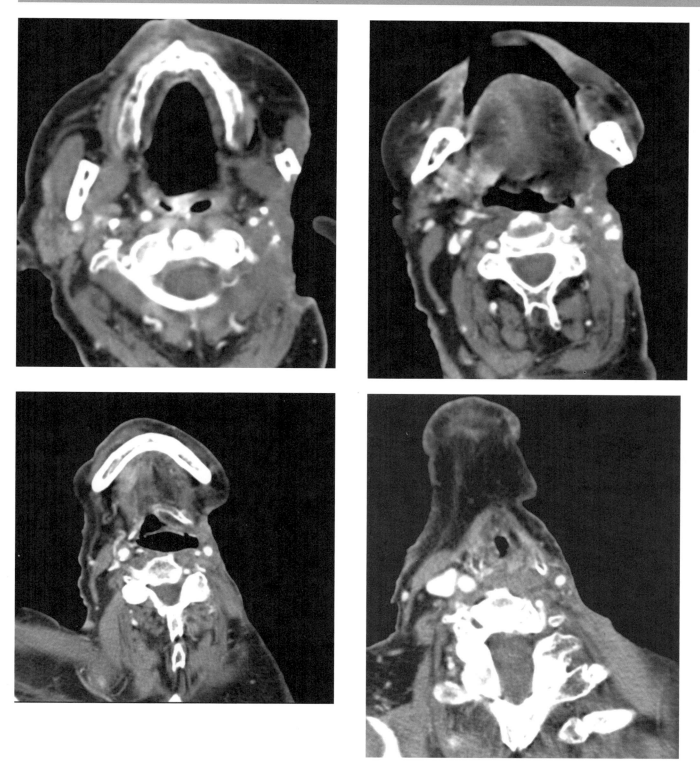

1. What cranial nerves are affected by the surgeries and radiation that this patient underwent?

2. List the findings for each nerve.

3. Name the most common cause of vocal cord paralysis.

4. What does a metallic foreign body in the upper eyelid imply?

Cranial Nerve Palsies after Therapy

1. V, VII, IX, X, XI, and XII.

2. Findings are as follows:

   V—muscles of mastication atrophy
   VII—platysma atrophy
   IX—uvula, pharyngeal atrophy
   X—vocal cord paralysis, pharyngeal atrophy
   XI—sternocleidomastoid atrophy, trapezius atrophy
   XII—tongue muscle atrophy

3. Iatrogenic from thyroid/parathyroid/neck surgery.

4. Facial nerve palsy.

Reference

Laine FJ, Underhill T: Imaging of the lower cranial nerves, *Neuroimaging Clin N Am* 14:595–609, 2004.

Cross-Reference

Neuroradiology: THE REQUISITES, pp 268–270.

Comment

This patient had extensive surgery for a retromolar trigone–tonsil–base of tongue tumor with radical neck dissection. The changes in the muscles of mastication may not be from cranial nerve V injury but may be from the primary tumor resection. Nonetheless the other cranial nerves were affected by the surgeries (cranial nerves IX, X, and XI by the neck dissection and cranial nerves IX and XII by the primary surgery). Radiation therapy also could cause cranial neuropathies.

Diabetes, uremia, and thyroid disease are the most common causes of metabolic neuropathies. Paraneoplastic syndromes also should be considered in some cases of unusual neuropathies in patients with cancers (see table).

Antigen-Target Relations

Hu	Neurons
Yo	Purkinje cells
Ri	Neurons
Tr	Purkinje cells
Voltage-gated calcium channel (VGCC)	Presynaptic neuromuscular junction

Syndromes

Sensory neuropathy

Anti-Hu	Group B streptococcus, chronic inflammatory demyelinating polyradiculopathy, motor neuron disease, subacute sensory neuropathy
	Hodgkin lymphoma, non-Hodgkin lymphoma, small cell lung carcinoma, sarcoma

Opsoclonus-myoclonus

Anti-Ri	Neuroblastoma in children, breast cancer, small cell lung carcinoma, bladder carcinoma in adults

Eaton-Lambert myasthenia

Anti-VGCC, anti-MysB, anti-synapto-tagmin	Small cell lung carcinoma, thymoma, non-Hodgkin lymphoma

Notes

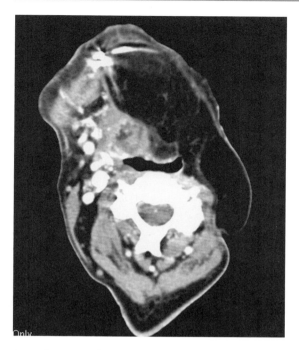

1. What are the most common sites in the head and neck to require free tissue flaps?

2. From which sites are the most free flaps taken?

3. For which sites are pedicled flaps used most commonly?

4. What type of flap is a pectoralis major flap (as seen here)?

Pectoralis Major Myocutaneous Flap

1. Oral cavity/oropharynx > hypopharynx > skin.

2. Radial forearm, fibula, iliac, and rectus.

3. Oral cavity/oropharynx > larynx/hypopharynx > parotid.

4. Pedicled myocutaneous flap.

Reference

Deschler D, Hayden RE, Yousem DM: Head and neck reconstruction, *Neuroimaging Clin N Am* 6:505–514, 1996.

Cross-Reference

Neuroradiology: THE REQUISITES, p 691.

Comment

The pectoralis major flap remains the most commonly employed reconstructive flap in head and neck surgery. It has been around a long time and has shown good results over time. This is a type of myocutaneous (muscle and skin)/myofascial flap also used with the platysma, pectoralis minor, trapezius, and latissimus dorsi muscles. Most pectoralis major flaps are tunneled under the clavicle after splitting the subclavius muscle. Flap failures occur in 6% to 10% of cases.

Free flaps have gained ascendancy since the 1990s with the use of radial forearm free flap with its arterial supply for oropharyngeal and hypopharyngeal defects and fibular grafts for reconstruction of the mandible. Other mandibular free flap reconstructions use the iliac crest or the scapula. These flaps with bone are often called *osteomyocutaneous flaps*. Overall, free flap failures occur in 2% to 6% of cases.

Flaps may be described as local (temporalis, sternocleidomastoid, and levator scapulae), regional (pectoralis, trapezius, and latissimus dorsi), or free flaps.

Notes

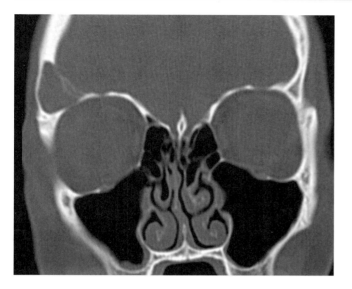 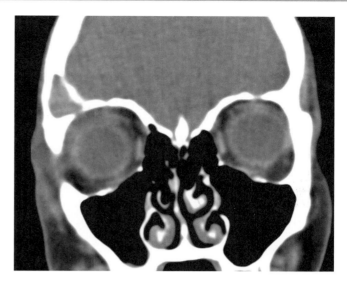

1. What does the differential diagnosis include?

2. Describe the characteristic features of an epidermoid of bone.

3. What is the ratio of benign to malignant skull lesions?

4. Name the most common primary bone tumor of the calvarium.

Epidermoid of Bone

1. Lytic metastasis, plasmacytoma, multiple myeloma, lymphoma, epidermoid, Langerhans cell histiocytosis, and giant cell reparative granuloma.

2. Lytic, well-defined, scalloped borders.

3. 1:4.

4. Osteoma.

Reference

Cummings TJ, George TM, Fuchs HE, McLendon RE: The pathology of extracranial scalp and skull masses in young children, *Clin Neuropathol* 23:34–43, 2004.

Cross-Reference

Neuroradiology: THE REQUISITES, pp 574–575.

Comment

While most neuroradiologists equate epidermoids with intracranial extraaxial masses within the cerebellopontine angle cistern, the most common site for an epidermoid is within the skull. When found within a skull, this is a lytic lesion with well-defined borders located in the diploic space. It typically does not show contrast enhancement and is dark on T1W scans and bright on T2W scans.

Epidermoids of bone have no significant threat of malignancy and should be considered a congenital rest rather than a neoplasm. They need not be in the midline, as opposed to dermoids in the CNS. Epidermoids usually manifest in childhood.

Notes

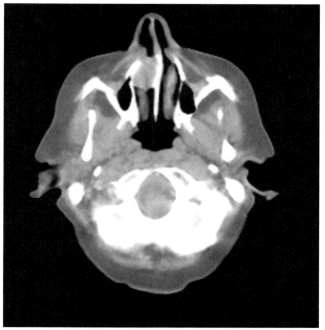

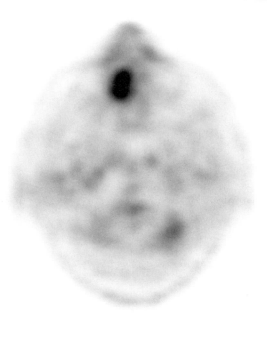

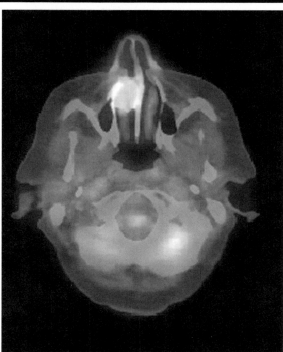

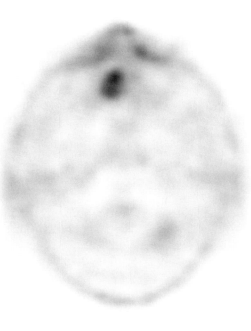

1. Where has the combination of positron emission tomography (PET) and CT scanning been the most helpful?

2. What normal structures show higher fluorodeoxyglucose (FDG) PET activity?

3. Can PET predict tumor responsiveness in the head and neck?

4. Looking retrospectively, in which percentage of cases would CT have been helpful in interpreting PET scans of the head and neck?

PET Scanning in Head and Neck Cancer

1. The head and neck, where the anatomy is so critical.

2. Muscles of mastication and phonation, lymphoid tissue, and salivary tissue.

3. Yes, to radiation therapy and to chemotherapy.

4. 25% to 30%.

Reference

Anzai Y, Minoshima S, Wolf GT, Wahl RL: Head and neck cancer: detection of recurrence with three-dimensional principal components analysis at dynamic FDG PET, Radiology 212:285–290, 1999.

Cross-Reference

Neuroradiology: THE REQUISITES, p 169.

Comment

Glucose metabolism in growing squamous cell carcinomas is enhanced and accounts for the increased uptake on FDG PET studies. The glucose analogue 2-deoxy-D-glucose is transported into the cell and metabolized in the glycolytic cycle. After phosphorylation with hexokinase to DG-6-phosphate, the compound remains in the malignant cells, where it can be used for imaging. FDG is used in part because of the longer half-life associated with the radiotracer and its well-known biokinetics. Neoplastic cells, because of their proliferation, incorporate more fluorine-labeled deoxyglucose, needed for nucleic acid synthesis.

Anzai et al compared the accuracy of FDG PET with MRI for the evaluation of patients after surgical treatment for squamous cell carcinomas. The study comprised 12 patients who were suspected clinically of having a recurrence. This selection criterion biased the sample in favor of positive studies. The authors found that FDG PET had a sensitivity of 88% (seven of eight) and a specificity of 100% (four of four). Conventional imaging (CT or MRI) was less sensitive (25% [two of eight]) and specific (75% [three of four]). The accuracy of PET after radiation therapy for subclinical recurrent head and neck cancer also has been reported to be high.

Posttreatment scanning 1 to 2 months after radiation therapy is insensitive in detecting residual disease. It is worrisome if there is persistent avid FDG uptake on the scans taken 1 to 2 months after treatment, but low activity is not as helpful. The posttreatment scans are more accurate if performed 4 months after treatment is completed, with a specificity of 100% and sensitivity of 83%.

Notes

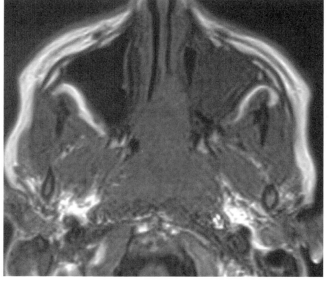
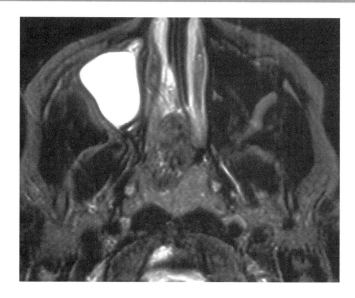
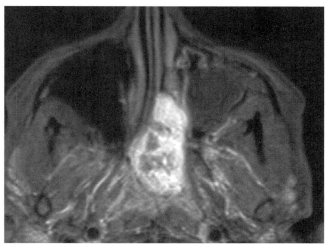
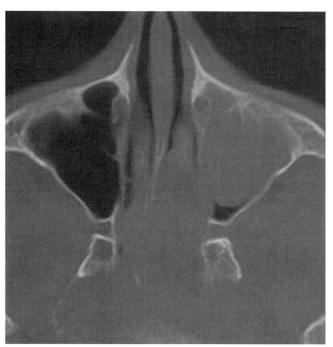

1. What is the ratio of males to females with this entity?

2. What does the differential diagnosis include?

3. What is the enhancement pattern of a juvenile nasopharyngeal angiofibroma?

4. If there is orbital invasion, what is the Fisch stage?

Juvenile Nasopharyngeal Angiofibroma

1. 19:1.

2. Lymphoma, hemangioma, venous vascular malformation, amyloidoma, and carcinoma.

3. Very strong enhancement.

4. Fisch III.

Reference

Paris J, Guelfucci B, Moulin G, et al: Diagnosis and treatment of juvenile nasopharyngeal angiofibroma, *Eur Arch Otorhinolaryngol* 258:120–124, 2001.

Cross-Reference

Neuroradiology: THE REQUISITES, pp 559–561.

Comment

Juvenile angiofibroma is a tumor characterized by its high vascularity and its propensity for bleeding. The typical patient is an adolescent boy who has recurrent epistaxis. The lesion has been said to arise from the sphenopalatine foramen (a medial egress from the pterygopalatine fossa). The tumor, although benign, often has aggressive growth with spread via the pterygopalatine fossa into the infratemporal fossa and the intracranial compartment.

Classification according to Sessions is as follows:

IA—tumor limited to posterior nares or nasopharyngeal vault

IB—extension into one or more paranasal sinuses

IIA—minimal lateral extension through sphenopalatine foramen into medial pterygomaxillary fossa

IIB—full occupation of pterygomaxillary fossa, displacing posterior wall of antrum forward; superior extension eroding orbital bones

IIC—extension through pterygomaxillary fossa into cheek and temporal fossa

IIIA—erosion of skull base, minimal intracranial spread

IIIB—extensive intracranial extension with or without cavernous sinus spread

Classification according to Fisch is as follows:

I—tumors limited to nasal cavity, nasopharynx with no bony destruction

II—tumors invading pterygomaxillary fossa, paranasal sinuses with bony destruction

III—tumors invading infratemporal fossa, orbit, or parasellar region remaining lateral to cavernous sinus

IV—tumors invading cavernous sinus, optic chiasmal region, or pituitary fossa

Notes

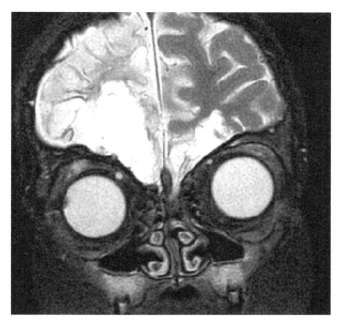
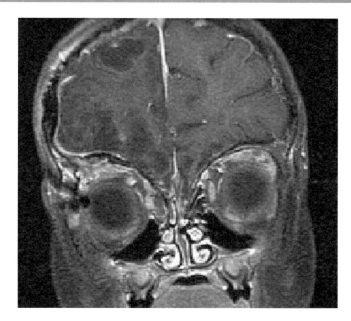

1. How much CSF is produced each day?

2. How much CSF is in the craniospinal axis?

3. What is the most common site of CSF leakage after functional endoscopic sinus surgery?

4. What chemical is tested for to determine if nasal fluid is CSF?

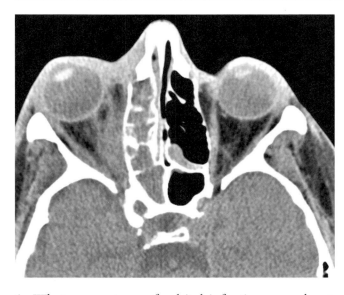
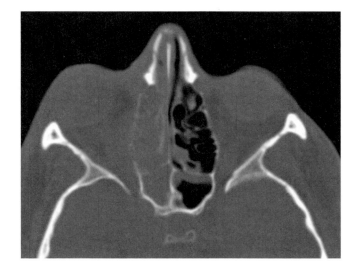

1. What percentage of orbital infections are due to sinusitis?

2. What are the most common bacteria?

3. Where does Pott's puffy tumor present?

4. What is the barrier to the spread of infection in ethmoid sinusitis–derived subperiosteal abscess?

CASE 134

CSF Leak after Trauma

1. 300 to 450 mL.

2. 150 mL (75 mL spinal, 50 mL ventricles, 25 mL intracranial subarachnoid space).

3. Cribriform plate/posterior ethmoid.

4. β_2-transferrin.

Reference

Hudgins PA, Browning DG, Gallups J, et al: Endoscopic paranasal sinus surgery: radiographic evaluation of severe complications, *AJNR Am J Neuroradiol* 13: 1161–1167, 1992.

Cross-Reference

Neuroradiology: THE REQUISITES, pp 624–629.

Comment

CSF leakage may occur spontaneously, in association with congenital cephaloceles, after trauma, or after surgery. With respect to the paranasal sinuses, CSF leak is usually in the cribriform plate region if it is caused by an iatrogenic etiology.

In the traumatic setting, the usual course of action is to place a lumbar drain and allow granulation tissue to form, sealing the leak. By reducing the pressure in the subarachnoid space to less than the usual value of 10 to 15 cm H_2O, the site of dehiscence stops leaking. Larger fractures tend to fare worse than small nondisplaced fractures. CT usually is employed to make the diagnosis, but occasionally MRI is helpful to exclude a posttraumatic encephalocele.

Spontaneous CSF leaks occur more commonly in women and may be associated with pseudotumor cerebri and elevated pressures. They may be located near the sphenoid sinus and sellar floor, which is often enlarged.

It is recommended to start the workup with a thin-section unenhanced CT scan. If CT shows a defect, and it correlates by the side and endoscopic evaluation, it is probably sufficient. For multiple defects or ambiguous active leaks, an intrathecally enhanced thin-section CT is performed to look for contrast accumulation. For intermittent leaks, an indium DTPA nuclear medicine study with pledgets may be warranted. When the nuclear imaging study points to a site, a dedicated CT study can be applied conservatively.

Notes

CASE 135

Sinusitis with Subperiosteal Abscess

1. 70%.

2. *Staphylococcus, Streptococcus,* and *Haemophilus influenzae.*

3. In the forehead.

4. Periorbita.

Reference

Skedros DG, Haddad J Jr, Bluestone CD, Curtin HD: Subperiosteal orbital abscess in children: diagnosis, microbiology, and management, *Laryngoscope* 103(1 Pt 1):28–32, 1993.

Cross-Reference

Neuroradiology: THE REQUISITES, 508–509.

Comment

The clinician should not wait to see an enhancing thick rim when dealing with a subperiosteal abscess associated with sinusitis. These abscesses occur most commonly along the lamina papyracea and lead to orbital symptoms. The periorbita provides a strong barrier to the spread of infection (or tumors) to the orbit, but one may see bowing of the periorbita and proptosis secondary to the infection.

Although immediate drainage has been the mainstay of therapy for subperiosteal abscess, some clinicians choose a trial of high-dose intravenous antibiotics as a first line of therapy.

Pott puffy tumor is a frontal osteomyelitis developing as a direct extension from the sinus or through thrombophlebitis in the diploic veins. The osteomyelitis erodes through the anterior table of the frontal bone, causing a subperiosteal abscess.

Notes

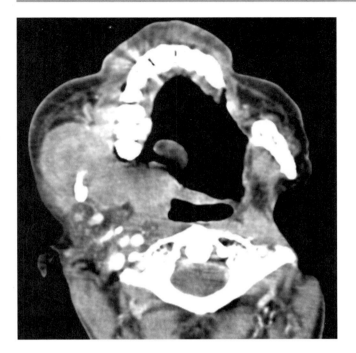
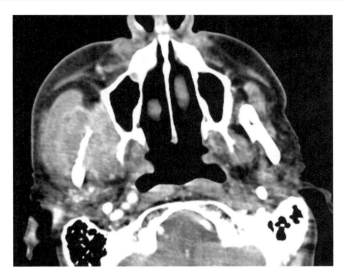

1. This patient already has undergone previous resection. Is this a tumor or postoperative change?

2. Where do recurrences occur in patients whose defects are reconstructed with flaps?

3. What features of tumors lead to the highest rate of recurrence?

4. In which head and neck site is repeat irradiation after recurrence most useful?

Recurrent Retromolar Trigone Cancer

1. It is a recurrent tumor.

2. Usually at the anastomosis and in the lymph nodes.

3. Perineural spread, irregular margins, vascular encasement, and high vascular growth factors.

4. Nasopharynx.

Reference

Bolzoni A, Cappiello J, Piazza C, et al: Diagnostic accuracy of magnetic resonance imaging in the assessment of mandibular involvement in oral-oropharyngeal squamous cell carcinoma: a prospective study, *Arch Otolaryngol Head Neck Surg* 130:837–843, 2004.

Cross-Reference

Neuroradiology: THE REQUISITES, pp 662–666.

Comment

The retromolar trigone resides behind the maxillary tuberosity and anterior to the ascending ramus of the mandible. It is a part of the oral cavity. Histologically, squamous cell carcinoma predominates as the malignancy of the retromolar trigone. Spread to the tonsil, pterygopalatine fossa, infratemporal fossa, and parapharyngeal space is rapid.

Mandibular or maxillary bone erosion is a risk of this tumor. In a review of the ability of MRI to detect mandibular invasion by oral cavity or orpharyngeal cancer, MRI was shown to have a sensitivity of 93%; specificity, 93%; accuracy, 93%; and negative and positive predictive values, 96% and 87.5%.

Surgery and radiation therapy are the mainstays of treatment.

Notes

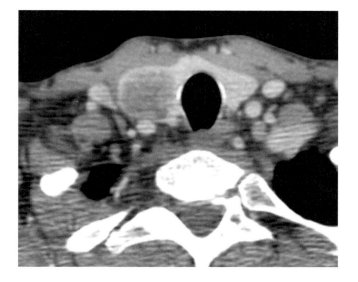
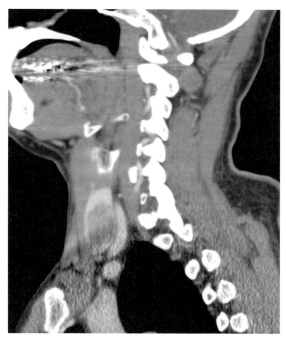
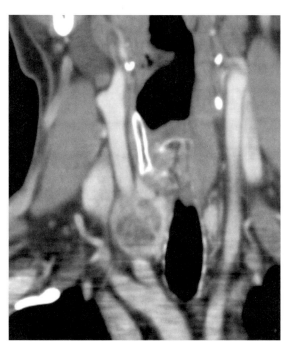
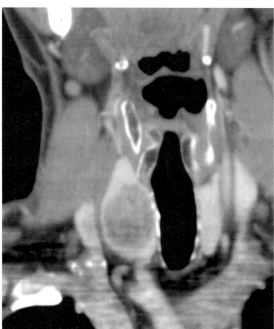

1. Which multiple endocrine neoplasia (MEN) syndrome is associated with medullary carcinoma of the thyroid gland?

2. What imaging findings favor medullary carcinoma over papillary carcinoma of the thyroid?

3. What is the rate of medullary as opposed to other thyroid carcinomas?

4. What nuclear medicine agent is optimal for medullary carcinoma of the thyroid?

Medullary Carcinoma of the Thyroid Gland

1. MEN IIa and IIb.

2. Stippled calcifications.

3. 10%.

4. Radioactive somatostatin analogues (octreotide), MIBG, DMSA or sestamibi. Fluorodeoxyglucose positron emission tomography can detect regional metastases.

Reference

Bustillo A, Telischi F, Weed D, et al: Octreotide scintigraphy in the head and neck, *Laryngoscope* 114:434–440, 2004.

Cross-Reference

Neuroradiology: THE REQUISITES, p 742.

Comment

Medullary carcinoma arises from the calcitonin-producing parafollicular cells of the thyroid gland. It is associated with MEN syndromes in 25% of cases, and it is sporadic in 75% of cases. Only 10% of all thyroid cancers are due to medullary carcinoma, with papillary and follicular the more common histologic types. MEN IIa consists of medullary carcinoma, pheochromocytoma, and hyperparathyroidism. MEN IIb does not have hyperparathyroidism but has mucosal ganglioneuromas and marfanoid appearance. Although women are more commonly affected than men in sporadic cases and present in their 50s, cases with MEN syndromes affect men and women equally, and patients usually present in their 30s.

Treatment is total thyroidectomy with neck dissections. Because this tumor is not from the thyroid hormone–producing cell, radioactive iodine is not useful in therapy.

Notes

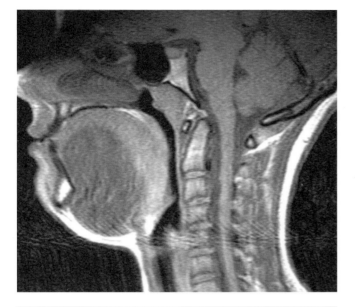

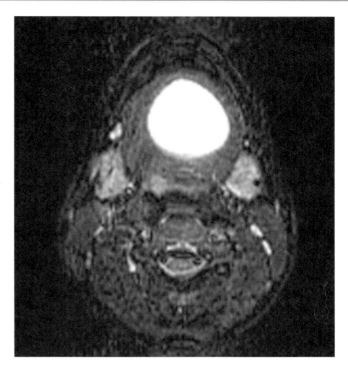

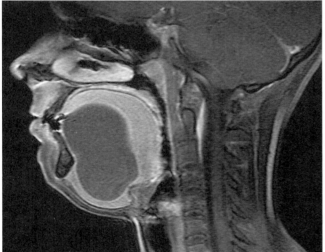

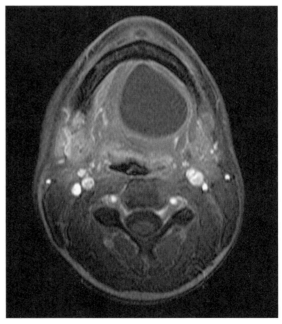

1. Name at least four cysts in the oral cavity.

2. What is the most common location for a dermoid/epidermoid cyst in the head and neck?

3. What percentage of all dermoid cysts occur in the head and neck?

4. Is a dermoid more like a tumor or a hamartoma?

Dermoid of the Tongue

1. Epidermoid/dermoid, thyroglossal duct cyst, ranula, lymphangioma, and mucus retention cyst.

2. Skin > nasal > orbit > tongue.

3. 7% (most are associated with the ovaries).

4. More like a hamartoma because it represents a "rest" of epidermal tissue and skin appendages.

Reference

Smirniotopoulos JG, Chiechi MV: Teratomas, dermoids, and epidermoids of the head and neck, *Radiographics* 15:1437–1455, 1995.

Cross-Reference

Neuroradiology: THE REQUISITES, p 660.

Comment

Dermoid cyst of the head and neck can arise in a variety of locations. Some common locations include around the lacrimal gland, along the nasion of the nose, in association with the maxilla, and within the tongue. Within the tongue, these lesions often are seen as midline abnormalities, which may be slightly hyperintense on T1W scan. Dermoid cysts of the tongue may truly be epidermoids because they rarely contain fatty material. The differential diagnosis of a dermoid cyst of the tongue includes a thyroglossal cyst, ranula, and lymphatic malformation. Other entities, such as a lingual thyroid gland, hemangioma, or venous vascular malformation, usually show contrast enhancement in portions of the lesion as opposed to the dermoid cyst.

Hair follicles, sebaceous cysts, sweat glands, and apocrine glands may be found in dermoids. Epidermoids (epidermal inclusion cysts) have only skin cells themselves. Surgery is the treatment of choice. Antibiotics may be required if the cyst becomes superinfected. Carcinomatous transformation has been known to occur with lingual dermoid cysts—usually to a squamous cell carcinoma.

Notes

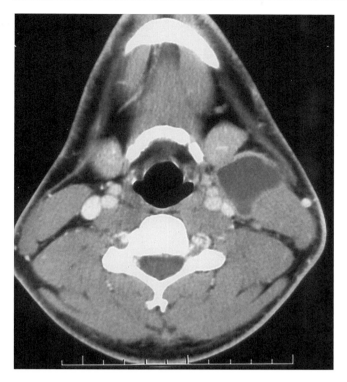

1. What type of branchial cleft cyst (BCC) is this?

2. If it developed a fistula internally, where would it drain?

3. Describe the Arnot classification of first branchial cleft cysts.

4. What percentage of BCCs are second BCCs?

Branchial Cleft Cysts

1. Bailey type II second BCC.

2. Palatine tonsil.

3. The Arnot classification is as follows:

   Type 1 first BCCs—cysts or sinuses in the parotid gland
   Type 2 first BCCs—in the anterior triangle of the
      neck, fistulous tract to the external auditory canal

4. 90% to 95%.

Reference

Mukherji SK, Fatterpekar G, Castillo M, et al: Imaging of congenital anomalies of the branchial apparatus, *Neuroimaging Clin N Am* 10:75–93, 2000.

Cross-Reference

Neuroradiology: THE REQUISITES, pp 746–748.

Comment

The second BCC is the most common of all the BCCs. These cysts are graded by the Bailey classification:

   Type I—cyst is superficial to the sternocleidomastoid
      muscle
   Type II—cyst is deep to the sternocleidomastoid
      muscle but superficial to the carotid bifurcation
   Type III—cyst invaginates between the external and
      internal carotid arteries at the carotid bifurcation
   Type IV—cyst is medial to the carotid bifurcation

Cysts usually present in young adulthood. Often they may become superinfected or traumatized, which may lead to their clinical presentation. Alternatively the presence of a palpable mass may lead to the imaging study, which clinches the diagnosis. Although the rim of the cyst may show minimal contrast enhancement after trauma or infection, there should not be nodular components to the cyst.

Differential diagnosis includes cystic lymph nodes, with tonsillar carcinoma, lymphoma, and thyroid carcinoma being the major culprits in that regard. Occasionally a plunging ranula extends below the floor of the mouth and simulates a BCC. One should be able to see the trailing edge leading to the sublingual space for the ranula.

Third and fourth BCCs are rare. Fistulas from the third and fourth branchial clefts go to the piriform sinuses from the lower anterior neck.

Notes

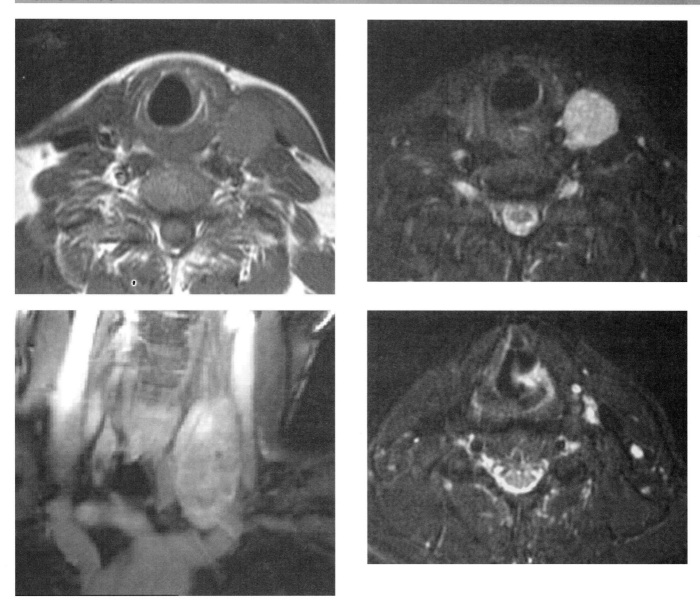

1. Name the most common mass in the carotid sheath.

2. What tumors arise from the vagus nerve?

3. Identify the complicating factor seen in the figure on the lower right.

4. Are necrosis and cystic change unusual for this tumor?

Vagus Schwannoma Causing Vocal Cord Paralysis

1. Schwannoma.

2. Schwannomas, paragangliomas, neurofibromas, and neurofibrosarcomas.

3. Vocal cord paralysis.

4. No.

Reference

Kehagias DT, Bourekas EC, Christoforidis GA: Schwannoma of the vagus nerve, *AJR Am J Roentgenol* 177:720–721, 2001.

Cross-Reference

Neuroradiology: THE REQUISITES, p 107.

Comment

The normal contents of the carotid space include the carotid artery; internal jugular vein; vagus nerve (cranial nerve X); sympathetic nervous plexus; branches of the ansa cervicalis/hypoglossi (C1-3 roots); and cranial nerves IX, XI, and XII. Lymph nodes abound around and within the carotid sheath. The carotid space courses down the entire length of the neck and begins at the skull base. Superiorly the carotid space is separated from the prestyloid parapharyngeal space by the styloid musculature, seen as small slips of the styloglossus and stylopharyngeus muscles just anterior to the carotid sheath but posterior to the parapharyngeal fat.

Most carotid space masses are benign. Of these, two classic lesions are the vagus schwannoma and the glomus tumor. Situated posterior to the carotid artery, vagus nerve lesions tend to displace the carotid artery and parapharyngeal fat in an anterior direction. Schwannomas of the vagus nerve usually are well-defined, rounded structures hypodense to muscle on CT that enhance moderately. The lesions are circumscribed on T1W scan because of the high signal intensity fat around the carotid sheath and around the parapharyngeal space. The border between the schwannoma and carotid artery or jugular vein may be indistinguishable on enhanced CT. On MRI, it is possible to identify the flow voids of the carotid artery and jugular vein as opposed to the enhancing solid tumor. On T2W scan, the signal intensity of schwannomas varies, depending on the content of Antoni A and Antoni B tissue. Occasionally, schwannomas may be cystic and show characteristic density and intensity features for cyst fluid. Schwannomas also may show intratumoral hemorrhage.

Notes

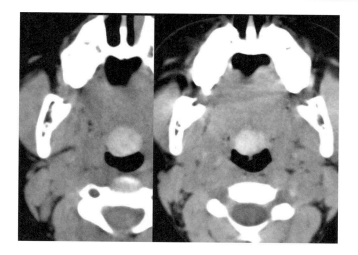

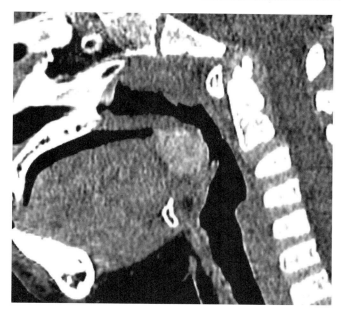

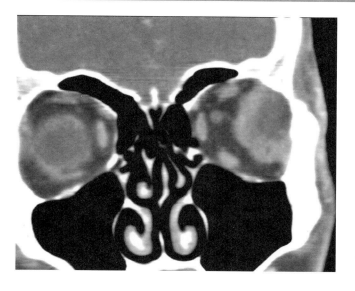

1. What are the hyperdense lesions of the tongue base?

2. At what stage in development does the thyroid gland descend from the foramen cecum?

3. Where in the tongue do most lingual thyroid glands arrest their migration?

4. What is the thyroid function status expected to be in this individual?

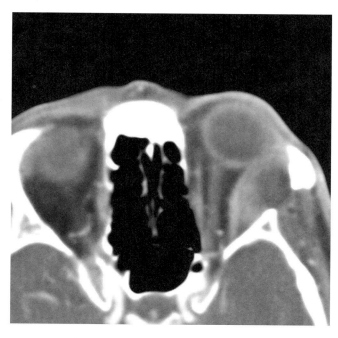

1. Name the most common epithelial tumor of the lacrimal gland.

2. What is the most common malignancy of the lacrimal gland?

3. What is the expected prognosis for lacrimal gland adenoid cystic carcinoma?

4. What is the most common symptom of lacrimal gland adenoid cystic carcinoma, and what does it imply?

Lingual Thyroid Tissue

1. Lingual thyroid gland, amyloidosis, hemangioma, and lymphoma.

2. In the first month of gestation.

3. 90% are on the dorsum of the tongue.

4. Hypothyroid > euthyroid.

Reference

Takashima S, Ueda M, Shibata A, et al: MR imaging of the lingual thyroid: comparison to other submucosal lesions, *Acta Radiol* 42:376–382, 2001.

Cross-Reference

Neuroradiology: THE REQUISITES, p 652.

Comment

When one finds a soft tissue mass in the base of the tongue, there is a broad differential diagnosis, which includes squamous cell carcinoma, lymphoma, lymphoid hyperplasia, hemangioma/venous vascular malformation, dermoid cyst, thyroglossal duct cyst, and lingual thyroid tissue. Only the lingual thyroid tissue shows marked hyperdensity on CT scan, a hyperdensity that simulates the thyroid gland.

In 80% of cases, the lingual thyroid glandular tissue is the only thyroid tissue in the individual's body. If one continues the scanning through the lower neck, one typically (80% of the time) finds absence of thyroid tissue on either side of the trachea, which should clinch the diagnosis. Because it represents normally functioning thyroid tissue, its gross removal would lead to acute hypothyroidism. In addition, the presence of this thyroid tissue leads to a possible occurrence of papillary cell carcinoma in the thyroid gland in the base of the tongue. Lingual thyroids occur four times more commonly in women than men; 70% present with hypothyroidism.

This lesion usually manifests during young adulthood and the adolescent surge of hormones. At that time, it is believed that the thyroid glandular tissue in the back of the tongue tends to enlarge, leading to the patient's feeling of dysphagia or airway obstruction. Often surgery to remove the thyroid glandular tissue is delayed until this adolescent surge has passed.

Notes

Lacrimal Gland Tumors

1. Pleomorphic adenoma.

2. Adenoid cystic carcinoma > adenocarcinoma.

3. Poor. Most people die of their disease.

4. Pain. It implies perineural spread of the tumor.

Reference

Esmaeli B, Ahmadi MA, Youssef A, et al: Outcomes in patients with adenoid cystic carcinoma of the lacrimal gland, *Ophthalmol Plast Reconstr Surg* 20:22–26, 2004.

Cross-Reference

Neuroradiology: THE REQUISITES, pp 510–511.

Comment

Lacrimal gland lesions typically are divided into three different varieties: (1) granulomatous/lymphomatous, (2) epithelial, and (3) congenital. Within the granulomatous category, lymphoma, pseudotumor, sarcoidosis, and Sjögren syndrome lesions are identified. Pseudotumor of the lacrimal gland may cause pain and increased tearing, called *epiphora*. Of the epithelial lesions, pleomorphic adenomas are the most common benign tumors of the lacrimal gland just as with minor salivary gland tumors, and adenoid cystic carcinoma is the most common malignancy to involve the lacrimal gland. Adenocarcinoma and undifferentiated carcinoma also may occur in this location.

Congenital lesions include the congenital rests that populate the lacrimal fossa. These include epidermoid and dermoid lesions of the lacrimal gland.

The lacrimal gland also may be inflamed secondary to viral illnesses, tuberculous and fungal infections, radiation adenitis, and adjacent cellulitis.

Adenoid cystic carcinoma of the lacrimal gland has early bone infiltration, perineural spread, and the possibility of intracranial dissemination. As with all adenoid cystic carcinomas, this tumor inexorably kills the patient with hematogenous metastases and perineural recurrences.

Notes

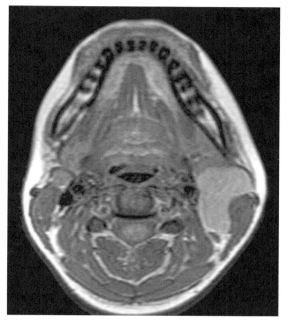

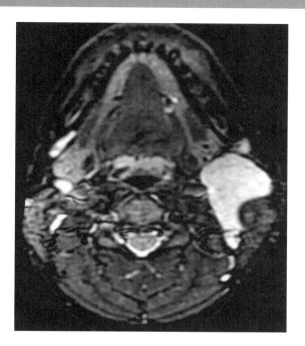

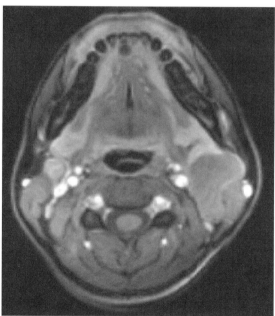

1. What percentage of these lesions occur in the neck versus the axilla?

2. What is the typical presentation?

3. What are classic MRI findings?

4. If a lymphatic malformation enhances, what should you think is the cause?

CASE 143

Cystic Hygroma/Lymphangioma/Lymphatic Malformation

1. 75% neck; 25% axilla.

2. Airway obstruction and neck mass.

3. Multiloculated mass with fluid-fluid levels, usually from bleeding or high protein, with some portions bright on T1W scan and without contrast enhancement.

4. Integration with a hemangioma (venous vascular malformation).

Reference

Breysem L, Bosmans H, Dymarkowski S, et al: The value of fast MR imaging as an adjunct to ultrasound in prenatal diagnosis, *Eur Radiol* 13:1538–1548, 2003.

Cross-Reference

Neuroradiology: THE REQUISITES, pp 498–500.

Comment

When one sees a multiloculated lesion in the posterior portion of the neck extending into the axilla that shows bright signal intensity on T1W scans and absence of contrast enhancement, one should lock down the diagnosis of cystic hygroma (lymphatic malformation). These lesions manifest in 90% of cases by age 2 years, and 65% are evident before or at birth. Cystic hygroma has an association with Turner syndrome, Noonan syndrome, and Down syndrome. Cystic hygromas often have a more infiltrated appearance because they invaginate into the various spaces of the head and neck region. These are located most commonly in the posterior triangle of the neck; however, rarely they may infiltrate deep to the sternocleidomastoid muscle. Lymphatic malformations may be combined with venous malformations to create mixed lesions that may show some element of contrast enhancement and a mixed density-intensity pattern.

Cystic hygroma is a diagnosis that should be made antenatally because there are amniotic fluid markers that point to the diagnosis (elevated alpha-fetoprotein). The recurrence rate after surgery is about 10%.

Notes

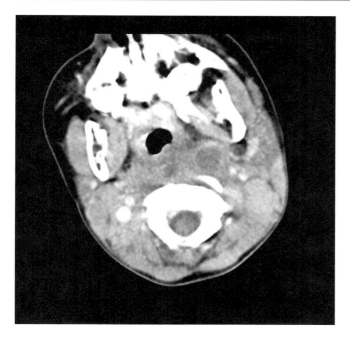

1. Name common microbes for this infection.

2. What is the name of the histiocytic necrotizing adenitis that occurs in the necks of young Korean women?

3. In the U.S., what is the most common cause of necrotic lymph nodes?

4. In the U.S., what is the most common cause of inflammatory necrotic lymph nodes?

Necrotizing Adenitis

1. *Streptococcus,* pneumococcus, and *Haemophilus influenzae.*

2. Kikuchi disease, which is typified by perinodal inflammation.

3. Squamous cell carcinoma.

4. Tuberculous adenitis.

Reference

Kwon SY, Kim TK, Kim YS, et al: CT findings in Kikuchi disease: analysis of 96 cases, *AJNR Am J Neuroradiol* 25:1099–1102, 2004.

Cross-Reference

Neuroradiology: THE REQUISITES, pp 730–731.

Comment

Necrotizing adenitis accounts for most necrotic-appearing inflammatory lesions in the retropharyngeal space. This entity is usually secondary to tonsillitis or pharyngitis with secondary spread to the lymph nodes. The lymph nodes become suppurative and enlarged. There may be associated cellulitis and inflammatory infiltration of the fat adjacent to the lymph node. The entity of retropharyngeal abscess has been largely discredited in most cases with the finding of lymphoid tissue adjacent to the purulent material. This finding suggests that the disease is within a lymph node rather than a de novo collection. Only when the collection is in the midline or crossing the midline should the definitive diagnosis be a "retropharyngeal abscess."

The retropharyngeal lymph nodes usually are classified as medial and lateral, depending on their location with respect to the carotid artery in the retropharyngeal space. The nodes by the classic terminology also are called the *nodes of Rouvière.* These are also the lymph nodes that may be associated with Grisel syndrome, which causes the subluxation of the C1 and C2 vertebral bodies on an inflammatory basis.

Notes

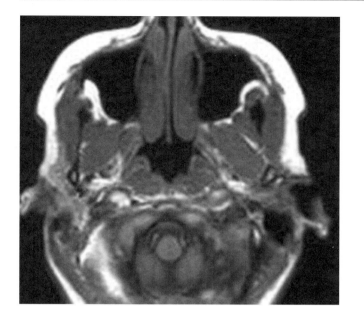

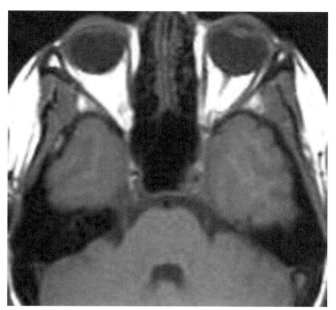

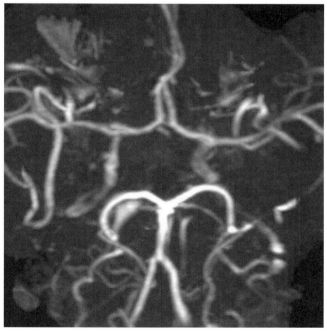

1. Identify the cause of this patient's Horner syndrome.

2. After amphetamine drops, what will this patient's pupils do?

3. What happens with amphetamine drops in patients with a Horner syndrome from a Pancoast tumor?

4. Where do most carotid dissections occur?

Bilateral Carotid Artery Dissections

1. Postganglionic sympathetic nervous system injury in association with carotid dissections.

2. Nothing—it is a postganglionic injury.

3. Pupils dilate.

4. The internal carotid artery, cervical portion.

Reference

Digre KB, Smoker WR, Johnston P, et al: Selective MR imaging approach for evaluation of patients with Horner's syndrome, *AJNR Am J Neuroradiol* 13: 223–227, 1992.

Cross-Reference

Neuroradiology: THE REQUISITES, pp 269, 735.

Comment

If one sees bilateral carotid artery dissections, one should consider the numerous potential predisposing syndromes for carotid dissections. Classically, bilateral carotid artery dissection has been described in patients with Marfan syndrome, homocystinuria, Ehlers-Danlos syndrome, fibromuscular dysplasia, cystic medial necrosis, and neurofibromatosis. It would be highly unusual for a traumatic or atherosclerotic event to cause bilateral simultaneous carotid dissections. Chiropractors certainly can do a "number" on a patient's neck, however, so one should not discount this possibility in patients who have been vigorously manipulated.

Many of the etiologies for dissections of the blood vessels also predispose patients to aneurysms and pseudoaneurysms (after the dissections). The appropriate vascular evaluation in a patient with dissection should include intracranial imaging to exclude aneurysm formation or strokes.

If the dissection is not associated with stroke or symptoms, the patient may be treated with antiplatelet medication alone. Patients who develop vascular stenosis and thromboembolic events or pseudoaneurysms may be treated endovascularly. Often a stent with supplemental antiplatelet medication is an effective strategy for complicated carotid dissections.

The understanding of the evaluation of a patient with Horner syndrome requires a modicum of clinical medical knowledge. Two clinical findings might suggest where a lesion is with respect to Horner syndrome. If the patient has anhydrosis, it implies that the sympathetic nervous system's first-order or second-order neurons are involved. The third-order neurons generally do not carry enervation to the sweat glands.

The other feature that helps localize Horner syndrome evaluation is the response of the eye to hydroxyamphetamine drops, which cause release of norepinephrine from presynaptic postganglionic neurons. In this case, the ganglion being referred to is the third-order ganglion at the superior cervical ganglion, located generally at the C4 level near the carotid bifurcation. With first-order and second-order neuron disease, use of hydroxyamphetamine drops causes the pupil to dilate. With third-order neuron disease, the eye does not dilate, as it should.

Reference to the orders of neurons assumes that one understands that the first-order neurons for the sympathetic system course from the hypothalamic region through the brainstem into the cervical spine and synapse at approximately the C7-T1 level. The second-order neurons leave from this synaptic junction and cross the stellate ganglion at the T1 rib compression. These second-order neurons synapse at the superior cervical ganglion in the neck after coursing along the carotid sheath. The third-order neurons are the ones that extend superiorly into the cavernous sinus and into the superior orbital fissure, where they help to innervate the muscles that control pupillary dilation and the eyelid. Carotid dissections affect the third-order neurons.

Although posterior inferior cerebellar artery infarctions are one of the most common etiologies for first-order neuron disease, and Pancoast tumors may affect second-order neurons, carotid dissections affect third-order neurons or distal second-order neurons. Cavernous sinus masses also affect the third-order neurons.

Nonetheless, despite this intricate anatomy, an interesting clinical pearl, there seems to be an intermediate rate of positive findings on imaging in patients who have primary Horner syndrome.

Notes

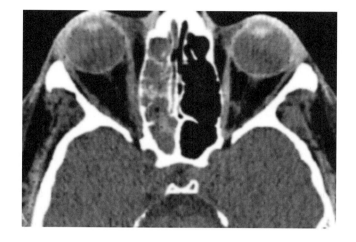

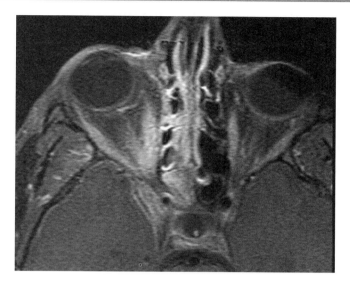

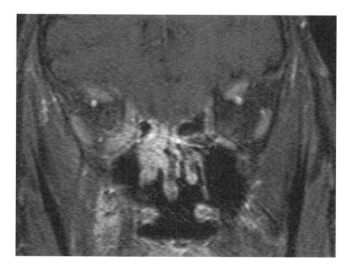

1. How often are the orbits and brain involved in invasive mucormycosis sinusitis?

2. What is the risk of cavernous sinus involvement with mucormycosis?

3. What is the characteristic finding on MRI of this infection?

4. Explain the significance of periantral soft tissue infiltration.

Mucormycosis of the Paranasal Sinuses Invading the Orbit

1. 80% orbital involvement; 11% intracranial.

2. Carotid arteritis, occlusion, and distal embolization.

3. Relatively low signal on T2W scan.

4. It is an early sign of invasive fungal infection.

Reference

Yousem DM, Galetta SL, Gusnard DA, Goldberg HI: MR findings in rhinocerebral mucormycosis, *J Comput Assist Tomogr* 13:878–882, 1989.

Cross-Reference

Neuroradiology: THE REQUISITES, p 627.

Comment

Mucormycosis is one of the most aggressive types of fungal sinusitis. It is characterized by the potential for aggressive infiltration to the orbit and the cavernous sinus. When mucormycosis infiltrates the cavernous sinus, thrombosis of the cavernous sinus, pseudoaneurysm formation of the carotid artery, or an inflammatory vasculitis involving the cavernous carotid artery may be seen.

When the cavernous carotid artery is involved, one may see an embolic phenomenon, which may be bland or mycotic, or one may see thrombosis of that blood vessel over time. Stenosis resulting from the inflammation on the wall also may be present, and the fungus may use the carotid artery as a vehicle into the intracranial space and subarachnoid space.

A clinical finding that is nearly pathognomonic for mucormycosis is a black eschar within the sinonasal cavity.

Notes

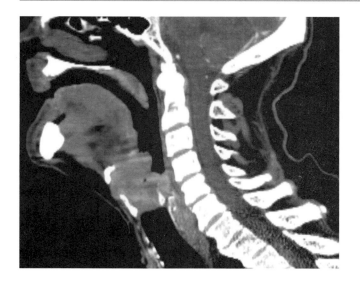
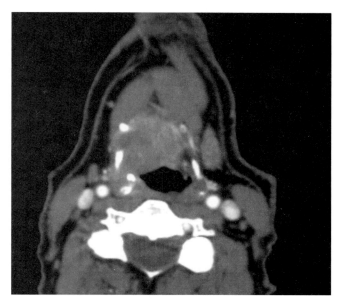

1. Explain the significance of tumor in this location.

2. Does tuberculosis affect the preepiglottic space?

3. What percentage of laryngeal carcinomas are supraglottic?

4. Explain the significance of preepiglottic space invasion with T staging of laryngeal carcinoma.

CASE 147

Preepiglottic Fat Invasion by Cancer

1. There is a 50% increased incidence of cervical adenopathy, it makes the advisability of doing supraglottic/supracricoid surgery for laryngeal voice conservation low, and it often means the supraglottic larynx and part of the tongue base would have to be removed for surgical cure.

2. No.

3. 30%.

4. It makes the cancer T3, high grade.

Reference

Loevner LA, Yousem DM, Montone KT, et al: Can radiologists accurately predict preepiglottic space invasion with MR imaging? *AJR Am J Roentgenol* 169:1681–1687, 1997.

Cross-Reference

Neuroradiology: THE REQUISITES, pp 672–676.

Comment

From the base of the tongue, a tumor may extend into the vallecula, the air space anterior to the epiglottis but posterior to the tongue base. When the vallecula is infiltrated, the critical space to be evaluated by the radiologist is the preepiglottic fat. When the preepiglottic fat space is infiltrated with tumor, it is surgically impossible to remove the fat while maintaining the integrity of the epiglottis' petiole (inferior stem). A tumor of the base of the tongue that does not involve the preepiglottic fat can be resected without requiring a portion of the supraglottic larynx to be included in the operative specimen. If the preepiglottic fat is invaded, the patient often requires an epiglottectomy, partial supraglottic laryngectomy, or, at worse, total laryngectomy. Often these must be combined with a base-of-tongue resection. The best way to evaluate the preepiglottic fat is with sagittal T1W scan and axial T1W scan in which soft tissue signal intensity within the fat suggests cancerous involvement. Occasionally, adjacent inflammation or peritumoral edema or partial volume effects might simulate preepiglottic fat invasion. Massive preepiglottic fat disease also often makes radiation therapy undesirable because of the bulk of the tumor, limiting curability. Preepiglottic invasion also predisposes to lymph node spread, so there is a worse prognosis associated with this feature.

Notes

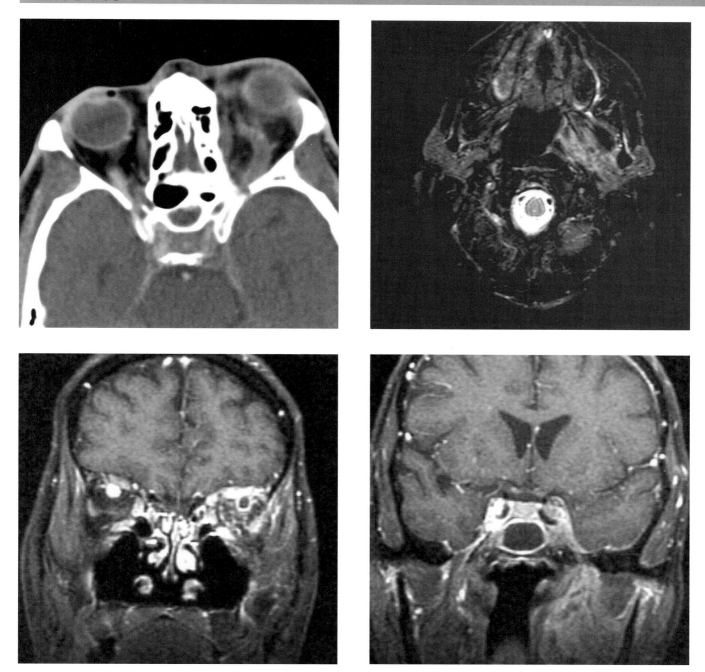

1. List the major findings of the case.

2. What is the most common source for this phenomenon?

3. Describe the typical findings in a cavernous carotid fistula with regard to the superior ophthalmic vein.

4. In what space would you put the T2W signal abnormality?

Superior Ophthalmic Vein Thrombosis

1. Superior ophthalmic vein thrombosis, cavernous sinus partial thrombosis, inflammation of the masticator space extending intracranially, and orbital edema.

2. Usually it is sinusitis. In this case, it was from a dental inflammation.

3. Ipsilateral and contralateral may be enlarged. They may become thrombosed before or with therapy or be used for access to the fistula.

4. The masticator space.

Reference

Schuknecht B, Simmen D, Yuksel C, Valavanis A: Tributary venosinus occlusion and septic cavernous sinus thrombosis: CT and MR findings, *AJNR Am J Neuroradiol* 19:617–626, 1998.

Cross-Reference

Neuroradiology: THE REQUISITES, p 553.

Comment

Cavernous sinus thrombosis has been described secondary to infections of the paranasal sinuses (especially fungal), middle ear and mastoid air cells, and facial or orbital cellulitis. Superior ophthalmic vein thrombosis may occur concomitantly or as an isolated phenomenon. Lemierre syndrome has been associated with superior ophthalmic vein thrombosis as well.

The superior ophthalmic vein is large in size, which might lead to a suspicion of a cavernous carotid fistula. In this case, the vein is usually patent and serves as a drainage pathway with retrograde flow from the fistula. The most common type of cavernous carotid fistula is the single hold direct connection between the carotid artery and the cavernous sinus. In some cases, this fistula is due to a carotid artery aneurysm rupture, but in most cases it is traumatic in origin. Dural vascular malformations and multiple feeders to a fistula comprise other types, with some having contributions from the external carotid artery as well.

Findings suggesting cavernous sinus thrombosis on enhanced CT include the following:

Alteration in density/signal intensity, size, and contour of the cavernous sinus
Absence of opacification with iodinated contrast material
Filling defects in an opacified cavernous sinus
Soft tissue in the sinus

Of cases of cavernous sinus thrombosis, 50% have associated superior ophthalmic vein thrombus.

Notes

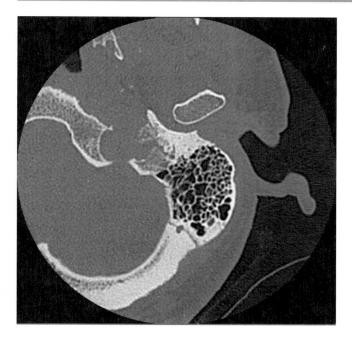

1. What is the difference between objective and subjective tinnitus?

2. Name the leading causes of objective tinnitus.

3. Name the one vascular diagnosis that causes pulsatile tinnitus that CT and MRI are least likely to make.

4. Can venous stenosis cause pulsatile tinnitus?

Glomus Jugulare

1. With objective tinnitus, the sound is perceived by the patient and the examiner.

2. Normal vascular variants, acquired vascular lesions (arteriovenous malformations, dural arteriovenous fistulas, aneurysms, stenosis), and temporal bone tumors.

3. Dural arteriovenous fistulas.

4. Yes.

Reference

Remley KB, Coit WE, Harnsberger HR, et al: Pulsatile tinnitus and the vascular tympanic membrane: CT, MR, and angiographic findings, *Radiology* 174:383–389, 1990.

Cross-Reference

Neuroradiology: THE REQUISITES, pp 584–588.

Comment

The work-up for a patient who has tinnitus depends in part on the clinician's assessment of whether the patient has subjective or objective tinnitus. Subjective tinnitus is less likely to be due to vascular abnormalities than objective tinnitus (tinnitus that can be heard with a stethoscope by the referring physician). In patients with objective tinnitus, one might begin with a thin section CT scan and CT angiography in the hopes of finding vascular stenosis, arteriovenous fistulas or malformations, hypervascular neoplasms such as glomus tumors, or significant vascular stenosis that may be causing the jet phenomena on the arterial or the venous side. In some cases, with a negative CT scan and CT angiography, the evidence and sound are compelling enough to the clinician that conventional arteriography is warranted. For subjective tinnitus, many clinicians advocate the use of MRI with contrast enhancement to evaluate the patient. There are many diagnoses to consider with an individual with subjective tinnitus; among these, many have few to no imaging findings, including pseudotumor cerebri, Ménière disease, and vascular migraines. To exclude intracranial pathology and inner ear pathology, MRI with gadolinium may be useful.

In 1990, Remley et al recommended, "All patients with subjective pulsatile tinnitus or a vascular retrotympanic mass should undergo high-resolution computed tomography of the temporal bone as the initial imaging study. Angiography is recommended for patients with objective tinnitus and a normal tympanic membrane. The role of MR imaging, even with the addition of gradient-echo techniques, remains limited and secondary."

In 2005, CT angiography and CT scanning may serve the needs of this patient population in most cases. As more temporal resolution CT angiography becomes available, conventional arteriography may not be needed at all as a diagnostic test.

Notes

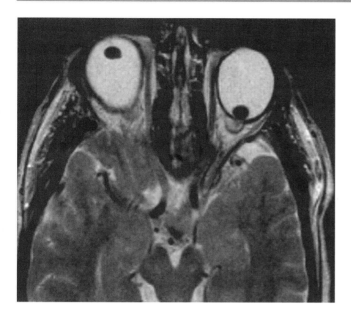

1. Name syndromes associated with this phenomenon.
2. In which direction does the lens dislocate in Marfan syndrome?
3. How often is the lens dislocated in Marfan syndrome?
4. Is the axial myopia seen here also characteristic of Marfan syndrome?

Lens Dislocation

1. Marfan syndrome, homocystinuria, ehlers-danlos syndrome, and aniridia.

2. Up and out with Marfan syndrome; down and in with homocystinuria.

3. 50% to 60%.

4. Yes.

Reference

De Paepe A, Devereux RB, Dietz HC: Revised diagnostic criteria for the Marfan syndrome, *Am J Med Genet* 62:417–426, 1996.

Cross-Reference

Neuroradiology: THE REQUISITES, pp 469–470, 477.

Comment

Intraocular lens dislocation after cataract surgery occurs as a complication in about 1% of surgical cases. The posterior capsule may rupture at the time of laser capsulotomy surgery.

Trauma to the lens of the eye may manifest as an acute cataract, displacement, dislocation, or rupture. In the acute setting, a traumatic cataract may appear less dense than the normal contralateral lens of the eye. Over time, the density increases, and there may be some loss of shape. Lens displacement may occur where one sees subtle changes in position of the lens within the globe. Often the lens may remain at the junction at the anterior chamber and posterior chamber but may be oriented in an abnormal fashion, still attached to the iris or its capsule or both. In some cases, one can identify the lens resting within the vitreous humor or freely floating within this substance. If the patient has a traumatic hyphema with blood in the anterior chamber, this may not be evident to the ophthalmologist, whose ability to visualize these structures is obscured by the hemorrhage. Rupture of the lens of the eye is least common and may be secondary to penetrating injuries. Iritis and glaucoma are complications of lens dislocation.

Marfan syndrome, aniridia, Ehlers-Danlos syndrome, and homocystinuria may be associated with lens dislocations (e.g., up and out with Marfan syndrome, downward with homocystinuria). The congenital causes of lens dislocation usually affect both eyes. This includes ectopia lentis syndrome, which has been mapped to mutations of the fibrillin-1 (*FBN1*) gene on chromosome 15 (as has Marfan syndrome).

The diagnosis of Marfan syndrome is a complicated clinical decision based on minor and major criteria (see table that follows).

For the index case, diagnostic requirements are as follows:

If the family/genetic history is not contributory, major criteria in at least two different organ systems and involvement of a third organ system

If a mutation known to cause Marfan syndrome in others is detected, one major criterion in an organ system and involvement of a second organ system

For a relative of an index case, diagnostic requirements are as follows:

Presence of one major criterion in the family history and one major criterion in an organ system and involvement of a second organ system

Notes

System	Major Criteria	Minor Criteria
Skeletal system	Presence of at least 4 of the following manifestations: Pectus carinatum Pectus excavatum requiring surgery Reduced upper-to-lower segment ratio or arm span-to-height ratio >1.05 Wrist and thumb signs Scoliosis >20° or spondylolisthesis Reduced extensions at the elbows (<170°) Medial displacement of the medial malleolus causing pes planus Protrusio acetabuli of any degree (ascertained on radiographs)	Pectus excavatum of moderate severity Joint hypermobility Highly arched palate with crowding of teeth Facial appearance (dolichocephaly, malar hypoplasia, enophthalmos, retrognathia, down-slanting palpebral fissures)
Ocular system	Ectopia lentis (dislocated lens)	Abnormally flat cornea (as measured by keratometry) Increased axial length of globe (as measured by ultrasound)
Cardiovascular system	Dilation of the ascending aorta with or without aortic regurgitation and involving at least the sinuses of Valsalva Dissection of the ascending aorta	Mitral valve prolapse with or without mitral valve regurgitation Dilation of the main pulmonary artery in the absence of valvular or peripheral pulmonic stenosis or any other obvious cause in patient <40 years old Calcification of the mitral annulus in patient <40 years old Dilation of dissection of the descending thoracic or abdominal aorta in patient <50 years old
Pulmonary system	None	Spontaneous pneumothorax Apical blebs (ascertained by chest radiography)
Skin and integument	None	Stretch marks not associated with marked weight changes, pregnancy, or repetitive stress Recurrent incisional hernias
Dura	Lumbosacral dural ectasia by CT or MRI	None
Family/genetic	Having a parent, child, or sibling who meets these diagnostic criteria independently Presence of a mutation in *FBN1* known to cause Marfan syndrome Presence of a haplotype around *FBN1,* inherited by descent, known to be associated with unequivocally diagnosed Marfan syndrome in the family	None

The criteria for Marfan syndrome are from the website for the National Marfan Foundation (http://www.marfan.org/nmf/GetSubContent RequestHandler.do?sub_menu_item_content_id=50&menu_item_id=3).

Challenge Cases

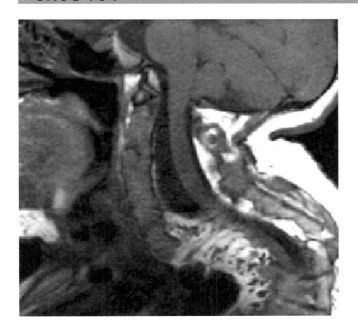 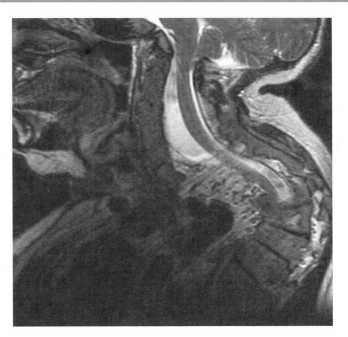

1. What is the value of the angle that is the critical determinant of platybasia?

2. Which lines make up the angle?

3. Name the intracranial finding that often is seen with platybasia.

4. What is the Chamberlain line, and what is it used for?

Platybasia

1. 143 degrees.

2. From the nasion to the dorsum sella, down the plane of the clivus to the anterior margin of the foramen magnum.

3. Chiari I malformation.

4. The Chamberlain line goes from the posterior margin of the hard palate to the posterior lip of the foramen magnum. If the dens is >5 mm above this line, there is basilar invagination.

Reference

Crockard HA, Stevens JM: Craniovertebral junction anomalies in inherited disorders: part of the syndrome or caused by the disorder? *Eur J Pediatr* 154:504–512, 1995.

Cross-Reference

Neuroradiology: THE REQUISITES, p 441.

Comment

Platybasia represents a flattening of the basal angle of the skull. The basal angle of the skull is measured from the nasion to the dorsum sella and down the plane of the clivus. Normally this angle should measure ≤143 degrees. If it is >143 degrees, it is said to represent platybasia. The causes of platybasia are similar to the causes of basilar invagination. Paget disease, rickets, osteomalacia, and Klippel-Feil syndrome all can cause platybasia and basilar invagination. With Klippel-Feil syndrome, one has abnormal segmentation of the vertebrae and an increase in skull base anomalies involving the occiput, C1, and C2 relationships.

Basilar invagination is diagnosed when the odontoid process extends >5 mm above the McGregor line or Chamberlain line. Both of these lines have their anteriormost point at the anterior margin at the foramen magnum. One extends to the midpoint of the posterior wall of the foramen magnum, whereas the other extends to the inferiormost margin of the foramen magnum. Usually the abnormality of the dens protruding above 5 mm is not so subtle so that either one of these lines needs to be used.

Notes

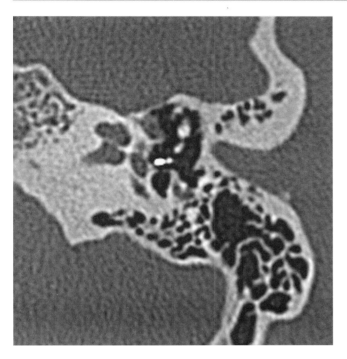

1. What is included in the differential diagnosis?

2. Name the types of tympanoplasties.

3. What is a PORP?

4. Define the pathophysiology of otospongiosis.

Stapes Prosthesis in a Patient with Otospongiosis

1. Otospongiosis, otosyphilis, and osteogenesis imperfecta.

2. In type 1, the procedure spares all the ossicles, and the graft rests on the malleus. In type 2, the graft rests on the incus; in type 3 (the most common), the graft rests on the head of the stapes; in type 4, the graft connects to the footplate of the stapes; and in type 5, the stapes is removed.

3. Partial ossicular replacement prosthesis (PORP). The hydroxyapatite head of the PORP extends from the tympanic membrane to the Plastipore shaft attaching to the capitulum of the stapes.

4. Conductive and sensorineural hearing loss.

Reference

Nelson EG, Hinojosa R: Questioning the relationship between cochlear otosclerosis and sensorineural hearing loss: a quantitative evaluation of cochlear structures in cases of otosclerosis and review of the literature, *Laryngoscope* 114:1214–1230, 2004.

Cross-Reference

Neuroradiology: THE REQUISITES, pp 596–599.

Comment

Otosclerosis is the most frequent cause of middle ear hearing loss in young adults, affecting about 10% of the population of the United States. Otosclerosis usually affects both ears and is seen more commonly in women than men in the teens and 20s.

The disease often shows a combined early conductive (the stapes becomes fixed at the oval window, unable to vibrate in response to sound waves) and late sensorineural (secondary to abnormal blood flow or enzymes produced by the otosclerostic process in the middle ear) hearing loss. Otosclerosis rarely causes sensorineural hearing loss without conductive loss.

Two genes have been associated with otospongiosis: the *OTSC1* gene on chromosome 15 and *OTSC2* on chromosome 7q. On average, a person who has one parent with otosclerosis has a 25% chance of developing the disorder. If both parents have otosclerosis, the risk increases to 50%.

Named ossicular prostheses include the Applebaum prosthesis (a synthetic prosthesis from the long process of the incus to the capitulum of the stapes), the Black oval top synthetic and Richards synthetic prostheses (from the tympanic membrane to the capitulum of the stapes or oval window), and the Goldenberg prosthesis (from the tympanic membrane to the capitulum of the stapes or oval window or the stapes to the malleus or the footplate to the malleus).

Notes

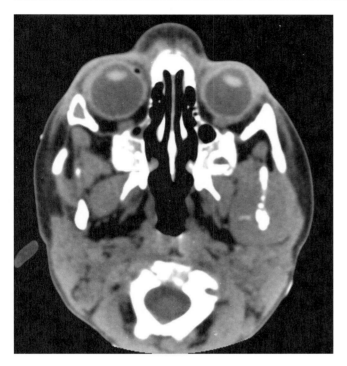

1. What percentage of pediatric malignancies are neuroblastomas?

2. Identify the usual site of origin.

3. Most neuroblastomas occur before what age?

4. What is the most common malignant neoplasm of infancy?

Mandibular Neuroblastoma

1. 7% to 8%.

2. Adrenal gland.

3. 3 years old (50% by age 2, 75% by age 4).

4. Neuroblastoma.

Reference

Kushner BH: Neuroblastoma: a disease requiring a multitude of imaging studies, *J Nucl Med* 45:1172–1188, 2004.

Cross-Reference

Neuroradiology: THE REQUISITES, pp 512, 735, 827.

Comment

There are several classic manifestations of head and neck neuroblastomas, as follows:

Sutural widening: This constitutes metastatic disease to the bone and can be seen in the skull or around the orbits.

Calcified lymph nodes in a child: In this case, the neuroblastoma may be a primary or secondary manifestation. The neck nodes may be jugular or posterior triangle in location.

Paraspinal masses: Classically these masses occur in the perivertebral space and may or not show calcification. More mature forms include ganglioneuroblastoma and ganglioneuroma, the latter of which is benign.

Bony mass in the facial or skull base location: This may be secondary to metastasis from the kidney with a lytic appearance.

High urinary catecholamine levels are present in 90% of cases and may allow a definitive diagnosis in an infant.

Staging is based on the International Neuroblastoma Staging System, a postoperative assessment, as follows:

1—localized tumor with complete gross excision, with or without microscopic residual disease; representative regional lymph nodes negative for disease (nodes attached to and removed with primary tumor may be positive)

2A—localized tumor with incomplete gross excision; identifiable ipsilateral and contralateral lymph nodes negative microscopically

2B—localized tumor with complete or incomplete gross excision; ipsilateral regional lymph nodes positive for tumor. Contralateral lymph nodes negative microscopically

3—unresectable tumor infiltrating across midline with or without regional lymph node involvement, localized tumor with contralateral regional lymph node involvement, or midline tumor with bilateral extension by infiltration (unresectable) or by lymph node involvement

4—any primary tumor with dissemination to distant lymph nodes, cortical bone, bone marrow, liver, or other organs (except as defined in stage 4S)

4S—localized primary tumor as defined for stage 1 or stage 2 with dissemination limited to liver, skin, or bone marrow; only applies to infants <1 year old

Notes

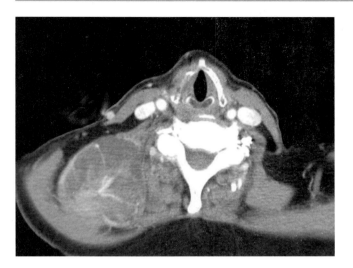 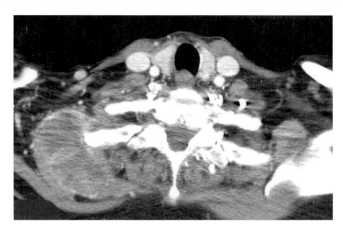

1. What is the most common malignant soft tissue sarcoma of adulthood?

2. On what is the prognosis of this tumor based?

3. Within the head and neck, what tissue shows the highest rate of occurrence of malignant fibrous histiocytoma (MFH)?

4. What is the enhancement pattern of MFH?

Malignant Fibrous Histiocytoma

1. MFH.

2. Size, histologic subtype, tumor grade, depth of spread, and metastases.

3. The muscles.

4. Peripheral and nodular.

Reference

Dalley RW: Fibrous histiocytoma and fibrous tissue tumors of the orbit, *Radiol Clin North Am* 37:185–194, 1999.

Cross-Reference

Neuroradiology: THE REQUISITES, p 512.

Comment

MFH is a sarcoma that usually presents in patients in their 50s or 60s as a painless enlarging mass. Men are affected twice as frequently as women. Several histologic subtypes of MFH exist, but the most common is the pleomorphic/storiform variety. Of all soft tissue sarcomas, 24% are MFH. The most common sites of metastases are to the lungs first and bone second. In the head and neck, nodal metastases occur in more than one third of cases. The overall 5-year prognosis is 40% to 70%, depending on the factors listed in answer 2. The rate of recurrence is about 40%.

This is a difficult diagnosis to make on fine-needle aspiration. Because of the fibrous tissue, it may be relatively acellular. When cells are retrieved, they may be "spindle cells," which has a broad diagnostic potential extending from a benign tumor, such as a schwannoma, to a malignant tumor, such as MFH, and many intermediate forms in between.

MFH may be induced by radiation after several years.

Notes

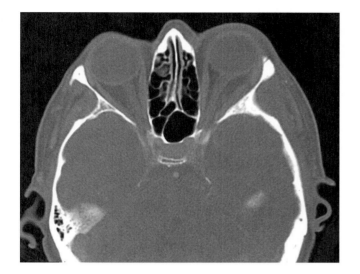 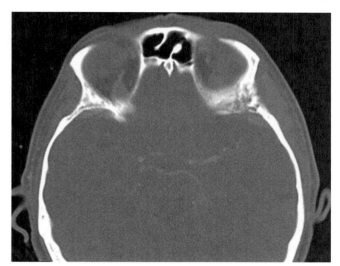

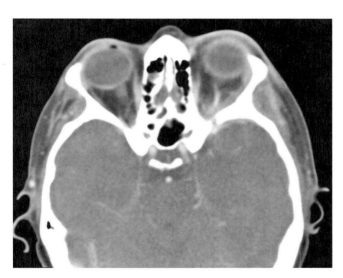

1. What is included in the differential diagnosis?
2. List typical musculoskeletal symptoms of SAPHO syndrome.
3. In the head and neck, what site is affected the most?
4. Is there a single site or multiple sites of bone involvement?

SAPHO Syndrome

1. Osteomyelitis, Paget disease, Langerhans cell histiocytosis, and aggressive neoplasms such as Ewing sarcoma and osteosarcoma.

2. Sternoclavicular arthritis, spondylitis, or sacroileitis.

3. Mandible.

4. Multiple.

Reference

Earwaker JW, Cotton A: SAPHO syndrome or concept? Imaging findings, *Skeletal Radiol* 32:311–327, 2003.

Cross-Reference

Neuroradiology: THE REQUISITES, p 660.

Comment

SAPHO syndrome comprises *s*ynovitis, *a*cne, *p*ustulosis, *h*yperostosis, and *o*steitis. Patients with SAPHO syndrome usually present with dermatologic abnormalities because of the pustule rash that occurs. When periosteal reaction of the bone occurs, it generally affects the long bones; however, involvement of the facial bones has been reported in several case reports and case series.

The etiology of SAPHO syndrome is unknown, and the cause of the periosteal reaction has not been elucidated. Symptoms associated with the periosteal reaction are more commonly due to the mass affect than to pain, discomfort, or pathologic fracture. Because of the subtle symptoms, the mean interval time between the patient's presentation and diagnosis of SAPHO averages 9 years. The more typical locations of bone reaction are the chest wall, proximal joints, or spine.

The pustulosis tends to be on the palms of the hands and the plantar surface of the feet.

Differential diagnosis of SAPHO syndrome includes osteomyelitis, Paget disease, and aggressive neoplasms such as Ewing sarcoma and osteosarcoma.

Treatment for SAPHO usually is directed toward the individual symptoms of acne, synovitis, osteitis, and periosteal reaction. Antibiotics and topical therapies are usually tried. The long-term prognosis of SAPHO syndrome is unknown.

Notes

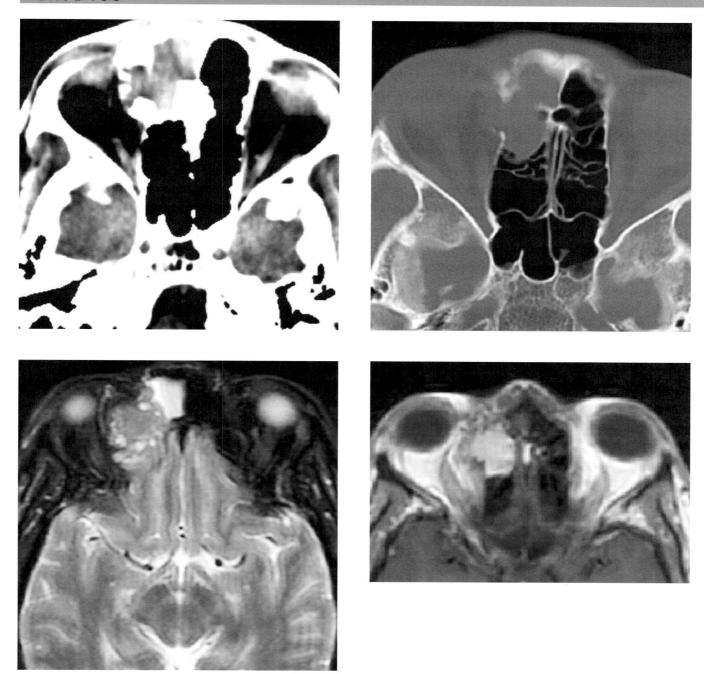

1. What is the most compelling imaging finding that suggests that this lesion is *not* inflammatory?

2. What benign sinonasal processes are dark on T2W imaging?

3. What are the most common head and neck sites for synovial sarcoma?

4. Name predisposing conditions for head and neck sarcomas.

CASE 156

Synovial Sarcoma of the Frontal Sinus

1. Solid gadolinium enhancement.

2. Fungal sinusitis, sarcoidosis, inspissated secretions, radiation fibrosis, inverted papillomas, osteomas, osteocartilaginous lesions, fibrous dysplasia.

3. Submucosa of the aerodigestive system, parapharyngeal space, masticator space.

4. Familial retinoblastoma, prior irradiation, Paget's disease, neurofibromatosis, Li Fraumeni syndrome, Ollier's syndrome, Thorotrast exposure.

Reference

Park JK, Ham SY, Hwang JC, Jeong YK, Lee JH, Yang SO, Suh JH, Choi DH: Synovial sarcoma of the head and neck: a case of predominantly cystic mass. *AJNR Am J Neuroradiol* 25:1103–1105, 2004.

Cross-Reference

Neuroradiology: THE REQUISITES, p 723.

Comment

Synovial sarcoma has no relationship to joints in the head and neck. The cell of origin resembles that of a synovial cell, hence its name. This is a spindle cell-like tumor. Synovial sarcomas populate the head and neck usually within the submucosa in the hypopharynx, the parapharyngeal space, or the masticator space. These lesions have a variable presentation radiographically in that they may show cyst formation, calcification, hemorrhage, or solid growth patterns. The frontal sinus is an unusual site for a synovial sarcoma but points out the lack of association with joints. This case is extremely uncommon.

As sarcomas go, synovial sarcomas have a more benign soft tissue than any of the other soft tissue sarcomas. In some cases they may be well encapsulated and can be removed in their entirety. Differential diagnosis will include soft tissue, rhabdomyosarcomas, and chondrosarcomas. Rarely, myositis ossificans may simulate a synovial sarcoma, but the latter would show progressive growth whereas over time myositis ossificans would become dormant.

T staging of sarcomas is by size (T1 < 5 cm, T2 > 5 cm) and depth (A, superficial; B, deep).

Notes

Case compliments of Minerva Becker, M.D, Geneva, Switzerland.

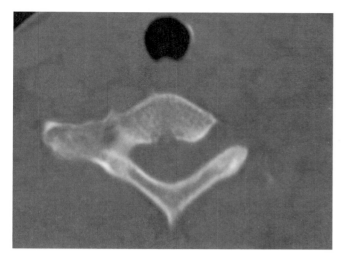
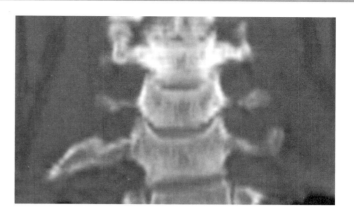

1. How does one differentiate a cervical rib from apophysomegaly?

2. In which direction do cervical ribs and first thoracic ribs point?

3. How often are cervical ribs bilateral, and if unilateral, which side predominates?

4. Which are more commonly symptomatic, complete or incomplete cervical ribs?

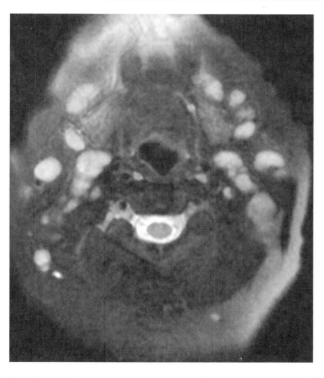
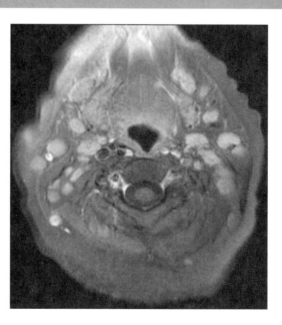

1. Given that this patient is a Japanese man with eosinophilia and subcutaneous nodules, what is the best (and most obscure) diagnosis?

2. What is Kikuchi disease?

3. What is Kawasaki disease?

4. What is Kussmaul disease?

CASE 157

Cervical Ribs

1. One is a bone that articulates with the vertebra, the other just a large transverse process.

2. Cervical ribs point downward, and T1 ribs point upward.

3. They are reported to be bilateral in 47% to 73% of cases. When unilateral, more are on the right.

4. Incomplete cervical ribs because they have a compressive fibrous band.

Reference

Gülekon N, Barut CD, Turgut HB: The prevalence of cervical rib in Anatolian population, *Gazi Med J* 10:149–152, 1999.

Cross-Reference

Neuroradiology: THE REQUISITES, pp 735–736.

Comment

Cervical ribs occur in approximately 3% of the population. They are more frequent in women than men, as is the brachial plexopathy associated with them. The significance of having the rib associated with the C7 vertebral body is the fact that it may create a predilection for brachial plexopathy. Complete cervical ribs that connect to the sternum and incomplete cervical ribs that extend only partially toward the sternum may cause a brachial plexopathy by compression at the anterior scalene level. Thoracic outlet syndrome may coexist with the brachial plexopathy—the former secondary to vascular compromise of the subclavian artery.

Cervical ribs are not the only bony abnormality that can cause a brachial plexus. Even if one has enlargement of the transverse process or apophyseal joint, compression phenomena can develop on the brachial plexus. Clavicle fractures with exuberant callus formation or hematomas are another source. Symptoms include pain and paresthesias in the shoulder and arm. Symptoms may be exacerbated by lifting the arms above the head. Surgical removal of the cervical rib or shaving of the transverse process can be performed if physical therapy does not solve the problem. Scalenectomy also has been performed to relieve pressure.

Other possible complications of cervical ribs include thrombus formation, aneurysm development, and embolism.

Notes

CASE 158

Kimura Disease

1. Kimura disease.

2. A necrotizing adenitis described in East Asian patients predominantly causing cervical adenopathy. It usually is self-limited.

3. Fever, rash, conjunctivitis, mucositis, and cervical adenitis resulting from a vasculitis. It can cause coronary thrombosis or aneurysms or both.

4. Recurrent sialadenitis secondary to ductal plugs, especially in dehydrated individuals.

References

Hiwatashi A, Hasuo K, Shiina T, et al: Kimura's disease with bilateral auricular masses, *AJNR Am J Neuroradiol* 20:1976–1978, 1999.

Takahashi S, Ueda J, Furukawa T, et al: Kimura disease: CT and MR findings, *AJNR Am J Neuroradiol* 17: 382–385, 1996.

Cross-Reference

Neuroradiology: THE REQUISITES, pp 684–685.

Comment

Kimura disease is endemic in the Asian population, particularly in Chinese and Japanese men. It manifests with multiple subcutaneous nodules, cervical adenopathy, and salivary gland adenitis. Muscular and skin inflammation may coexist. The disease also is termed *eosinophilic lymphogranuloma* because of the presence in the blood smear of eosinophilia, elevated serum IgE, and the lymphadenopathy. Spontaneous remission is the rule, but the episodes may recur in 25% of cases. If renal disease occurs, treatment is with steroids because the etiology is thought to be an allergic reaction by virtue of the eosinophilia and IgE.

Kimura disease causes intense enhancement of lymph nodes.

Notes

Case compliments of Bill Dillon, UCSF.

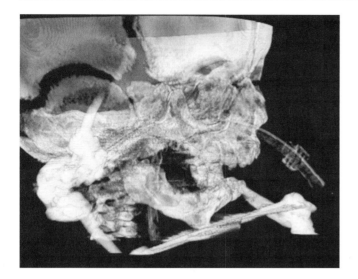

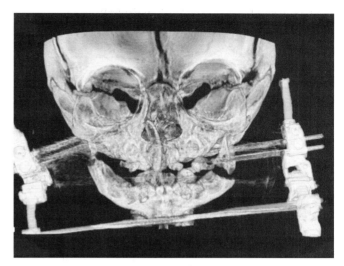

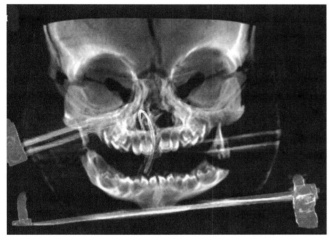

1. Describe the facial manifestations of Treacher Collins syndrome.

2. What is the mode of inheritance?

3. What finding in the mandible is pathognomonic for Treacher Collins syndrome?

4. Which branchial arches are affected?

Treacher Collins Syndrome with Mandibular Advancement

1. Hypoplasia of the face, small ear, small mandible, possible external auditory canal atresia, hypoplastic malar eminence, and cleft palate.

2. Autosomal dominant.

3. Downward curve of the horizontal portion of the ramus of the mandible—bowing of its inferior cortical surface.

4. Usually first and second.

Reference

Binaghi S, Gudinchet F, Rilliet B:. Three-dimensional spiral CT of craniofacial malformations in children, *Pediatr Radiol* 30:856–860, 2000.

Cross-Reference

Neuroradiology: THE REQUISITES, pp 266–269.

Comment

Treacher Collins syndrome, also known as mandibulo-facial dysostosis or Franceschetti-Klein syndrome, has been mapped to a mutation in the "treacle" gene (*TCOF1*) on chromosome 5q32. Inheritance is autosomal dominant. The manifestations of the disease include antimongoloid slant of the eyes, coloboma of the lid, micrognathia, microtia and other deformity of the ears, hypoplastic zygomatic arches, and macrostomia. Conductive hearing loss secondary to the malformed external auditory canal and ossicles is commonly seen. Patients also may have cleft lip with or without cleft palate, heart defects, and strabismus.

The ear anomalies associated with Treacher Collins syndrome are usually bilateral and symmetric. The external auditory canal is atretic or stenotic. The middle ear cavity is small, and the ossicles are either missing or malformed. The inner ears are normal. The zygomatic arch may be short, and the temporomandibular joint may be dislocated.

This child was having a mandibular advancement procedure to improve the micrognathia.

Notes

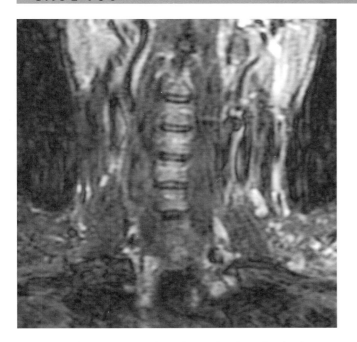 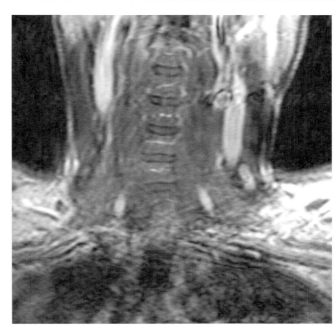

1. Behind what muscles does the brachial plexus course?

2. What artery does the brachial plexus surround?

3. At what level do the cords converge with the branches?

4. What is the differential diagnosis of bilateral bright nerve roots?

Brachial Plexopathy: Chronic Inflammatory Demyelinating Neuropathy

1. Anterior scalene muscle.

2. Subclavian artery.

3. At the clavicle.

4. Brachial plexitis, chronic inflammatory demyelinating neuropathy (CIDP), neurofibromatosis, multiple schwannomas, Charcot-Marie-Tooth disease hereditary sensory motor neuropathies, sarcoidosis, Guillain-Barré syndrome, Dejerine Sottas syndrome, and cytomegalovirus polyradiculopathy.

Reference

Oguz B, Oguz KK, Cila A, Tan E: Diffuse spinal and intercostal nerve involvement in chronic inflammatory demyelinating polyradiculoneuropathy: MRI findings, *Eur Radiol* 13(Suppl 4):L230–L234, 2003.

Cross-Reference

Neuroradiology: THE REQUISITES, p 822.

Comment

CIDP is an immune-mediated polyneuropathy that may be related to Guillain-Barré syndrome. The disease often has an antecedent viral infection, which may send the cascade of immune reactivity down this untoward pathway. It may coexist with HIV infection. Usually patients have paresthesias at the start, but this may progress to anesthesia, loss of reflexes, fatigue, and subsequent motor weakness. The disease usually begins in the feet and progresses to involve the upper extremities. The CSF shows elevated protein concentrations, and electromyography/nerve conduction study shows slowing of conduction and prolonged latencies. Biopsy specimens of the nerves show demyelination and variable T cell–mediated inflammation, but because this disease is characterized by "skip lesions," random biopsy specimens may be less useful. Imaging using a magnetic resonance neurography sequence may be a useful alternative.

The nerves on MRI, when abnormal, are usually hyperintense, enlarged, and enhancing.

Treatment for CIDP is usually conservative at first with the hope that the condition will spontaneously resolve. A relapsing course is seen in 30%, and a chronic progressive course is seen in 70%. For patients with chronic or progressive disease, plasmapheresis, immunoglobulin therapy, and steroids are employed. Recovery may take months to years, but complete remission eventually is seen in 80% of cases.

Notes

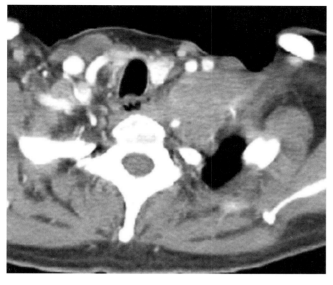
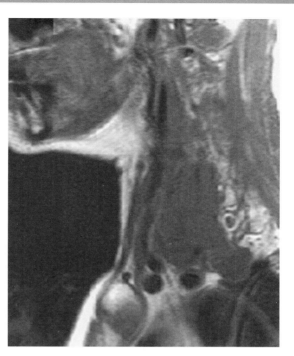
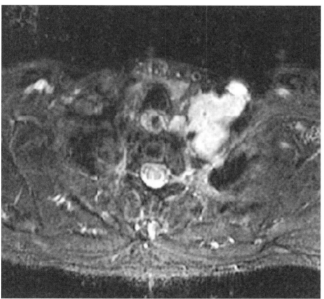
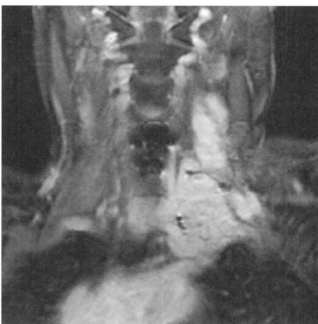

1. What is included in the differential diagnosis?

2. Of those listed in the differential diagnosis, which lesions grow fastest?

3. In the head and neck, what is the most common early childhood fibrous lesion?

4. What are the usual symptoms associated with nodular fasciitis?

Nodular Fasciitis

1. Nodular fasciitis, myxoma, fibrous histiocytoma, lymphoma, fibrosarcoma, malignant fibrous histiocytoma, and benign lymph node.

2. Fibrosarcoma, malignant fibrous histiocytoma, and nodular fasciitis.

3. Nodular fasciitis.

4. Soft tissue mass in a 20- to 40-year-old; 50% have pain.

Reference

Shin JH, Lee HK, Cho KJ, et al: Nodular fasciitis of the head and neck: radiographic findings, *Clin Imaging* 27:31–37, 2003.

Cross-Reference

Neuroradiology: THE REQUISITES, pp 733–735.

Comment

In histologic series, nodular fasciitis represents a large number of the masses in the head and neck. Nodular fasciitis represents one form of fibromatous lesions in the neck, including aggressive fibromas, malignant fibrous histiocytomas, and benign fibromas. In many cases, the presentation of nodular fasciitis is that of a palpable or asymptomatic mass composed of fibroblastic tissue. Masses may occur in the muscles, subcutaneous tissue, and skin. Because of mass effect on adjacent nerves, one may develop neurologic symptoms or discomfort or both. Nonetheless, the differential diagnosis includes a benign lymph node.

After the upper extremity, the head and neck are the second most common sites of nodular fasciitis. It tends to border the mandible and zygomatic regions. The lesion enhances with contrast administration.

Notes

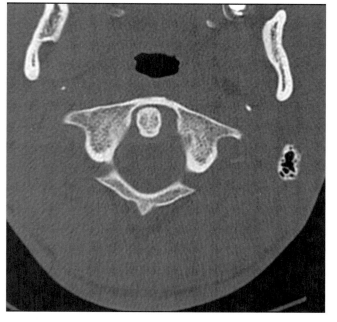

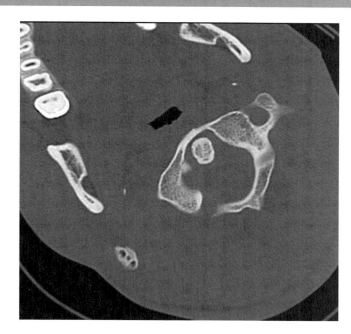

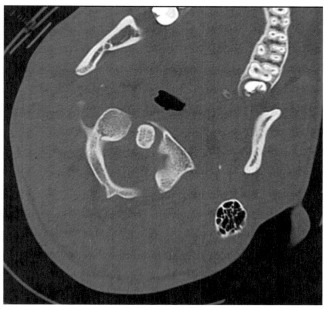

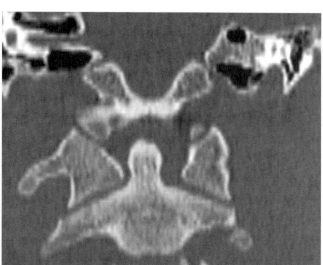

1. What is the definitive way to make this diagnosis?

2. Does this entity occur in children or adults?

3. What are the typical symptoms?

4. How is rotatory subluxation classified?

Rotatory Subluxation of C1-2

1. Perform CT scans in the neutral, head to the left, and head to the right positions and show persistent malposition of the dens and C1 arch.

2. It occurs more commonly in children (80%).

3. Torticollis after a pharyngitis or minor trauma.

4. Type 1, no anterior displacement; type 2, 3- to 5-mm anterior displacement of C1 on C2; type 3, >5 mm anterior displacement of C1 on C2; type 4, posterior displacement of C1 on C2.

Reference

Harth M, Mayer M, Marzi I, Vogl TJ: Lateral torticollis on plain radiographs and MRI: Grisel syndrome, *Eur Radiol* 14:1713–1715, 2004.

Cross-Reference

Neuroradiology: THE REQUISITES, p 733.

Comment

Rotatory subluxation may be a cause of torticollis in children. It is diagnosed by CT when there is a malposition of the odontoid process with respect to the C1 arch that is persistent in all head positions (fixed rotatory subluxation). This entity sometimes is seen as a complication of a pharyngitis/tonsillitis (Grisel syndrome), a muscular spasm owing to a local irritant, or a traumatic event. The inappropriate laxity of the alar and transverse ligaments supporting the odontoid process induced by the inflammation or trauma seems to be at fault. Simple muscle spasm could be the etiology as well—this is still being debated.

Most cases resolve spontaneously with physical therapy, use of a soft collar, and pain control. Sometimes halter traction is required, particularly if the vertebral arteries are deemed to be compromised. This happens with >45 degrees of rotation or >5 mm of anterolisthesis. The longer a patient goes before a diagnosis or before presenting for treatment, the less likely conservative management will succeed. Chronic cases may require fusion.

Notes

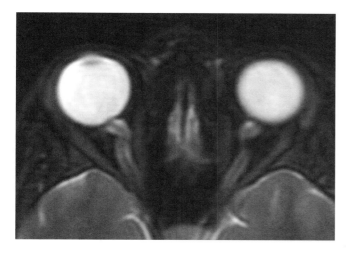
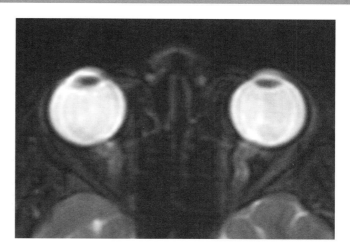

1. What is a normal CSF pressure?

2. What entity is associated with elevated CSF pressure, obesity, visual changes, and headaches?

3. What is the suspected etiology for this condition?

4. Identify the sequelae of long-standing papilledema.

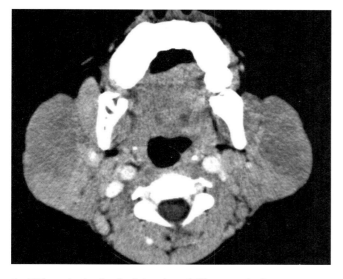
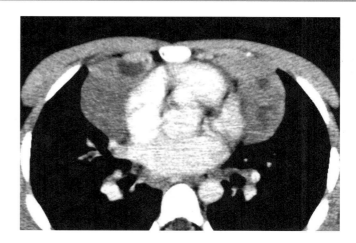

1. What is included in the differential diagnosis?

2. What are the usual symptoms?

3. Name the classic histologic feature of this entity.

4. What is the incidence of extranodal disease?

Papilledema

1. 80 to 150 mm H_2O; some extend to 50 to 180 mm H_2O.

2. Idiopathic intracranial hypertension (pseudotumor cerebri).

3. Venous outflow stenosis or obstruction versus increased resistance to CSF outflow at the arachnoid granulations.

4. Optic atrophy and visual loss.

Reference

Biousse V, Ameri A, Bousser MG: Isolated intracranial hypertension as the only sign of cerebral venous thrombosis, *Neurology* 53:1537–1542, 1999.

Cross-Reference

Neuroradiology: THE REQUISITES, pp 378–379, 490–491.

Comment

The finding of reversed indentation of the optic nerve at its insertion site with the globe suggests papilledema. Another ancillary finding of papilledema is enlargement of the optic nerve sheath complex.

When a clinician observes papilledema on ophthalmologic examination in an acutely ill patient, there is immediate concern for increased intracranial pressure. The pressure is transmitted from the subarachnoid space within the brain to the communicating subarachnoid space around the optic nerve sheath complex. This increased pressure results in dilation of the optic nerve sheath and the transmission of the pressure to the optic nerve head insertion, causing the reversed cupping that is evident on the CT or MRI cross-sectional scans.

Numerous causes of reverse cupping and pallor to the optic nerve head insertion may simulate papilledema. These are usually termed *pseudopapilledema.* Inflammatory causes include papillitis, which has a viral etiology. Occasionally, multiple sclerosis demyelinating plaques or idiopathic optic neuritis of the nerve near the insertion may cause swelling that simulates papilledema. Finally, optic nerve head drusen may cause the elevation of the optic nerve head insertion.

The neuroradiologist should proceed in evaluating the intracranial structures. With enlargement of the lateral ventricles out of proportion to sulci or the finding of transependymal CSF flow (interstitial edema), the diagnosis of hydrocephalus in association with increased intracranial pressure should be made. Occasionally one finds that the lateral ventricles and basal cisterns are effaced with flattening of the sulci throughout. This is another manifestation of increased intracranial pressure causing papilledema.

Notes

Sinus Histiocytosis with Massive Lymphadenopathy (Rosai-Dorfman Disease)

1. Mastocytosis, sinus histiocytosis, Rosai-Dorfman disease, lymphoma, mononucleosis, amyloidosis, PTLD, and sarcoidosis.

2. Neck mass, fevers, and fatigue.

3. Rosai-Dorfman bodies, an S-100 protein-expressing histiocyte with pale cytoplasm showing leukoerythrophagocytosis.

4. 30% to 40%.

Reference

McAlister WH, Herman T, Dehner LP: Sinus histiocytosis with massive lymphadenopathy (Rosai-Dorfman disease), *Pediatr Radiol* 20:425–432, 1990.

Cross-Reference

Neuroradiology: THE REQUISITES, p 684.

Comment

This is a disease entity of cervical adenopathy with associated fevers. Although fairly dramatic in the extent of lymph node enlargement and distribution, it usually has a benign course and spontaneously regresses. It affects African Americans more commonly than whites and is generally a disease affecting individuals before age 30.

Extranodal disease has been reported in many locations, most notably the mediastinum, orbit, eyelid, upper aerodigestive tract, and retroperitoneum. CNS involvement has been reported even in the absence of nodal pathology and is generally intracranial and leptomeningeal. Nonetheless, dural involvement in the spinal canal also has been reported. It usually simulates a lymph node.

Notes

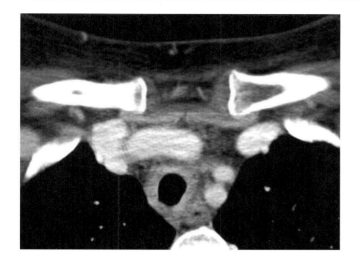

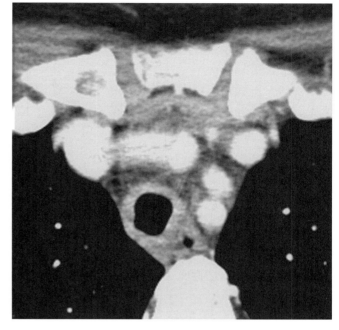

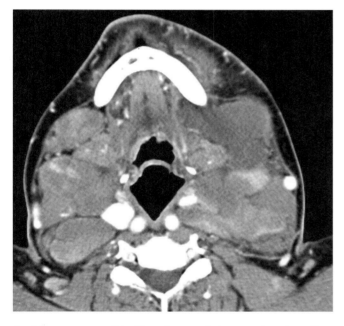

1. List causes of infiltrations of the tracheal walls.

2. How often is amyloidosis a single-organ disease?

3. Which organs does relapsing polychondritis affect in the head and neck?

4. Identify the classic stain for amyloidosis.

Amyloidosis

1. Infections (tuberculosis, papillomatosis, croup, histoplasmosis), neoplasms (lymphoma, squamous cell carcinoma, minor salivary gland lesions), metabolic/acquired (amyloidosis, asthma, tracheopathia osteochondroplastica), radiation, postoperative granulation, Wegener granulomatosis, and sarcoidosis.

2. 10%.

3. Ears, nose, larynx, and trachea.

4. Congo red showing apple-green birefringence.

Reference

Kirchner J, Jacobi V, Kardos P, Kollath J: CT findings in extensive tracheobronchial amyloidosis, *Eur Radiol* 8:352–354, 1998.

Cross-Reference

Neuroradiology: THE REQUISITES, pp 653–654, 672.

Comment

This case shows a relatively unusual manifestation of amyloidosis—tracheal infiltration and diffuse lymphadenopathy. In this example, the disease is in its systemic form, but amyloidomas in a single location also may exist. The patient's symptoms may include hemoptysis, asthma, and pneumonia. The bronchial walls also may be involved and may show calcification on histology or on high-resolution CT. Congo red staining shows the typical birefringent pattern from the bronchial specimen. Other names for this type of pattern are "light chain deposition disease" and "amyloidosis of light chain origin." The former does not stain with Congo red but is periodic acid–Schiff positive instead.

Primary amyloidosis is a systemic disorder of uncertain origin but may be related in part to multiple myeloma. Secondary amyloidosis may occur as a result of chronic infections such as tuberculosis, familial Mediterranean fever, and connective tissue disorders. There is also a hereditary form of amyloidosis.

Notes

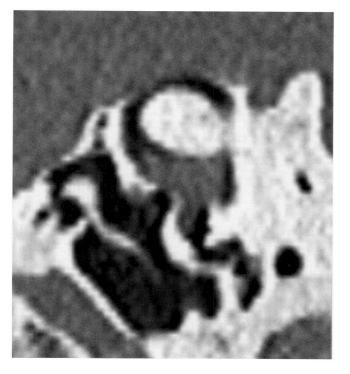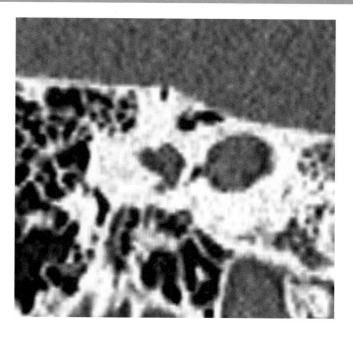

1. Which semicircular canal is the last to form and hence the most likely to be congenitally dysplastic?

2. What is Tulio syndrome?

3. What is the most common example of labyrinthine maldevelopment causing sensorineural hearing loss?

4. What are the causes of semicircular canal dehiscences?

Superior Semicircular Canal Dehiscence

1. Lateral.

2. A syndrome in which vertigo and imbalance are triggered by loud noises or pressure in the affected ear. These symptoms are due to an opening in the bone overlying one of the inner ear balance canals.

3. Enlarged vestibular aqueduct syndrome.

4. Trauma, cholesteatoma, cephaloceles, congenital/ idiopathic, surgical, and chronic otitis media.

Reference

Belden CJ, Weg N, Minor LB, Zinreich SJ: CT evaluation of bone dehiscence of the superior semicircular canal as a cause of sound- and/or pressure-induced vertigo, *Radiology* 226:337–343, 2003.

Cross-Reference

Neuroradiology: THE REQUISITES, pp 592–595.

Comment

Dehiscence of the superior semicircular canal is a phenomenon that was born from multidetector CT technology. Before this era, the subtle discontinuities of the superior semicircular canal along the arcuate eminence were invisible to CT. With submillimeter scan thicknesses, however, one can show this disease entity more readily. Thin slices coupled with multiplanar and especially radial reconstructions render this finding simple. More recent studies suggest a 1.5% to 9% rate of superior semicircular canal dehiscence in normal subjects.

This history is classic. Patients feel dizzy and nauseated and have a sensation that the room is moving when there are loud sounds or when they perform the Valsalva maneuver. With the loud sounds, the eyes show nystagmoid features up and away from the loud noise. Bilateral disease has been reported in 17%. Even without dehiscence bilaterally, the bone is thinned contralaterally at a high rate, suggesting a mesodermal defect.

In some disabling cases, surgical plugging of the opening in the affected superior semicircular canal may be beneficial.

Notes

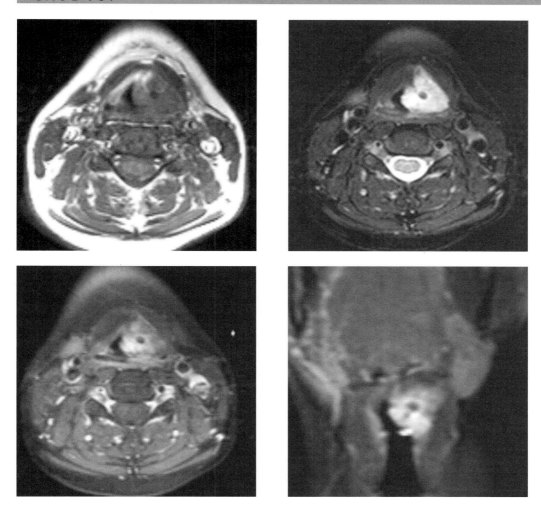

1. What is the likely source of the low-intensity area in this lesion on T1W, T2W, and postcontrast scans?

2. Given the answer to no. 1, provide a differential diagnosis.

3. What iatrogenic causes of low signal in the vocal cord could be possible?

4. What is the blue rubber bleb nevus syndrome?

Venous Vascular Malformation
of the Larynx

1. Calcification.

2. Venous vascular malformation with phleboliths, chondroid lesion, amyloidoma, post-traumatic dystrophic calcification.

3. A vocal cord implant (silastic, gelfoam, Teflon, cartilage).

4. The syndrome associated with multiple cutaneous venous malformations, mucosal and visceral hemangiomas/venous vascular malformations, often with a coagulopathy.

Reference

Hendrickx S, Hermans R, Wilms G, Sciot R: Angiomatosis in the neck and mediastinum: an example of low-flow vascular malformations, *Eur Radiol* 13:981–985, 2003.

Cross-Reference

Neuroradiology: THE REQUISITES, pp 671–672.

Comment

This patient shows a lesion that is dark on T1W imaging, bright on T2W imaging, intensely enhancing, and has a low-intensity area centrally on all pulse sequences. The lesion was bright red on endoscopy and represents a venous vascular malformation. Formerly called hemangiomas, these lesions occur in the glottic and supraglottic region, as opposed to the childhood true capillary hemangiomas, which are more frequently seen in a subglottic location. They may be pedunculated, and they may appear red or blue at endoscopy. Whereas childhood subglottic hemangiomas affect females more than males, supraglottic venous vascular malformations affect males more than females.

No treatment is the best option unless the patient becomes symptomatic. Nd YAG laser ablation may be attempted.

The blue rubber bleb nevus syndrome, also known as Bean syndrome, has been reported to be a source of some cases of laryngeal vascular malformations. However, more commonly, the bowel and upper gastrointestinal tract are affected. Phleboliths may be evident (as in this case), and the patient may develop a consumptive coagulopathy from platelet trapping. Chronic anemia due to slowly leaking gastrointestinal vascular malformations is the rule.

Notes

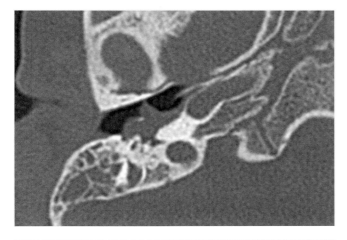

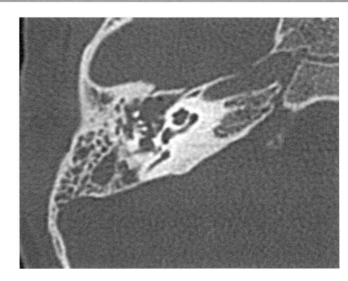

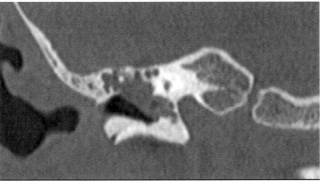

1. In what space would you put this lesion?

2. What is included in the differential diagnosis?

3. If the mass is red, what are the most likely diagnoses?

4. What is another name for heterotopic tissue in this location?

Glial Choristoma

1. Middle ear cavity.

2. Cholesteatoma, cholesterol granuloma, epidermoid, schwannoma, glomus tympanicum, and aberrant vessel.

3. Cholesterol granuloma, glomus tympanicum, glomus jugulare, and aberrant vessel.

4. A choristoma.

Reference

Lee JI, Kim KK, Park YK, et al: Glial choristoma in the middle ear and mastoid bone: a case report, *J Korean Med Sci* 19:155–158, 2004.

Cross-Reference

Neuroradiology: THE REQUISITES, pp 426–428.

Comment

This patient had a blue mass behind the tympanic membrane. The lesion was characterized as an admixture of mature neuroglial tissue and choroid plexus with melanin production. The neuroglial tissue was immunoreactive for glial fibrillary acidic protein (GFAP), and the choroid plexus component was immunoreactive for GFAP (focal), synaptophysin, and cytokeratin. The pathogenesis of glial choristomas of the middle ear likely involves an encephalocele, in which communication with the CNS has undergone fibrous obliteration. In other words, this is a "nasal glioma" of the ear—effectively heterotopic brain.

By choristoma, we mean normally organized tissue in the wrong place as opposed to a hamartoma, where the tissue is a disorganized mass. Most are grayish white, not blue. GFAP positivity argues strongly for the glial origin of the mass. Some middle ear choristomas may be of salivary gland origin. All choristomas of the middle ear have a propensity to involve the middle ear ossicles.

Notes

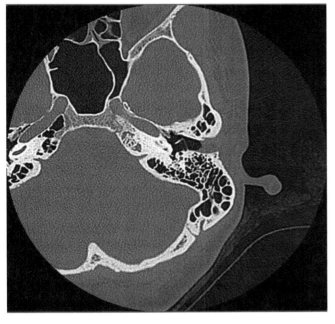
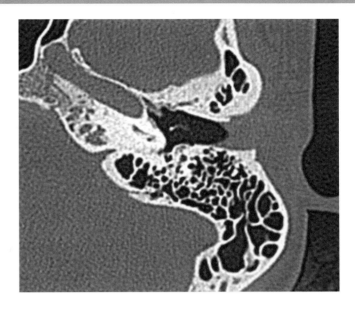
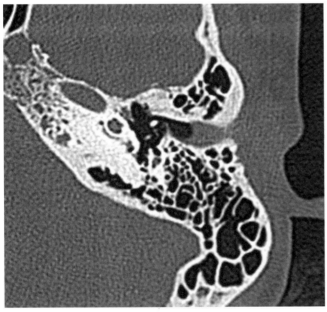
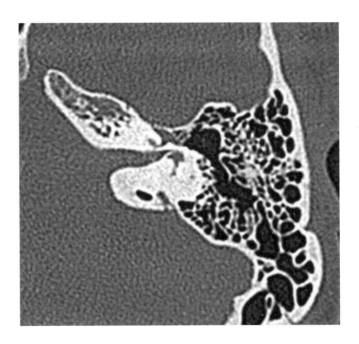

1. What are the etiologies for this entity?

2. What are the implications regarding cochlear implantation?

3. How is this diagnosis different from otosclerosis?

4. Could this be Paget disease?

Labyrinthitis Ossificans

1. Typically a complication of meningitis, chronic infectious labyrinthitis, or trauma.

2. The cochlea would have to be drilled out, and there may be failure of full implant placement.

3. Otosclerosis typically involves the bone around the cochlea, not within the scala vestibuli and tympani.

4. No. Labyrinthine involvement with Paget disease occurs in the last stages.

Reference

Woolford TJ, Roberts GR, Hartley C, Ramsden RT: Etiology of hearing loss and cochlear computed tomography: findings in preimplant assessment, *Ann Otol Rhinol Laryngol* 166(Suppl):201–206, 1995.

Cross-Reference

Neuroradiology: THE REQUISITES, pp 594–597.

Comment

Labyrinthitis ossificans is a late complication of bacterial meningitis (most frequently pneumococcal), severe otitis media with perilymphatic fistulas, chronic infectious labyrinthitis, radiation osteitis, or trauma in which there is ossification of the cochlea and in severe forms of the vestibule and semicircular canals. The result is a conductive and sensorineural hearing loss.

In some cases, the obliteration may be fibrous and not ossific. In these cases, CT findings may be falsely negative. For this reason, some radiologists at progressive institutions advocate use of MRI with high resolution and three-dimensional reformatting of T2-weighted scans to depict the "lumen" of the cochlea. The demonstration of cochlear patency is helpful in planning cochlear implantation. If one side is obliterated and the other less involved, the otologist implants the patent ear.

This is not otosclerosis, which is seen more typically as rarefaction of the bone around the cochlea or anterior to the oval window. It is only in its late stages or after fluoride therapy that one may see it as a truly "sclerosing" entity that may encroach on the perilymphatic and endolymphatic channels of the cochlea.

Of patients with hearing loss after meningitis, 40% have a positive CT scan for labyrinthitis ossificans. Labyrinthitis ossificans is usually the sequela of meningitis in which there is inflammatory exudate that extends into the labyrinth in structures. This incites a sclerotic osteogenic response, which leads to obliteration of the perilymphatic and endolymphatic spaces within the labyrinthine system or within the cochlea.

Notes

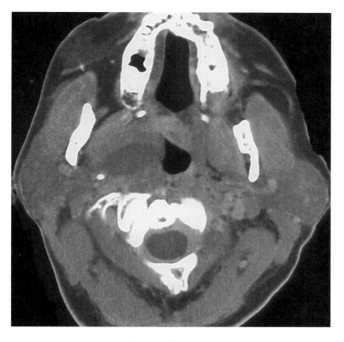
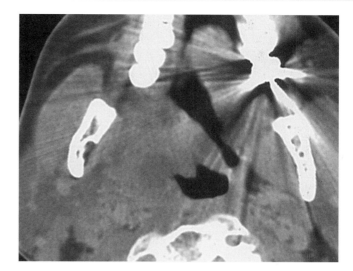

1. In a patient with an allograft renal transplant, what should be included in the differential diagnosis?
2. What are the manifestations of posttransplant lymphoproliferative disorder (PTLD) in the neck?
3. Is necrosis seen in PTLD?
4. Besides the lymph nodes, what is the most common site of PTLD in the head and neck?

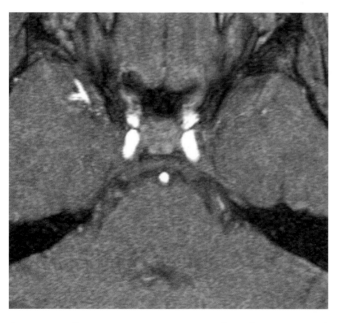
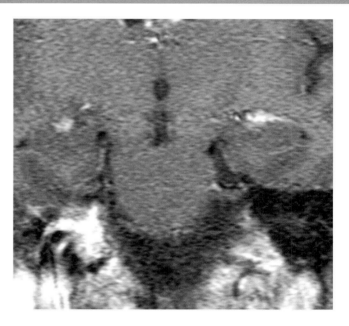

1. Name the symptoms associated with trigeminal neuralgia.
2. What is the most common imaging finding associated with this lesion?
3. What is the best pulse sequence for the evaluation here?
4. What vessel is most commonly implicated?

CASE 170

Posttransplant Lymphoproliferative Disorder

1. Abscess, lymphoma, posttransplant lymphoproliferative disorder, schwannoma, and necrotizing adenitis.

2. Cervical adenopathy, Waldeyer ring enlargement diffusely or focally, and lymphoma.

3. Yes.

4. The tonsils.

Reference

Loevner LA, Karpati RL, Kumar P, et al: Posttransplantation lymphoproliferative disorder of the head and neck: imaging features in seven adults, *Radiology* 216: 363–369, 2000.

Cross-Reference

Neuroradiology: THE REQUISITES, pp 507, 685–686.

Comment

PTLD is a complication of solid-organ transplantation related to infection with Epstein-Barr virus in an immunocompromised host in which B cell proliferation becomes unrestricted. It is most common after intestine > lung > kidney/pancreas > heart transplants. T cell–depleted bone marrow transplant patients also are at risk. Rates of involvement range from 1% to 8% of cases. Cyclosporine and tacrolimus (FK506) therapy may predispose to PTLD development.

Manifestations include lymphoid hyperplasia, a polymorphous polyclonal lymphoma, or an aggressive monoclonal lymphoma.

Treatment is with reduction of the immunosuppressive therapy so that the body can regulate the Epstein-Barr virus infection and B cell pathology. This treatment leads to a higher chance of rejection of the transplant.

Cytomegalovirus infection, in patients who are seronegative for Epstein-Barr virus, may be an additional risk factor.

The Harris classification of PTLD is as follows:

Early lesions: reactive plasmacytic hyperplasia (infectious mononucleosis)

PTLD polymorphic: polymorphic B cell hyperplasia/ lymphoma

PTLD monomorphic: diffuse large B cell lymphoma > peripheral T cell lymphoma

PTLD other: T cell–rich/Hodgkin disease–like PTLD and plasmacytoma-like PTLD

Notes

CASE 171

Trigeminal Neuralgia

1. Pain in cranial nerve V distribution, often with facial spasms.

2. Normal.

3. Magnetic resonance angiography raw data so that you can see the nerve and vessel.

4. Superior cerebellar artery.

Reference

Yoshino N, Akimoto H, Yamada I, et al: Trigeminal neuralgia: evaluation of neuralgic manifestation and site of neurovascular compression with 3D CISS MR imaging and MR angiography, *Radiology* 228:539–545, 2003.

Cross-Reference

Neuroradiology: THE REQUISITES, pp: 107–108.

Comment

Trigeminal neuralgia, although classically caused by vascular compression of the cisternal trigeminal nerve, also may be caused by masses in the cerebellopontine angle, by demyelinating plaques in the brainstem, by brainstem astrocytomas, and by no known etiology. Patients usually present in their 40s or 50s, and the pain can become so unbearable that some individuals are driven to suicide.

The vascular lesion may be seen well on high-resolution MRI or magnetic resonance angiography. Nearly 90% of patients with symptoms related to the maxillary division can be shown to have vascular compression at the medial side of the root entry zone of the trigeminal nerve, and nearly three fourths of patients with pain in the mandibular division have compression at the lateral aspect of the root entry zone of the trigeminal nerve. The superior cerebellar artery > anterior inferior cerebellar artery > both arteries > veins > basilar arteries seem to be the culprits in most cases.

Microvascular decompressions, gamma knife radiation therapy, radiofrequency ablation, and botulinum toxin injections have been used as therapy.

Notes

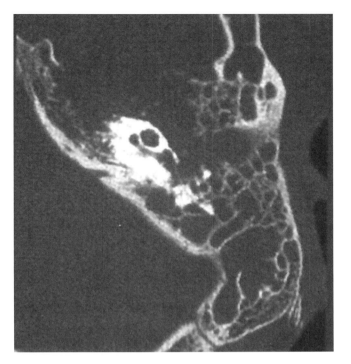
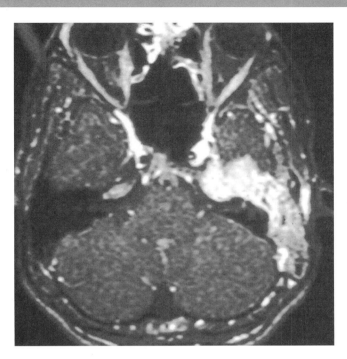

1. Identify the features here that suggest a malignancy as opposed to infection.

2. What should be included in the differential diagnosis?

3. What is the average age of onset of rhabdomyosarcomas?

4. What percentage of pediatric rhabdomyosarcomas occur in the head and neck?

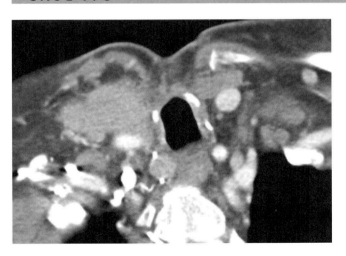
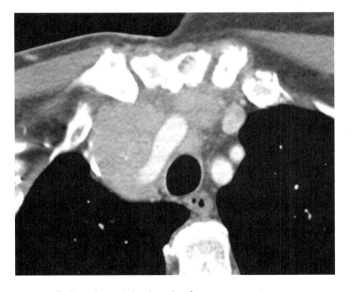

1. What is the best way to follow differentiated carcinomas of the thyroid gland after surgery?

2. List the factors that are most important for predicting differentiated thyroid cancer recurrence.

3. Name risk factors related to nodal metastases in papillary cancer.

4. What is the role of sestamibi scanning in a patient after thyroidectomy for surveillance for metastases?

Rhabdomyosarcoma

1. The large amount of bone destruction and spread to the cavernous sinus, solid enhancement.

2. Rhabdomyosarcoma, skin cancer, Langerhans cell histiocytosis, malignant fibrous histiocytoma, lymphoma and metastatic carcinoma (neuroblastoma).

3. 4 to 6 years old.

4. 30%.

Reference

Durve DV, Kanegaonkar RG, Albert D, Levitt G: Paediatric rhabdomyosarcoma of the ear and temporal bone, *Clin Otolaryngol* 29:32–37, 2004.

Cross-Reference

Neuroradiology: THE REQUISITES, pp 569–570, 650–651, 731–732.

Comment

Rhabdomyosarcomas are the most common pediatric head and neck tumors. They usually are separated into tumors that are parameningeal versus tumors that are not parameningeal. In general, parameningeal sarcomas do worse prognostically than nonparameningeal rhabdomyosarcomas. Tumors that are considered parameningeal include those at the skull base, orbit, and nasopharynx. Soft tissue rhabdomyosarcomas lower down in the neck are the nonparameningeal variety.

Rhabdomyosarcomas also are separated based on histology, with the most common variety being the embryonal histologic subtype > alveolar. The alveolar cell type is less responsive to chemotherapy and radiation treatment.

Although these tumors may be approached surgically, in general radiation and chemotherapy are effective in dealing with them.

On imaging, one may see hemorrhage within the rhabdomyosarcoma in approximately one fourth of cases. Rhabdomyosarcomas often have heterogeneous signal intensity because of the presence of hemorrhage, hypercellularity, or tumor necrosis.

With contrast administration, rhabdomyosarcomas generally uniformly enhance. The meningeal extension of rhabdomyosarcomas also shows avid enhancement. With these tumors, one also should look for enhancement of cranial nerves or tumor along the skull base foramina because of direct spread via these foramina into the intracranial compartment.

Temporal bone rhabdomyosarcomas usually present with symptoms suggesting otitis media or mastoiditis or both with hearing loss and otorrhea. Facial palsy is present in more than half of patients at presentation. Five-year survival, even without surgery, is approximately 80%.

Notes

Papillary Carcinoma of the Thyroid Gland

1. Iodine 131 scans.

2. (1) Family history of thyroid cancer, (2) extent of surgical treatment needed (i.e., total thyroidectomy), (3) advanced initial T stage of disease, (4) older age, (5) nodal metastases at presentation, and (6) male sex.

3. Tumor multifocality, extension beyond the thyroid capsule, and a diffuse sclerosing histology.

4. None.

Reference

Fernandes JK, Day TA, Richardson MS, Sharma AK: Overview of the management of differentiated thyroid cancer, *Curr Treat Options Oncol* 6:47–57, 2005.

Cross-Reference

Neuroradiology: THE REQUISITES, pp 740–745.

Comment

Papillary carcinoma of the thyroid gland has many different manifestations, primarily in the thyroid gland and with respect to its metastases. This tumor may show adenopathy that is bright on T1W scans because of the presence of colloid in the lymph node or from hemorrhage. In addition, cystic, hypervascular, and calcified lymph nodes may be seen.

The primary tumor may show the psammomatous calcifications represented as microcalcifications in the lesion, or it may show more chunky calcifications. Another primary manifestation of papillary carcinoma is a nodule within a cyst in the thyroid gland; this nodule also may show small calcifications.

Hematogenous metastases from papillary carcinoma may be hemorrhagic or cystic. Micrometastasis in a papillary fashion in the lungs also has been described.

Notes

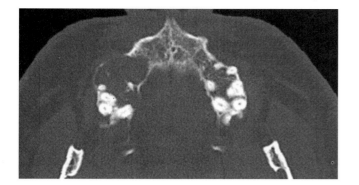
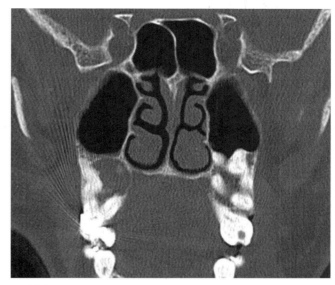

1. Is this tumor more common in the maxilla or the mandible?

2. Does this tumor have malignant potential?

3. What are its imaging characteristics?

4. What benign odontogenic lesion does this most closely resemble?

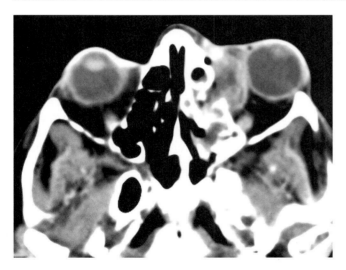
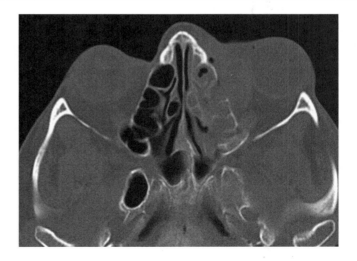

1. Is this lesion more likely to represent a complication of sinusitis or a chloroma in a patient with leukemia?

2. What is a chloroma, and why is it called that?

3. When do chloromas develop with respect to leukemias?

4. Why are sinus CT scans performed on leukemia patients before bone marrow transplant?

Adenomatoid Odontogenic Tumor (AOT)

1. Maxilla.

2. No.

3. A unilocular cystic lesion in the anterior maxilla often associated with the crown of an unerupted tooth. Some dense areas may be associated with the crown of the tooth in the lesion.

4. Dentigerous cyst.

Reference

Hicks MJ, Flaitz CM, Batsakis JG: Adenomatoid and calcifying epithelial odontogenic tumors, *Ann Otol Rhinol Laryngol* 102:159–161, 1993.

Cross-Reference

Neuroradiology: THE REQUISITES, pp 660–662.

Comment

Cystic adenomatoid odontogenic tumor is a tumor that appears in the anterior maxilla usually in association with the crowns of the lateral incisor or canine teeth. Most of these masses present in females in the teens or 20s. It represents 3% of all odontogenic tumors. In 74% of cases the AOT is associated with impacted teeth. The maxilla is affected three times more often than the mandible. AOTs are usually unilocular masses for which conservative excision is the best treatment.

Odontogenic keratocysts (OKCs) typically are found in the mandible. They may be unilocular and tend to have scalped margins. As opposed to dentigerous and radicular cysts, it has been said that OKCs are oriented in the plane of the mandible when they occur there. Their orientation is more along the anteroposterior plane than the dentigerous and radicular cysts, which are more oriented in a superioinferior plane.

OKCs are the dental lesions that are associated with Gorlin syndrome, also known as basal cell nevus syndrome, nevoid basal cell carcinoma, and Gorlin-Goltz syndrome. From a neuroradiologic standpoint, this diagnosis is made when the OKC is seen in association with heavy falcian calcification, dermal lesions representing the basal cell carcinomas, and the rare coexistent medulloblastoma. The syndrome has numerous other manifestations, including bifid ribs, dysmorphic facies with frontal bossing, flattened nasal bridge, hypertelorism, mental retardation, and palmar and plantar pits, which are irrelevant to the head and neck radiologist.

Notes

Leukemia and the Sinus

1. Sinusitis complication.

2. A chloroma, also known as granulocytic sarcoma, is a soft tissue mass that is associated with a myeloblastic leukemia; it is an uncommon malignant tumor that rarely involves the breast. It is essentially a solid mass composed of granulocyte precursor cells. It is called *chloroma,* similar to *chlorophyll,* because it has a green hue caused by high levels of myeloperoxidase in the immature cells.

3. At onset, relapse, and remission.

4. There is a high incidence of unsuspected sinusitis, and the existence of the infection bodes for a less successful outcome.

Reference

Billings KR, Lowe LH, Aquino VM, Biavati MJ: Screening sinus CT scans in pediatric bone marrow transplant patients, *Int J Pediatr Otorhinolaryngol* 52:253–260, 2000.

Cross-Reference

Neuroradiology: THE REQUISITES, pp 637–638.

Comment

The most common finding with respect to paranasal sinus disease and leukemia is bland sinusitis. Patients commonly are screened for the presence of sinusitis before bone marrow transplantation (BMT) for leukemia because it has been shown that the prognosis of an individual who has sinusitis at the time of BMT is worse (78% death rate at 2 years) than the prognosis of an individual who has no evidence of active sinus inflammatory disease (69% death rate at 2 years). Screening BMT patients in advance and treating them for active sinusitis is part of the pretransplant protocol. In addition, whenever a leukemic patient or a patient who has undergone BMT has a fever of unknown origin, screening CT scans through the paranasal sinus are performed to exclude that source of infection. The issue arises in pretransplant and posttransplant cases when one identifies chronic inflammatory changes, such as mucus retention cyst or mere mucosal thickening. Depending on the extent, a course of antibiotics or decongestants may be applied with rescanning after therapy. White blood cell counts are lower in patients who develop sinusitis after BMT, and patients frequently progress to chronic sinusitis.

In children undergoing BMT for leukemia, the pre-BMT CT scans through the sinuses showed severe disease in nearly 17%, and 67% of these developed chronic sinusitis after BMT.

Notes

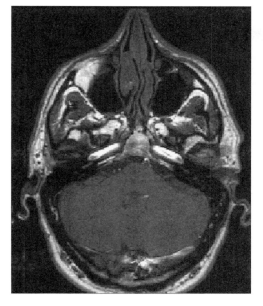
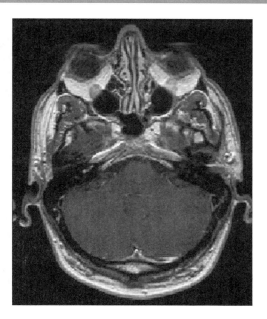

1. What is the finding?

2. What are possible causes?

3. What is the expected outcome if this is hemorrhage?

4. Identify common sources of hemorrhage in the cochlea.

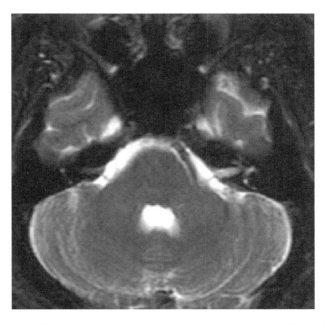
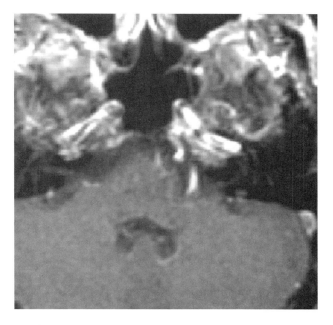

1. What vessel is usually implicated in hemifacial spasm?

2. What percentage of patients have contralateral neurovascular compression of a nerve (on the asymptomatic side)?

3. How often do the MRI findings correspond with the surgical findings with respect to the identification of the correct vessel?

4. How often is vascular compression simply not identified at all at surgery?

Hemolabyrinth

1. High signal in the basal turn of the cochlea before contrast administration.

2. Blood versus fat, therefore trauma versus cholesterol granuloma versus dermoid/lipoma/Pantopaque.

3. There is a high rate of permanent hearing loss.

4. Surgery, trauma, anticoagulants, and barotraumas.

Reference

Hegarty JL, Patel S, Fischbein N, et al: The value of enhanced magnetic resonance imaging in the evaluation of endocochlear disease, *Laryngoscope* 112:8–17, 2002.

Cross-Reference

Neuroradiology: THE REQUISITES, pp 594–600.

Comment

Trauma to the temporal bone may result in hemolabyrinth. This is a potential mistaken diagnosis in institutions where precontrast T1W scans are not performed in evaluations with patients with sensorineural hearing loss with MRI scanning. Because the hemolabyrinth looks bright on a T1W scan owing to the methemoglobin in the labyrinth, if one performs only contrast-enhanced scans, one might assume that the bright signal within the labyrinth is due to gadolinium enhancement. In contrast, if a pre–gadolinium-enhanced T1W scan had been performed, it would have been noticed that the labyrinth was bright beforehand. Without the precontrast scan, a radiologist may suggest a diagnosis of labyrinthitis or, worse, labyrinthine schwannoma.

In most cases, the labyrinth is transgressed by a vertically oriented fracture. Horizontal fractures usually do not carry across the plane of the semicircular canals or vestibule. In either case, the patient may develop conductive and sensory hearing loss as a result of the effects of the fracture, hematoma in the middle ear, and toxic effect of the blood on the sensorineural structures of the labyrinth of the cochlea as they intermix.

Although lipomas occur in the internal auditory canal, they are rare in the labyrinth. When they occur there, they are associated with sensorineural hearing loss. These labyrinthine lipomas are associated with cerebellopontine angle lipomas in more than half of cases. Occasionally, one may see hemolabyrinth without evidence of a fracture, and this is thought to be due to barotrauma in deep-sea divers or patients undergoing hyperbaric oxygen treatment.

Notes

Hemifacial Spasm

1. The anterior inferior cerebellar artery > posterior inferior cerebellar artery.

2. 15%.

3. 85% to 90%.

4. 10% to 15%.

Reference

Hastreiter P, Naraghi R, Tomandl B, et al: Analysis and 3-dimensional visualization of neurovascular compression syndromes, *Acad Radiol* 10:1369–1379, 2003.

Cross-Reference

Neuroradiology: THE REQUISITES, p 226.

Comment

Hemifacial spasm is usually the result of compression of cranial nerve VII by an arterial vascular structure. In most cases, the artery that compresses the nerve is the anterior inferior cerebellar artery, vertebral artery, or posterior inferior cerebellar artery, any of which may be torturous. Vascular impression seen at MRI is shown in almost 67% to 87% of patients with hemifacial spasm, but also may be seen in 15% on the normal contralateral side. The nerve may be compressed within the cerebellopontine angle cistern or, less likely, the anterior auditory canal.

The treatment of hemifacial spasm is similar in concept to that of trigeminal neuralgia, with an attempt to remove the artery from the position where it compresses the nerve.

The best pulse sequence for evaluating the subject for hemifacial spasm is the raw data from magnetic resonance angiography. On this T1W time-of-flight pulse sequence, one is able to detect cranial nerve VII as it courses through the cerebellopontine angle cistern and the bright-appearing blood vessel. The maximum intensity projection images are less useful; although they show the blood vessels, they do not show the cranial nerves to show the site of compression. High-resolution, thin-section T2W scans may show black blood vascular structures opposed to the dark signal intensity cranial nerve and may substitute for the raw data of magnetic resonance angiography.

Many cases of hemifacial spasms are not due to vascular compression. These may be secondary to multiple sclerosis, meningitis, arteriovenous malformations, Paget disease, neoplastic causes, or inflammatory causes.

Botulinum toxin (Botox) injection seems to relieve the symptoms.

Notes

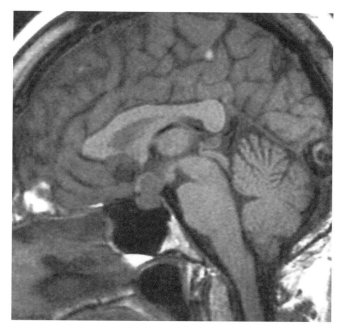
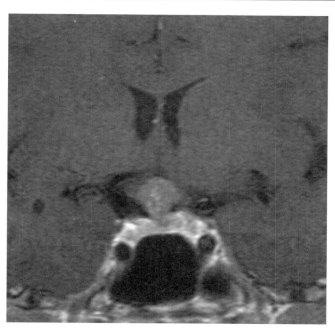

1. What should be included in the differential diagnosis?

2. What primary tumors are most likely to metastasize to the sella?

3. If you have a sellar mass with extraocular muscle palsy, is it more or less likely to be a pituitary adenoma?

4. How often are pituitary metastases seen at autopsy in patients with end-stage breast cancer?

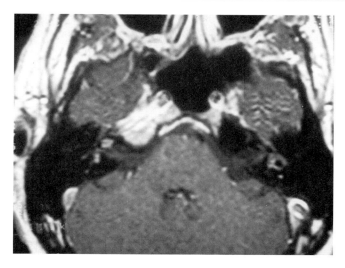

1. Name the most common cause of the imaging findings seen.

2. What does enhancement of the basal turn of the cochlea correlate with clinically?

3. What is the difference in the course of the disease from autoimmune labyrinthitis?

4. Identify the best diagnostic test for autoimmune inner ear disease.

CASE 178

Breast Metastasis to the Sella

1. Craniopharyngioma, Langerhans cell histiocytosis, Erdheim Chester disease, hypothalamic glioma, meningioma, metastasis, pituitary adenoma, sarcoidosis, tuberculosis, and germinoma.

2. Breast cancer and small cell lung carcinoma.

3. Less likely. That is classic for a metastasis.

4. 6% to 29%.

Reference

Fassett DR, Couldwell WT: Metastases to the pituitary gland, *Neurosurg Focus* 16:E8, 2004.

Cross-Reference

Neuroradiology: THE REQUISITES, pp 537–540.

Comment

The pituitary gland, because of its inherent high vascularity, is a potential source for accumulation for metastatic disease; this is rarely identified clinically but can be found in greater instances on autopsy cases. More frequent than a metastasis to the pituitary gland is a metastasis around the sella. In this case, breast cancers and lung cancers are the most common. Breast cancer is the most common lesion to cause pituitary metastases. Metastases to the pituitary gland seem to favor the posterior pituitary (57%) because of its direct arterial supply, but breast cancer metastases favor the anterior pituitary gland (75%), perhaps because of hormonal attraction factors.

Symptoms include compromise of the optic nerves via the optic canal or due to compromise of the optic chiasm upward from the sella. Occasionally, patients present with hormonal abnormalities, including pituitary insufficiency if the pituitary stalk is compromised by the neoplastic process. Excessive stalk enhancement may indicate neoplastic infiltration; however, this is more common with lesions such as lymphoma or granulomatous infections. Diabetes insipidus can occur from posterior pituitary involvement.

Notes

CASE 179

Autoimmune Inner Ear Disease

1. Viral labyrinthitis.

2. High-frequency hearing loss.

3. It progresses much more rapidly, and the sensorineural hearing loss is bilateral in 80%.

4. A trial of immunosuppressives that cures the patient.

Reference

Mark AS, Fitzgerald D: Segmental enhancement of the cochlea on contrast-enhanced MR: correlation with the frequency of hearing loss and possible sign of perilymphatic fistula and autoimmune labyrinthitis, *AJNR Am J Neuroradiol* 14:991–996, 1993.

Cross-Reference

Neuroradiology: THE REQUISITES, pp 599–600.

Comment

When one sees enhancement of portions of the labyrinthine inner ear structures, one should consider inflammatory etiologies over neoplastic etiologies. The most common condition to cause enhancement of the cochlea, vestibule, or semicircular canals is viral labyrinthitis. There are no unique viruses that have predilections for inner ear structures other than the herpesvirus family, which can cause Ramsay Hunt syndrome and Bell's palsy. Bacterial infections are less common but include Lyme disease, syphilis, tuberculosis, or spread of a more typical otomastoiditis (*Streptococcus*) via a perilymphatic fistula.

Among the noninfectious inflammatory etiologies, one should consider sarcoidosis and autoimmune labyrinthitis. The latter is distinguished by the presence of anticochlear antigen antibodies, which cause a self-inflicted reaction against the inner ear structures. This is one of the entities that may cause bilateral enhancement of portions of the inner ear, including the cochlea, vestibule, and semicircular canals. Usually this disease process is self-limited, but occasionally it requires intervention with immunosuppressives.

Notes

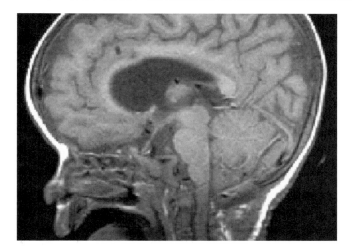

1. Based on the findings (list), what is the best diagnosis?

2. Do magnetic resonance venograms show jugular vein stenoocclusive disease in achondroplasia?

3. What causes large ventricles in achondroplastic patients?

4. Explain the significance of cervicomedullary compression seen on MRI in a patient with achondroplasia.

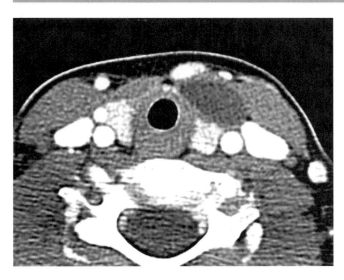

1. What percentage of thymic cysts have mediastinal extension?

2. State the four theories regarding the origins of cervical thymic cysts.

3. What are the demographics of this lesion?

4. What is included in the differential diagnosis?

CASE 180

Achondroplasia

1. Large head, frontal bossing, small foramen magnum, cervical spinal stenosis, dwarfism = achondroplasia.

2. Yes, frequently.

3. CSF or venous outflow obstruction at the foramen magnum and jugular fossa or both.

4. They are at risk for sudden death.

Reference

Rollins N, Booth T, Shapiro K: The use of gated cine phase contrast and MR venography in achondroplasia, *Childs Nerv Syst* 16:569–577, 2000.

Cross-Reference

Neuroradiology: THE REQUISITES, pp 441, 595.

Comment

Numerous imaging findings may be evident on films of patients with achondroplasia. In addition to the frontal bossing that may be evident on the scalp film, patients with achondroplasia have a small foramen magnum. This small foramen magnum potentially can lead to syringomyelia formation. Additionally the cervical spine may show evidence of stenosis. There may be some redundancy of the tissues around the cervicomedullary junction from ligament thickening.

Other skull base findings include a J-shaped sella and foreshortened temporal bones. There is also a short clivus and a small sphenoid bone. The posterior fossa and the angulation of the petrous portions of the temporal bone are more horizontal. A prominent mandible is noted. Platybasia also may coexist.

Notes

CASE 181

Thymic Cysts

1. 50%.

2. The four theories are as follows:

   Remnants of embryologic thymopharyngeal ducts
   Sequestration products of thymic involution
   Degeneration of Hassal corpuscles
   Connective tissue, lymph nodes, and blood vessels arrested in various stages of thymic development

3. Males > females; <20 years old; left side of neck.

4. Branchial cleft cyst, epidermoids, plunging ranula, thyroid/parathyroid cyst, thyroglossal duct cyst, external laryngocele, esophageal diverticulum, and lymphatic malformation.

Reference

Burton EM, Mercado-Deane MG, Howell CG, et al: Cervical thymic cysts: CT appearance of two cases including a persistent thymopharyngeal duct cyst, *Pediatr Radiol* 25:363–365, 1995.

Cross-Reference

Neuroradiology: THE REQUISITES, p 746.

Comment

Thymic cysts constitute a small portion of all of the congenital cysts of the head and neck. These lesions usually occur in a paramedian location and may be present anywhere from the upper neck to the anterior mediastinum. They usually are seen in the anterior aspect of the neck as opposed to the posterior triangle or posterior mediastinal structures. Thymic cysts usually do not show evidence of mass effect or of contrast enhancement or have signal intensity and density characteristics similar to those of pure fluid.

The differential diagnosis includes thyroglossal duct cysts, branchial cleft cysts, and lymphoceles that may arise at the thoracic duct region. These lymphoceles may result from trauma to the thoracic duct, particularly after neck dissections, or may arise de novo. The thoracic duct lymphoceles may occur at the junction of the jugular vein with the subclavian vein, and there is a propensity for the left side more than the right side.

Thymic cysts are pretty rare. They are thought to arise congenitally from the thymopharyngeal ducts or as a result of inflammatory degeneration of the thymus. The cysts often are multiloculated, thin walled, and paratracheal or intramediastinal. The coronal T1W scan best shows that this is not a thyroid lesion but an exophytic thyroid cyst that probably should be included in the differential diagnosis.

Remember the association of thymomas and myasthenia gravis and thymomas and red blood cell aplasia. The thymus may appear as a large mediastinal mass after the use of steroids or after the relief of severe body stress ("thymic rebound"). It is also enlarged in patients with hyperthyroidism, Addison's disease, lymphoma, leukemia, and Langerhans cell histiocytosis. It is absent in DiGeorge syndrome.

Notes

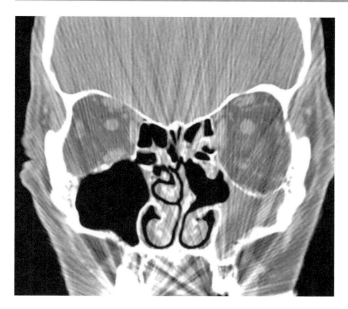

1. What do the findings of a small maxillary sinus, enophthalmos, and hypoglobus imply?

2. Is the left maxillary antrum under higher pressure or lower pressure compared with the right maxillary antrum?

3. Describe the typical position of the uncinate process in this syndrome.

4. Is the sinus usually filled or empty in this entity?

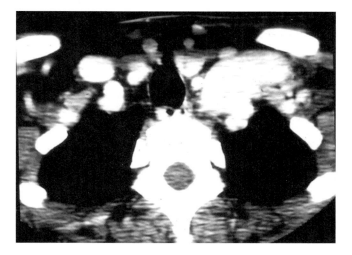

1. Identify causes of intensely enhancing lymph nodes.

2. Which is the more benign form of Castleman disease, hyaline vascular or plasma cell type?

3. What percentage of patients with Castleman disease have involvement in the head and neck?

4. Besides a lymph node, what else should be considered here?

Silent Sinus Syndromes

1. Silent sinus syndrome.

2. Lower pressure.

3. There is apposition of the uncinate process against the inferomedial aspect of the orbital wall with lateral displacement of the uncinate process.

4. Filled.

Reference

Illner A, Davidson HC, Harnsberger HR, Hoffman J: The silent sinus syndrome: clinical and radiographic findings, *AJR Am J Roentgenol* 178:503–506, 2002.

Cross-Reference

Neuroradiology: THE REQUISITES, p 616.

Comment

The silent sinus syndrome is a cause of enophthalmos and ocular depression with lid retraction. This entity seems to show chronic reduction in the volume of maxillary sinus. It is associated with depression of the floor of the orbit, accounting for the enophthalmos and sometimes diploplia. In addition, the posterior lateral wall of the maxillary antrum appears to be caved inward, and there is proliferation of the fat posterior to the maxillary sinus. The walls of the sinus may be thickened, and the ipsilateral sinus may be completely opacified.

The exact etiology of the silent sinus syndrome is unclear; however, it is thought to be due to chronic obstruction of the osteomeatal complex leading to negative pressure effects in the sinus. When one sees a complete opacified paranasal sinus with decreased volume, one should consider silent sinus syndrome.

Maxillary sinus hypoplasia is in the differential diagnosis, but this usually is a more symmetric decrease in the volume of the maxillary sinus and does not have the characteristics of the fat that silent sinus syndrome has.

Notes

Castleman Disease

1. Castleman disease, angioimmunoblastic lymphoma, Kaposi sarcoma, thyroid carcinoma metastases, and Kimura disease.

2. Hyaline vascular.

3. 10%.

4. Paraganglioma, schwannoma, and hemangioma.

Reference

Koslin DB, Berland LL, Sekar BC: Cervical Castleman disease: CT study with angiographic correlation, *Radiology* 160:213–214, 1986.

Cross-Reference

Neuroradiology: THE REQUISITES, pp 599–600.

Comment

Castleman disease is also known as angiofollicular hyperplasia. This entity is thought to represent a premalignant lesion, which may be associated with lymphoma. Of cases, 80% are associated with the more indolent, less progressive hyaline vascular form, which rarely progresses, as opposed to the plasma cell type. Multicentric Castleman disease may have liver and spleen involvement. This is considered a B cell lymphoproliferative disorder.

Castleman disease is much more common in the mediastinum and abdomen than it is in the neck. Characteristically, it presents as a solitary node or multiple lymph nodes that show avid contrast enhancement. The lymph nodes are often quite large and need not progress in a stepwise pattern of spread the way squamous cell carcinoma metastases do.

There is a broad differential diagnosis for the enhancing lymph nodes, which includes thyroid carcinoma lymph nodes, lymphoma, Kaposi sarcoma, and Castleman disease.

Notes

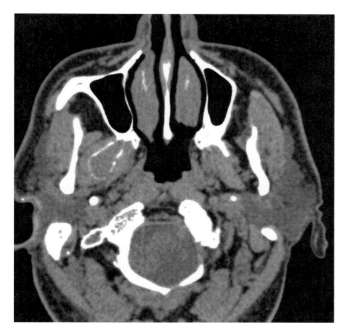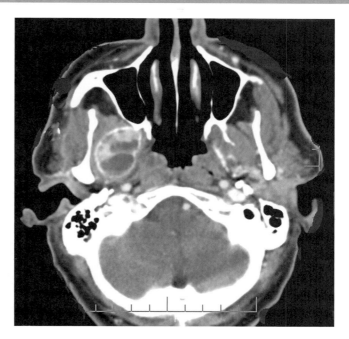

1. What is included in the differential diagnosis of this lesion?

2. Where in the head and neck do giant cell reparative granulomas occur most commonly?

3. How are giant cell tumors and giant cell reparative granulomas distinguished radiographically?

4. What percentage of aneurysmal bone cysts occur in the skull or face?

Giant Cell Tumor of the Pterygoid Plate

1. Giant cell tumor, nonosseous fibroma, chondroblastoma, chondromyxoid fibroma, unicameral bone cyst, giant cell reparative granuloma, aneurysmal bone cyst, synovial sarcoma, brown tumor of hyperparathyroidism, osteosarcoma, osteoblastoma, and eosinophilic granuloma.

2. Mandible and maxilla.

3. More extraosseous mass, potential for metastases in giant cell tumors.

4. 2%.

Reference

Harris AE, Beckner ME, Barnes L, Kassam A, Horowitz M: Giant cell tumor of the skull: a case report and review of the literature. *Surg Neurol* 61:274–277, 2004.

Cross-Reference

Neuroradiology: THE REQUISITES, p 661.

Comment

Ninety percent of giant cell tumors (GCTs) are observed at the ends of long bones in patients aged 20 to 40 years. Giant cell reparative granulomas (GCRGs) are seen both in a younger age group involving the mandible and an older age group (50–60 years old) affecting other sites. GCTs are true neoplasms, whereas GCRGs reflect a reactive inflammatory process related to trauma, iatrogenic manipulation, and/or intraosseous hemorrhage. Giant-cell tumors originate in the bone marrow, whereas GCRGs arise from periosteal connective tissue. GCT comprise about 4% to 7% of all primary bone tumors, and 90% of these cases involve the epiphysis of major long bones. Less than 2% of giant cell tumors present in the craniofacial region. GCTs show malignant degeneration in 3% to 5% of cases.

On radiologic evaluation, GCTs and GCRGs are indistinguishable. Both types of tumor are lytic and expansile. They usually do not produce new bone and do not have matrixes within them. They both enhance. GCTs may devolve into an appearance of an aneurysmal bone cyst with blood fluid levels, a pattern less frequently seen in GCRGs. In close to one third of cases, GCTs may show an extraosseous soft tissue component on MR. MR also demonstrates a hypointense rim in most cases of GCT and GCRG, usually attributable to hemosiderin or dense collagen deposition in the wall.

GCRG occurs in many bones, with the mandible, maxilla, and temporal bone being the most common in the head and neck. GCRGs have no malignant potential compared to GCTs, and they have a lower rate of recurrence. The main distinguishing features are the younger age of occurrence for some GCRGs compared with GCTs and the more frequent appearance of GCTs at the end of long bones.

Notes

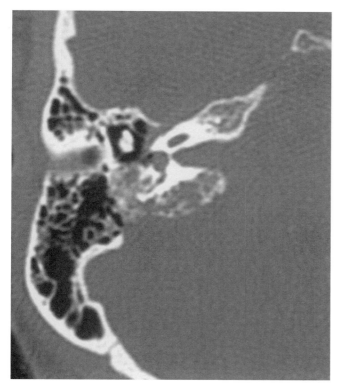

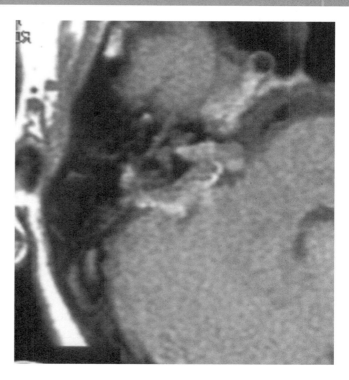

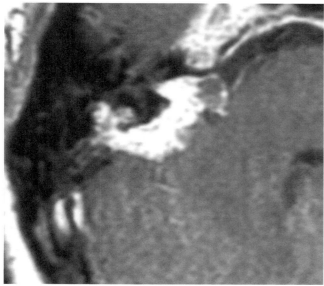

1. What syndrome is this entity linked to?

2. What should be included in the differential diagnosis?

3. What percentage of endolymphatic sac tumors (ELSTs) have high signal foci on T1W scans?

4. What percentage of ELSTs have calcification in the matrix?

Endolymphatic Sac Tumor

1. von Hippel–Lindau disease.

2. Cholesterol granuloma, metastasis, glomus tumor, and epidermoid.

3. 80%.

4. 100%.

Reference

Lonser RR, Kim HJ, Butman JA, et al: Tumors of the endolymphatic sac in von Hippel-Lindau disease, *N Engl J Med* 350:2481–2486, 2004.

Cross-Reference

Neuroradiology: THE REQUISITES, pp 604–605.

Comment

ELSTs arise within the vestibular aqueduct/endolymphatic sac of the temporal bone. This tumor causes bony erosion of the mastoid and petrous portions of the temporal bone. Imaging findings include a calcified matrix and lytic destruction of the bone. On MRI, one may see bright signal intensity on T1W scans, possibly representing hemorrhage, new bone formation, or calcified matrix. Mild enhancement is characteristic.

ELSTs arise sporadically but also are associated with von Hippel–Lindau syndrome with multiple hemangioblastomas. The von Hippel–Lindau gene is found on chromosome 3, and reports are that ELSTs occur in 7% to 15% of patients with von Hippel–Lindau syndrome. Bilateral disease is seen in 30% of cases. Almost all patients present with hearing loss, tinnitus, and dizziness.

Generally the orientation of the ELST is along the same axis as the vestibular aqueduct, which should help with the differential diagnosis. One also might consider chondrosarcomas and metastatic disease in the differential diagnosis. Because of the similarity in the cellular appearance, these lesions previously were thought to represent a metastatic lesion from papillary carcinoma of the thyroid gland or to be of minor salivary gland origin.

Notes

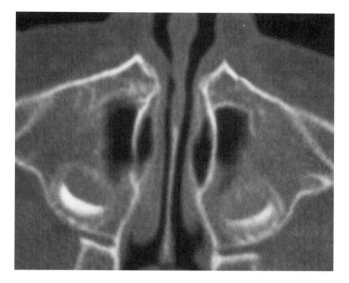

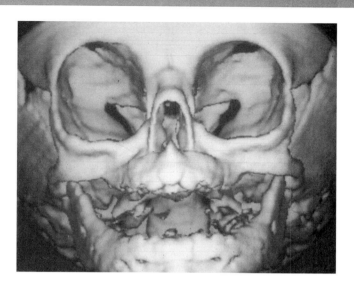

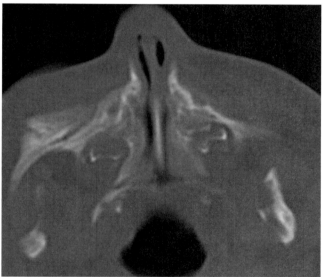

1. In this child with difficulty breathing, where is the area of airway narrowing?

2. What is the lower limit of normal width for a piriform aperture in a term infant?

3. Describe the ancillary dental findings.

4. Which is more common as a cause of airway obstruction in the neonate, choanal atresia/stenosis or nasal aperture stenosis?

Nasal Piriform Aperture Stenosis

1. In the nasal cavity, piriform aperture.

2. 11 mm.

3. A single large central incisor with a narrow palate with a downward hanging bony ridge.

4. Choanal atresia.

Reference

Belden CJ, Mancuso AA, Schmalfuss IM: CT features of congenital nasal piriform aperture stenosis: initial experience, *Radiology* 213:495–501, 1999.

Cross-Reference

Neuroradiology: THE REQUISITES, p 615.

Comment

This is a little known entity that may be a source of nasal airway obstruction in a neonate. No patients in the series by Belden et al had an aperture >8 mm, whereas all normal subjects had apertures >11 mm. A simple measurement should do the trick.

The pathogenesis may be due to a deficiency of the primary palate or bony overgrowth of the nasal processes of the maxilla during facial development.

Encephaloceles, holoprosencephaly, Dandy Walker syndrome, and other CNS anomalies may coexist. Hypopituitarism also may be present.

Notes

Case compliments of Mauricio Castillo, Wake Forrest, NC.

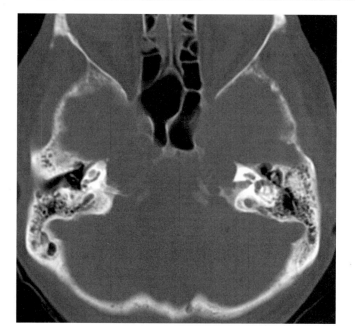
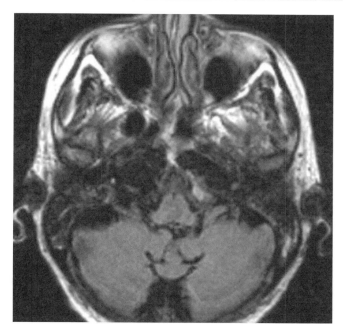
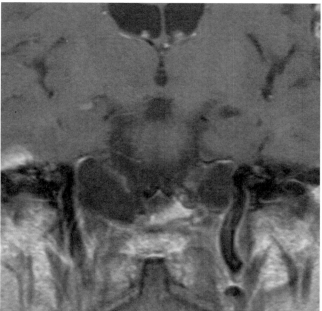

1. What is the abnormality seen?

2. Is this an arachnoid cyst or meningocele or neither?

3. How would you prove it?

4. How often is the petrous apex pneumatized?

Meckel Cave Meningocele

1. Enlarged CSF space at the petrous apex/Meckel cave.

2. It is thought to be a meningocele.

3. Use intrathecal contrast material. If it flows into the lesion readily, it is more likely a meningocele than an arachnoid cyst.

4. 30% of the time.

Reference

Moore KR, Fischbein NJ, Harnsberger HR, et al: Petrous apex cephaloceles, *AJNR Am J Neuroradiol* 22: 1867–1871, 2001.

Cross-Reference

Neuroradiology: THE REQUISITES, pp 459–461, 558–561.

Comment

The Meckel cave region is a potential source for dilation of the subarachnoid space. The size of the Meckel cave and trigeminal cistern varies from person to person. Some people have capacious Meckel cave regions, whereas others seem to have very little CSF space present with dominance of the trigeminal ganglia. Herniation of the meninges into Meckel cave leads to the entity called Meckel cave meningoceles (or petrous apex cephaloceles). Typically, one sees CSF herniating from the middle cranial fossa into the region of the Meckel cave/petrous apex at the trigeminal impression. One rarely sees brain tissue herniating along with the meninges. When that happens, there is the potential for seizure development.

The differential diagnosis includes arachnoid cyst, (which would not be expected to communicate with the subarachnoid space openly), petrous apex cholesterol granulomas, and epidermoids. One should look for the signal intensity and density that are identical to CSF to make the diagnosis of the meningocele. Smooth excavation and nonaggressive bone growth characterize this lesion.

Notes

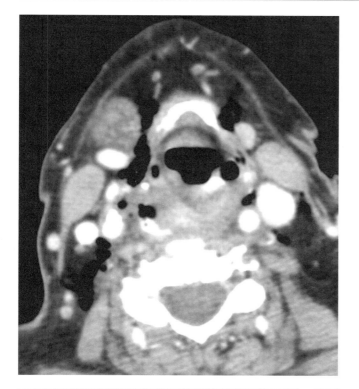
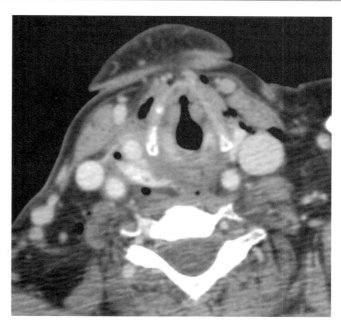
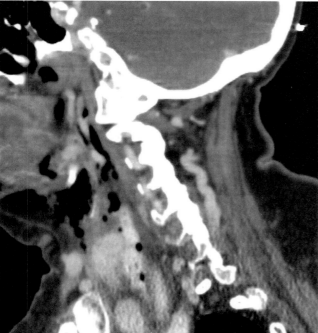

1. Where is the extraluminal air coming from?

2. Identify the most common causes of esophageal perforation.

3. What part of the esophagus is most likely to be perforated?

4. What is the prognosis?

Perforated Esophagus

1. A perforated esophagus.

2. Iatrogenic (64%), foreign bodies (17%), and trauma (14%).

3. Cervical > thoracic > abdominal regions.

4. Poor—death in 14% within 30 days.

Reference

Eroglu A, Can Kurkcuogu I, Karaoganogu N, et al: Esophageal perforation: the importance of early diagnosis and primary repair, Dis Esophagus 17:91–94, 2004.

Cross-Reference

Neuroradiology: THE REQUISITES, p 733.

Comment

Any time one has air leaking into the neck one should be concerned about the grave implications of a perforated viscus. Probably the most common cause for air accumulation in the neck is a postoperative case in which one sees residual air after reconstructive surgery. The next most common etiology is spread of air from a pneumomediastinum or pneumothorax up into the neck. This etiology would show a gradation of air from inferior to superior in the neck because the source comes from below. With respect to perforated viscus, one should be concerned about traumatic injury to the larynx, trachea, or esophagus. In this case, the etiology was a perforated esophagus. This entity may occur because of surgery on an iatrogenic basis or may be due to rupture of the esophagus lower down with excessive vomiting, retching, or coughing. A tear may occur at the lower esophageal sphincter. Alternatively, air may be leaking from the larynx. The most common etiology of a laryngeal air leak is a motor vehicle accident with a crush injury to the laryngeal cartilage, which may be associated with a mucosal tear.

Patients present with pain and dyspnea and require immediate surgical intervention. Mediastinitis may cause death early. Patients with spontaneous perforation seem to do worse.

Notes

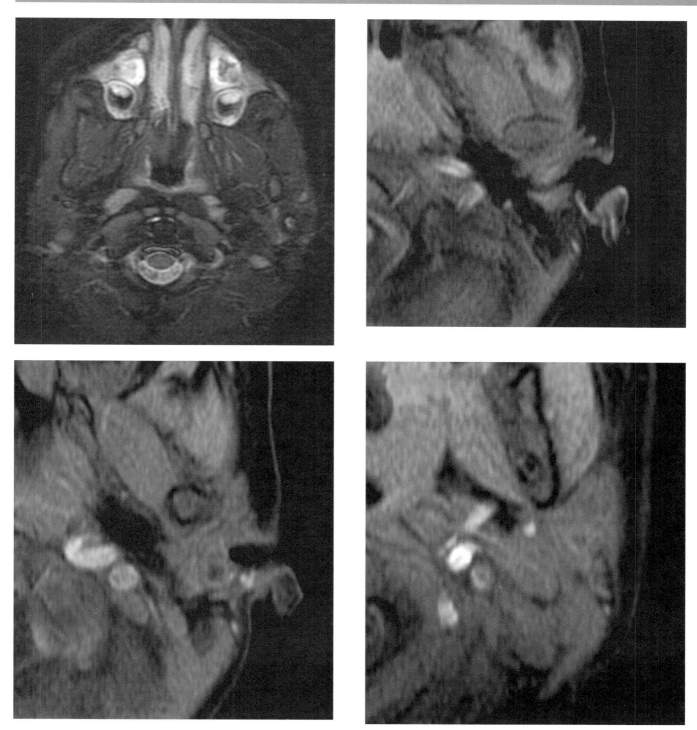

1. What is the cause of this fistulous tract to the ear?

2. Identify the facial infection that has a predilection for fistula formation.

3. Which of the four branchial cleft lesions are more commonly cysts than fistulas?

4. Which branchial apparatus makes the superior parathyroid glands?

First Branchial Cleft Fistulas

1. First branchial cleft fistula.

2. Actinomycosis.

3. First and second are more commonly cysts. Third and fourth branchial clefts make fistulae more commonly.

4. Fourth pharyngeal pouch.

Reference

Sichel JY, Halperin D, Dano I, et al: Clinical update on type II first branchial cleft cysts, *Laryngoscope* 108: 1524–1527, 1998.

Cross-Reference

Neuroradiology: THE REQUISITES, pp 567, 700–701.

Comment

The first branchial cleft is responsible for the formation of the external auditory canal. When one identifies a fistula leading from or to the external auditory canal, one should consider a first branchial cleft as the etiology.

There is a classification for first branchial cleft cyst similar to the various classifications for second brachial cleft cyst. The Work classification has superceded the Arnot classification:

Work type I anomaly: ectodermal duplication of the membranous external auditory canal. The lesions reside in the preauricular space.

Work type II lesions: duplications of the membranous external auditory canal and pinna that contain skin (ectoderm) and cartilage (mesoderm). The lesions lie posterior and inferior to the mandible.

First branchial cleft sinuses open below the external auditory canal, posterior to the mandibular mentum, and above the hyoid bone.

The lesions correspond to the extent to which the first branchial cleft cyst is within the parotid tissue.

Second branchial cleft fistulas drain to the palatine tonsils, whereas third and fourth branchial cleft fistulas drain to the piriform sinus and piriform sinus apex.

Notes

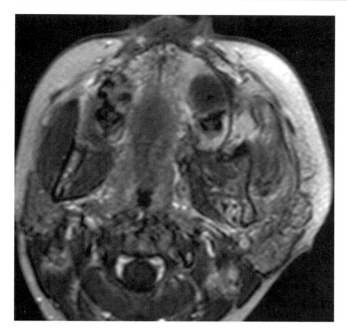

1. Identify the abdominal tumor that is associated with hemihypertrophy.

2. What is Friedreich disease?

3. Name the entity of facial hemihypertrophy with epidermal nevi.

4. Name the entity of port-wine stains, hemihypertrophy, and venolymphatic vascular malformations.

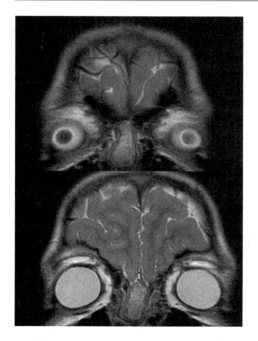

1. What percentage of these lesions are extranasal?

2. What percentage have a fibrous connection to the dura?

3. What is a better name for this lesion?

4. Which has a better prognosis, nasal glioma or meningocele, and why?

Facial Hemihypertrophy

1. Wilms tumor.

2. Facial hemihypertrophy, which may be generalized.

3. Solomon syndrome.

4. Klippel-Trénaunay syndrome.

Reference

Cohen MM Jr: Perspectives on craniofacial asymmetry: IV. hemi-asymmetries, *Int J Oral Maxillofac Surg* 24: 134–141, 1995.

Cross-Reference

Neuroradiology: THE REQUISITES, pp 236, 719.

Comment

Numerous syndromes are associated with hemihypertrophy; these include a hemihypertrophy associated with Wilms tumor of the kidney, Solomon syndrome, Friedreich disease, Beckwith-Wiedemann syndrome, Proteus syndrome, neurofibromatosis, and Klippel-Trénaunay syndrome. The last-mentioned is a syndrome associated with hemihypertrophy, vascular cutaneous malformations, and arteriovenous malformations.

The role of three-dimensional postprocessing for the evaluation of craniofacial anomalies has grown significantly through the use of multidetector CT scanning. Surface reconstructions of the face and cutaway views of the bony anatomy assist the plastic surgeon in determining how much of the asymmetry is secondary to soft tissue abnormality versus a bony process. Additionally, reconstructive implants can be fashioned from three-dimensional data, comparing the normal side with the abnormal side and reconstructing using implants that stimulate the normal symmetric anatomy.

Notes

Nasal Glioma

1. 60%.

2. 15%.

3. Extranasal heterotopia.

4. Nasal glioma because there is no risk of meningitis.

Reference

Rahbar R, Resto VA, Robson CD, et al: Nasal glioma and encephalocele: diagnosis and management, *Laryngoscope* 113:2069–2077, 2003.

Cross-Reference

Neuroradiology: THE REQUISITES, pp 616–617.

Comment

Nasal glioma is a misnomer for many reasons. This lesion is not a glioma. It does not represent neoplastic tumor. It actually represents heterotopic brain tissue, which presents outside the intracranial compartment. There is no potential for growth or metastases.

The second reason it is a misnomer is that nasal gliomas may occur intranasally or extranasally. One may see the lesion under the skin or lateral to the nasal ala or in other perplexing locations.

In many cases, there is a fibrous attachment of the nasal heterotopic brain tissue to the dural compartment. This is in contrast to a dermal sinus tract or a cephalocele in that there is not an opening between the nasal glioma and the intracranial space. No CSF connection is present. No patent tract is present.

The density and signal intensity of the nasal glioma may be similar of that of gray matter tissue, or it may show heterogeneous signal intensity on contrast to that of normal brain tissue.

Notes

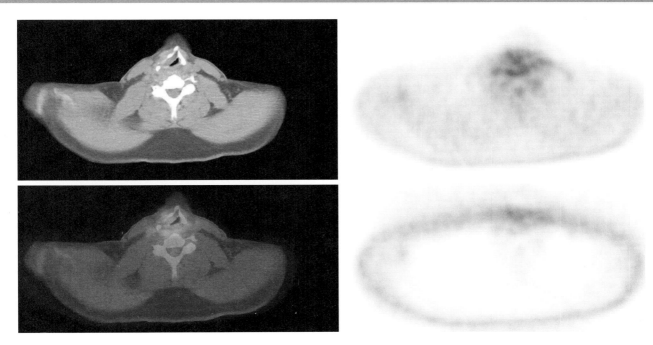

1. What is created when the larynx is removed?

2. What is removed in a supracricoid laryngectomy?

3. Why use positron emission tomography in the postoperative setting?

4. What is left behind in the lateral neck after a radical neck dissection?

Normal Postoperative Appearance of the Larynx

1. A neopharynx.

2. Thyroid cartilage and either all or most of the epiglottis with supraglottis and glottis, sparing arytenoids.

3. To detect residual or recurrent disease and second primary tumors.

4. Carotid arteries and vagus nerves.

Reference

Maroldi R: Imaging of postoperative larynx and neck, *Semin Roentgenol* 35:84–100, 2000.

Cross-Reference

Neuroradiology: THE REQUISITES, p 677.

Comment

The larynx has many different appearances after laryngeal surgery, depending on the type of procedure that has been performed. After a total laryngectomy, one is left with absence of laryngeal cartilages and the hyoid bone with the only "tube" that is seen being the neopharynx. The patient breathes through a tracheostomy and swallows through the neopharynx. The neopharynx consists of the cut edges of the pharynx and mucosa and supporting tissue, which have been joined together in the midline to create the swallowing tube.

Often a hemithyroidectomy is performed at the time of a laryngectomy to allow exposure for the laryngectomy. Alternatively the thyroid tissue may be flipped to one side of the neck to the other, creating a confusing picture for the thyroid tissue; however, this should not be mistaken for a lymph node.

Recurrences around the stoma of the tracheostomy are difficult to treat. If there is extension inferiorly into the mediastinum, this is unresectable, incurable disease. Alternatively, radiation therapy, chemotherapy, or revision reconstruction with resection may be contemplated.

Notes

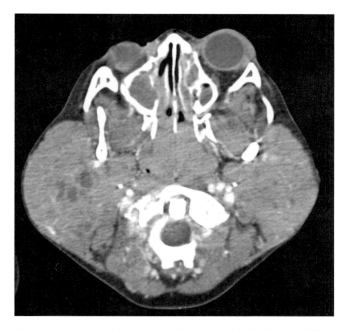

1. Identify the characteristic parotid lesion in Sjögren syndrome.

2. What would happen to the apparent diffusion coefficient in a parotid gland of a patient with Sjögren syndrome compared with that of a normal patient?

3. Name three connective tissue diseases linked to Sjögren syndrome.

4. Do calcifications in parotid glands imply Sjögren syndrome?

Sjögren Syndrome

1. Benign lymphoepithelial lesion.

2. It goes up; less glandular stroma.

3. Rheumatoid arthritis, lupus, and scleroderma.

4. Yes, they are frequently present and punctate in appearance.

Reference

Patel RR, Carlos RC, Midia M, Mukherji SK: Apparent diffusion coefficient mapping of the normal parotid gland and parotid involvement in patients with systemic connective tissue disorders, *AJNR Am J Neuroradiol* 25:16–20, 2004.

Cross-Reference

Neuroradiology: THE REQUISITES, pp 703–704.

Comment

Sjögren syndrome represents a form of the sicca syndrome in which the patient has dry mouth and dry eyes in association with a systemic collagen vascular disease. In most cases, this collagen vascular disease is rheumatoid arthritis; alternatively, one may have mixed connective tissue disorders or even scleroderma. The manifestations in the parotid glands are multiple lymphoepithelial lesions analogous to the lesions in HIV-positive patients. These benign lymphoepithelial lesions are usually bilateral and dominate the entire parotid gland.

Sjögren syndrome also is a risk factor for the development of lymphoma of the parotid gland. This may be primary or secondary lymphoma with systemic disease.

Occasionally, with late-stage Sjögren syndrome, one may find a small fibrotic gland without the cyst and nodules. This would correspond to the sclerosis of the ductal system within the parotid gland, which on sialography looks like the pruned tree effect that has been described previously. The related entity to Sjögren syndrome is Mikulicz disease, which essentially is Sjögren syndrome without the systemic collagen vascular disease.

Notes

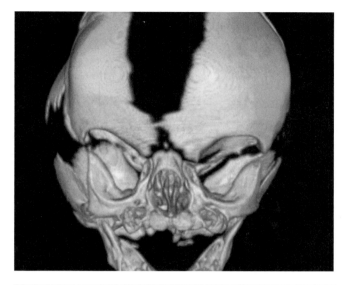
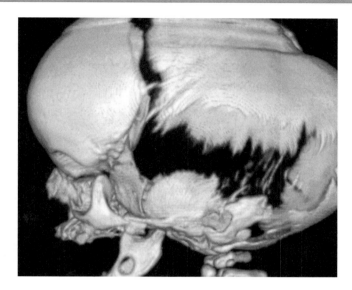
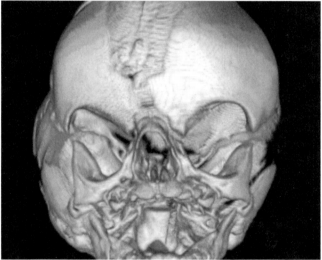

1. In this infant, who has had strip cranioplasties for multiple sutural closures, syndactyly with broad inwardly deviated toes and thumbs, and midface hypoplasia, what is the best diagnosis?

2. Why are strip cranioplasties performed?

3. Which sutures are most commonly affected in Pfeiffer syndrome?

4. Which suture closes first in humans?

Pfeiffer Syndrome after Strip Cranioplasties

1. Pfeiffer syndrome.

2. To allow brain growth and relieve pressure effects.

3. Sagittal and coronal.

4. Metopic.

Reference

Tokumaru AM, Barkovich AJ, Ciricillo SF, Edwards MS: Skull base and calvarial deformities: association with intracranial changes in craniofacial syndromes, *AJNR Am J Neuroradiol* 17:619–630, 1996.

Cross-Reference

Neuroradiology: THE REQUISITES, pp 438–440.

Comment

Pfeiffer syndrome type I is also known as acrocephalosyndactyly type V and is due to a disorder of fibroblast growth factor receptor I or II. Patients have craniosynostosis with broad thumbs and toes. The calvaria has a cloverleaf or pointed (turricephaly) appearance and brachycephaly. The face shows shallow orbits and midface underdevelopment. Because of the shallow orbital development, the globes seem to bulge. The maxilla is small, the mandible protrudes, and the eyes are widely spaced. Cleft palate is not unusual.

The temporal bones of patients with Pfeiffer syndrome may show stenosis or atresia or both of the external auditory canal and hypoplasia of the middle ear cavity and its ossicles.

The entity is transmitted in an autosomal dominant fashion, but most cases are sporadic. Children with Pfeiffer syndrome type I are intellectually normal.

Notes

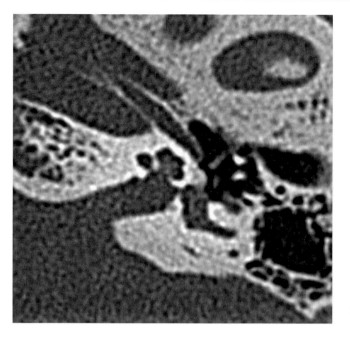 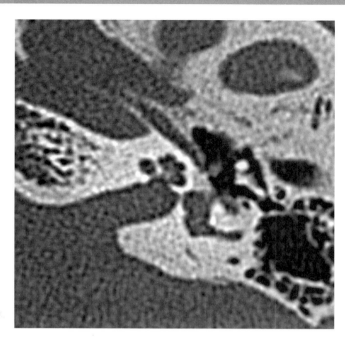

1. Define fissula ante fenestram.

2. Why should this entity not be called otosclerosis?

3. What is the typical age range of patients with the disease?

4. What is the treatment?

Otospongiosis

1. The area in between the oval window and the spot where the tensor tympani tendon makes its turn laterally to connect to the malleus neck. (Just look anterior to the oval window.)

2. It causes demineralization of bone, not sclerotic bone.

3. 15 to 35 years old.

4. Fluoride treatment, stapedectomy, and stapes prosthesis.

Reference

Guneri EA, Ada E, Ceryan K, Guneri A: High-resolution computed tomographic evaluation of the cochlear capsule in otosclerosis: relationship between densitometry and sensorineural hearing loss, *Ann Otol Rhinol Laryngol* 105:659–664, 1996.

Cross-Reference

Neuroradiology: THE REQUISITES, pp 598–599.

Comment

Otospongiosis is an unusual disorder in which the extremely dense bone of the labyrinth around the cochlea and the vestibule is replaced by spongiotic, less dense bone. This disease is quite frequently bilateral and generally occurs in young adults. It causes sensorineural hearing loss and conductive hearing loss. The conductive hearing loss seems to be most common in the retroocular or fenestral form of otospongiosis, in which the most common site is the anterior margin of the oval window. At this site, the spongiotic bone causes fixation of the stapes footplate within the oval window, preventing conduction of stapes motion to the oval window. This causes the conductive hearing loss.

Sensorineural hearing loss associated with otospongiosis seems to be due to the enzymatic process around the cochlea in which proteins extend into the perilymph or endolymph leading to a toxic effect on the hair cells on the organ of Corti. Otospongiosis may be arrested in its course by fluoride treatment. The fluoride treatment itself causes increased density to the bone, leading to a more sclerotic appearance and a more appropriately named entity of otosclerosis. In most cases, otosclerosis is a misnomer because the bone is not sclerotic but more spongiotic, which is why we teach trainees to use the term *otospongiosis.*

The differential diagnosis for demineralization around the otic capsule is otosyphilis, osteogenesis imperfecta, and late-stage Paget disease.

Fenestral otosclerosis is seen at the anterior margin of the oval window in 81% of cases, at the round window niche in 36%, and at the cochlear walls in 22%. Otospongiosis is bilateral in 76% of cases.

The disease is likely hereditary. It affects women more than men and whites more than blacks. Histologically, it affects 10% of the overall population, but only 1% are symptomatic.

Notes

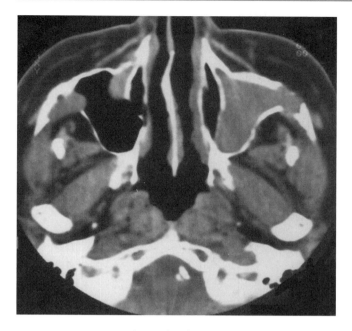

1. In a patient with multiple myeloma, what should be included in the differential diagnosis?

2. What is the typical classification of plasmacytomas in the head and neck?

3. How often do plasmacytomas progress to multiple myeloma?

4. Identify the most common site for extramedullary plasmacytomas in the head and neck.

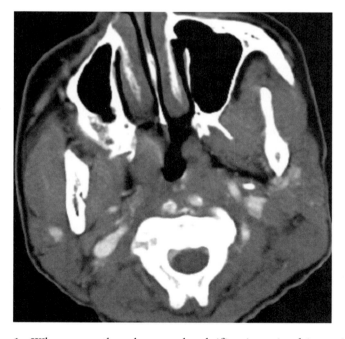 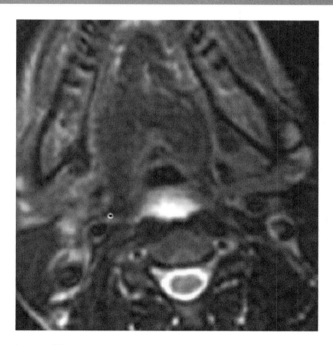

1. Where are the abnormal calcifications in this patient's neck?

2. What is the implication of their presence?

3. What should be included in the differential diagnosis?

4. Identify causes of retropharyngeal edema.

CASE 196

Multiple Myeloma of the Paranasal Sinuses

1. Multiple myeloma, invasive fungal sinusitis, lymphoma, Langerhans cell histiocytosis, mastocytosis.

2. Extramedullary plasmacytoma, solitary plasmacytoma of bone, and multiple myeloma.

3. 33%, but less in extramedullary plasmacytomas (58% in solitary plasmacytoma of bone, 20% in extramedullary plasmacytoma).

4. The submucosa of the sinonasal cavity.

Reference

Nofsinger YC, Mirza N, Rowan PT, et al: Head and neck manifestations of plasma cell neoplasms, *Laryngoscope* 107:741–746, 1997.

Cross-Reference

Neuroradiology: THE REQUISITES, pp 830–831.

Comment

In my experience, multiple myeloma is more likely to affect the walls of the paranasal sinuses than is metastatic disease from other causes. This is particularly noticeable in the case of the walls of the maxillary antrum, which, because of their thinness, might be expected to be relatively hypovascular. Multiple myeloma manifests in the paranasal sinuses as it does in other bones with punched-out lytic lesions. In some cases, these findings may be relatively subtle because of the thinness of the bone, but in other cases, soft tissue masses are associated with them, which may project into or along the wall of the paranasal sinus.

This diagnosis may be difficult to make with nuclear medicine scanning because of the low activity of the multiple myeloma and because inflammatory disease adjacent to the bone may stimulate neoplasm.

When one does have metastasis to the paranasal sinus, the most common primary tumor is renal cell carcinoma. These lesions may be hemorrhagic and could present with epistaxis.

The most common manifestation of multiple myeloma in the paranasal sinuses is inflammatory sinusitis. Multiple myeloma is one of the diagnoses besides leukemia, lymphoma, and other hematopoietic diseases for which scanning of the paranasal sinuses before bone marrow transplantation is common.

Notes

CASE 197

Calcific Tendinitis Longus Musculature

1. The longus colli muscles.

2. Calcific tendinitis.

3. Calcific tendinitis, pseudogout, tumoral calcinosis, myositis ossificans, ochronosis, calcium-phosphorus dysmetabolism, scleroderma, and gout.

4. Adjacent inflammation from pharyngitis, tonsillitis, or tendinitis; anasarca; lymph node necrosis and spread of lymphadenitis; lymphedema; radiation changes; and abscess formation.

Reference

Eastwood JD, Hudgins PA, Malone D: Retropharyngeal effusion in acute calcific prevertebral tendinitis: diagnosis with CT and MR imaging, *AJNR Am J Neuroradiol* 19:1789–1792, 1998.

Cross-Reference

Neuroradiology: THE REQUISITES, pp 730–731.

Comment

Patients with longus colli tendinitis present with neck pain, odynophagia, or dysphagia and may have a low-grade fever. There is usually no limitation in the range of motion. Men are affected more commonly than women, and the typical age range is 30 to 60 years old. Other names for this entity include calcific retropharyngeal tendinitis, calcific tendinitis of the longus colli, and calcific prevertebral tendinitis. Because the longus musculature is not part of the retropharyngeal space but is considered within the prevertebral compartment, calcific retropharyngeal tendinitis is the least accurate name.

CT scans reveal calcifications (calcium hydroxyapatite) anterior to the cervical spine within the longus colli muscle or tendon or both with thickening of the muscle. The calcifications occur most commonly at the C1-2 levels (where the superior oblique tendon fibers of the longus colli muscle abound). Rarely one may see edema or fluid in the retropharyngeal soft tissues. This fluid may extend even into the thoracic region as part of the potential space of the retropharyngeal compartment or the "danger space" or both.

This is a self-limited entity that usually resolves with nonsteroidal antiinflammatory drugs within 1 month.

Notes

Case compliments of Laurie A. Loevner, Philadelphia, PA.

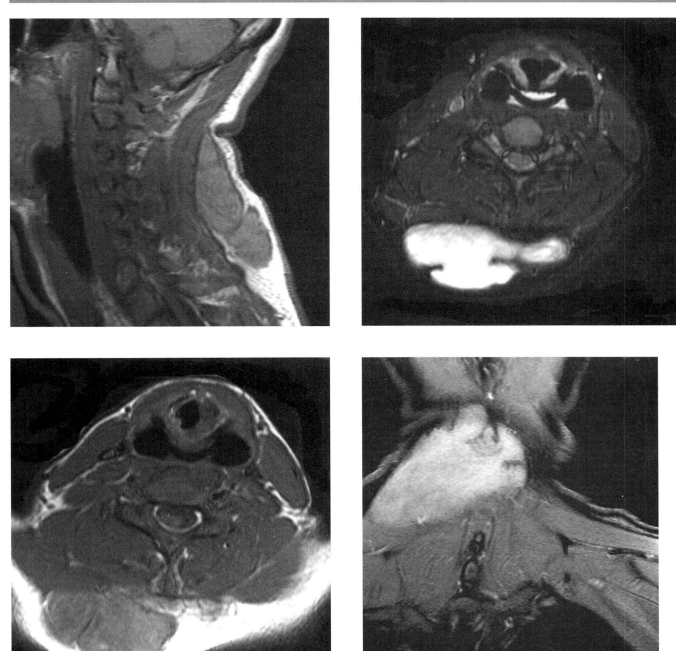

1. What should be included in the differential diagnosis?

2. What is the origin of hibernoma tumors?

3. Identify the most common sites of hibernomas.

4. Is there malignant potential in hibernomas?

Hibernoma

1. Lymphangioma, venous vascular malformation, liposarcoma, hibernoma, lymphoma, hemangiosarcoma, angiolipoma, atypical lipoma, nodular fasciitis, resolving hematoma, abscess, seroma, and myxoid liposarcoma.

2. Brown fat from fetal tissue.

3. Shoulder, back, neck, axilla, mediastinum, and thigh.

4. No.

Reference

Baskurt E, Padgett DM, Matsumoto JA: Multiple hibernomas in a 1-month-old female infant, *AJNR Am J Neuroradiol* 25:1443–1445, 2004.

Cross-Reference

Neuroradiology: THE REQUISITES, pp 117–118, 431–432.

Comment

Hibernomas are benign tumors of the brown fat that is present during fetal life. This fat predominates in the neck and upper chest—hence the locations of most hibernomas. Despite their derivation from fetal tissue, the tumors usually do not present until the 20s or 30s (mean age 38), typically as a nonpainful, slowly growing mobile mass. At the time of resection, the average size is >9 cm.

The lesion does *not* have the imaging characteristics of typical fat, as seen in this case as well. The signal intensity is usually between that of fat and muscle on T1W scans and bright on T2W scans. In a similar fashion, the density on CT is usually between that of fat and muscle. The lesion is usually lobulated and loculated. One feature that is particularly unexpected is that the mass enhances quite prominently. On ultrasound, the lesion is hyperechoic.

Notes

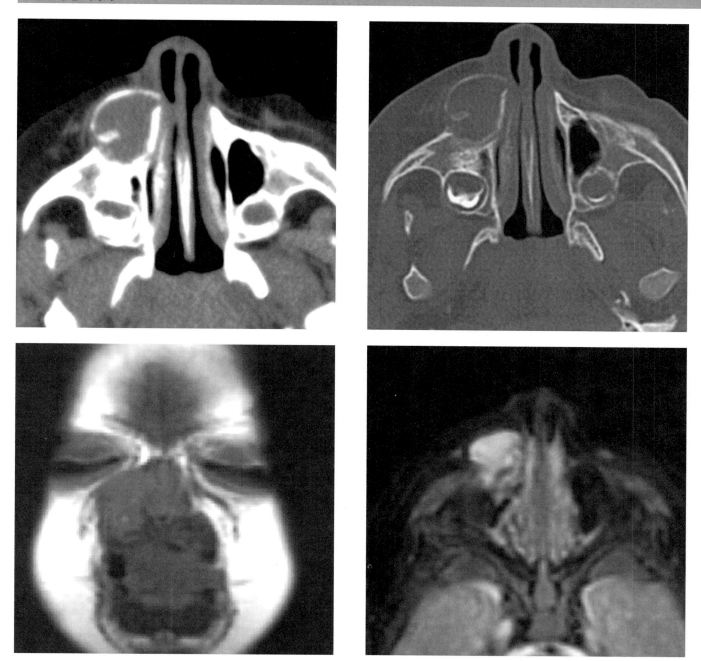

1. What is the most common site of an odontogenic myxoma?

2. What should be included in the differential diagnosis?

3. Is a myxoma more commonly multilocular or unilocular?

4. Do myxomas cross the midline?

(Case continued)

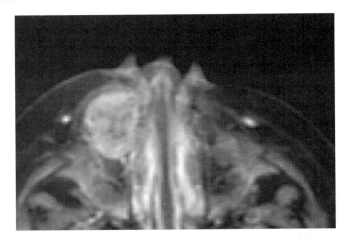

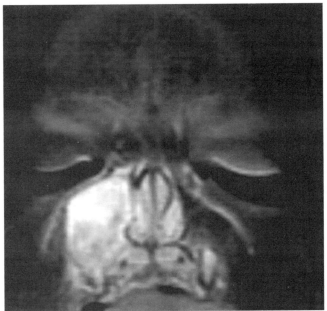

Odontogenic Myxoma

1. The mandible (2:1 ratio over maxilla).

2. Ameloblastoma, synovial sarcoma, chondromyxoid fibroma, sarcoma, and giant cell granuloma.

3. Multilocular.

4. No.

Reference

Simon EN, Merkx MA, Vuhahula E, et al: Odontogenic myxoma: a clinicopathological study of 33 cases, *Int J Oral Maxillofac Surg* 33:333–337, 2004.

Cross-Reference

Neuroradiology: THE REQUISITES, pp 660–662.

Comment

The odontogenic source of myxomas has come under debate; however, in most cases, the lesions are associated with the tooth-bearing portions of the maxilla and mandible. Occasionally, odontogenic epithelium is present histologically, and the thought is that these arise from the mesenchyme of developing teeth. When fibrous/collagenous tissue coexists, the lesion may be termed a *myxofibroma*.

Myxomas usually present as painless masses that create symptoms based on their mass effect. Most arise in adults in their 20s and 30s. Women are affected more commonly than men. In most series, myxomas are the second most common odontogenic tumors after ameloblastomas. The tumors may recur, but they have no known malignant potential, and no cases of metastases have been reported. Treatment is radical surgery.

On imaging, these lesions are usually multiloculated and are characterized by their avid solid enhancement characteristics, which would be unusual for any of the odontogenic cysts. This is a lytic lesion that expands the bone, as in this case. Although this lesion suggests slow growth, local recurrence is common. This lesion does not cross the midline and is characterized by its "soap bubble" or "honeycomb" appearance with obvious septa. Perforation of the cortex of the bone with soft tissue beyond the bony confines on CT scan has been reported at high frequency.

Notes

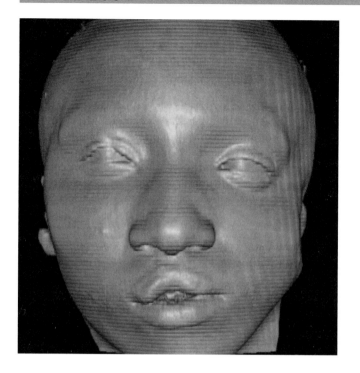 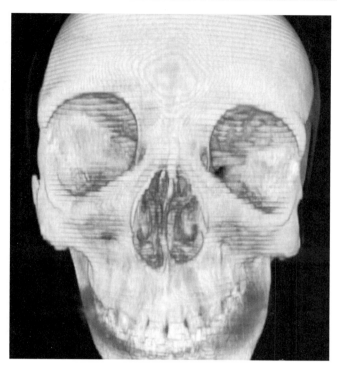

1. What is the finding on the soft tissue views of the face?

2. Name some causes of this phenomenon.

3. Name the neuroradiologic features of Parry-Romberg syndrome.

4. When do these patients present?

Parry-Romberg Syndrome

1. Hemifacial atrophy.

2. Parry-Romberg syndrome, amniotic band syndrome, Sturge-Weber syndrome, hemifacial microsomia of Padwa, Dyke-Davidoff-Masson syndrome, Goldenhar syndrome, and scleroderma (saber slash).

3. Wasting of the soft tissues of the face, microtia, enophthalmos, small mandible with delayed dentition, and hemiatrophy of the hemispheres.

4. 10 to 20 years old.

Reference

Moko SB, Mistry Y, Blandin de Chalain TM: Parry-Romberg syndrome: intracranial MRI appearances, J Craniomaxillofac Surg 31:321–324, 2003.

Cross-Reference

Neuroradiology: THE REQUISITES, pp 590–592.

Comment

Parry-Romberg syndrome usually presents in the adolescent/young adult period with progressive facial hemiatrophy. As seen in this case, the findings are usually more dramatic with respect to the soft tissue wasting, seen here on the left side. The maxillomandibular region and the nasolabial fold region are the first areas to be affected. The eyes may droop or become enophthalmic, and the mandible is deformed with delayed eruption of the teeth. Microtia with deformed temporal bone also is possible. The tongue may be small. Skin and hair discoloration is often present.

The patient may present with seizures, and one may see hemiatrophy of the ipsilateral hemisphere. Trigeminal neuralgia is another common symptom associated with this disorder. Some reports of "hypermyelination" of the white matter are noted.

Notes